Data Monitoring in Clinical Trials

David L. DeMets
Curt D. Furberg
Lawrence M. Friedman
Editors

Data Monitoring in Clinical Trials

A Case Studies Approach

With 40 Illustrations

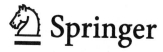 Springer

David L. DeMets
Department of Biostatistics and Medical
  Informatics
University of Wisconsin Medical School
Madison, WI 53972-4675
USA

Curt D. Furberg
Department of Public Health Sciences
Wake Forest University School
  of Medicine
Winston-Salem, NC 27157
USA

Lawrence M. Friedman
Bethesda, MD
USA

ISBN-10: 0-387-20330-3   Printed on acid-free paper.
ISBN-13: 978-0387-20330-0

Printed in the United States of America.   (MP)

9 8 7 6 5 4 3 2 1

springeronline.com

Preface

Monitoring of clinical trials for early evidence of benefit and harm has gotten considerable attention.[1] More formal guidelines and requirements[2-4] have evolved in recent years, but in fact monitoring of trials is a practice that has been going on for almost four decades.[5] For trials that involved conditions or interventions with serious risks, such as mortality or major morbidity, the tradition and policy has been to have an independent monitoring committee to review accumulating data for evidence of harm or convincing benefit that would require modifying or terminating a trial early. During the past four decades, many trials have had monitoring committees to assume this responsibility. With the new emphasis on monitoring, this type of activity is increasing dramatically as the number of clinical trials being conducted to evaluate new interventions for patients or participants with serious risk or serious outcomes also increases. For example, policies of the National Institutes of Health (NIH) in the United States (US) call for monitoring committees for all phase III trials.[2] Guidelines of the US Food and Drug Administration suggest such committees for trials of high-risk interventions or patients at high risk.[3]

As the number of monitoring committees increases, the challenge exists to pass along the experiences and best practices of the monitoring process to colleagues who are assuming this responsibility for the first time. Textbooks such as the one by Ellenberg, Fleming, and DeMets[6] provide many of the basic principles for monitoring committees. Other texts such as those by Friedman, Furberg, and DeMets;[7] Meinert;[8] Pocock;[9] Jennison and Turnbull;[10] and Piantidosi[11] provide statistical fundamentals and methods for the design, monitoring, and analysis of clinical trials. This text is intended to complement those texts by providing a collection of examples or case studies of monitoring experiences from a variety of trials across different disease disciplines. Each case study will describe the background of the individual trial, summarize the overall results, review the critical issues that emerged in the monitoring of the trial, and finally reflect on the lessons learned from that trial. All of the examples presented share the complexity of the process of monitoring and the lesson that no single rule or algorithm can replace the wisdom and judgment of a monitoring committee. Through these examples, we hope to share the experience of these past committees and pass along some of their sometimes hard-earned wisdom.

Selection of the case studies was largely based on the collective experiences of the editors and their interactions with colleagues involved with clinical trials. Many of the 29 examples are from the field of cardiology, where the practice of monitoring committees was established early. However, there are examples from other disciplines. Regardless of the disease, many of the lessons learned and practices are useful for any trial. Individual colleagues were invited to present the monitoring experience of a trial they were involved with as they saw it and experienced it. Their presentations and discussions do not necessarily represent the official view of either the trial sponsor, the trial investigators, or the trial monitoring committee. We have tried to get representation from each of these constituencies on many of the trials when possible.

For most of the past four decades, the existence and practice of monitoring committees has not been widely recognized or understood. Our belief is that clinical research will benefit with better understanding of the process by both the research community and the interested public. The intended audience for this book are those who are planning to serve on a monitoring committee or are already on one and wish to gain further insight into the monitoring and decision-making process. We also believe that these examples will be useful to investigators as they design their trials and propose monitoring procedures; to sponsors, who typically receive monitoring committee recommendations, and to regulatory agencies, who often must review the results of trials that have been monitored by a committee. In addition, Institutional Review Boards may benefit from these case studies since they ultimately have responsibility for protecting participants at the local level but must rely on the monitoring committee process for most multicenter trials and increasingly for institutional trials. Journal editors, sciences writers, and practicing physicians may also find these case studies instructive.

Over the past four decades, many individuals have served on monitoring committees and participated in the monitoring of many challenging studies. We wish to thank all of those individuals who have contributed directly or indirectly to the practice of monitoring and from whose experience we all have benefitted. We have listed in Appendix 1 the individuals who have served on the committees for the trials presented as case studies in this book and wish to thank them in particular.

ACKNOWLEDGMENTS

We also want to thank the many contributors to the drafting of these case studies. We have listed them in the section which follows. They contributed their experiences because of their commitment to clinical trials, the monitoring process, and to teaching the next generation of clinical trial researchers about the important process of monitoring trials for early evidence of benefit or harm. We are grateful that they accepted our invitation and persevered through the drafts and editing process.

We would also like to acknowledge the substantial contributions by Ms. Suzanne Parman for her editorial and logistical support. Without her dedication this text could not have been completed in a timely fashion.

David L. DeMets

Curt D. Furberg

Lawrence M. Friedman

REFERENCES

1. Shalala D: Protecting research subjects–what must be done. 2000. *N Engl J Med* 343: 808–810.
2. National Institutes of Health. 2000. Further Guidance on a Data and Safety Monitoring for Phase I and Phase II Trials, NIH Guide, June 5, 2000. http://grants.nih.gov/grants/guide/notice-files/NOT-OD-00-038.html
3. US Food and Drug Administration. 2001. Draft Guidance for Clinical Trial sponsors on the establishment and operation of Clinical Trial Data Monitoring Committees. Rockville, MD: FDA. http://www.fda.gov/cber/gdlns/clindatmon.htm
4. Food and Drug Administration, Department of Health and Human Services. 1998. International Conference on Harmonisation: Guidance on statistical principles for clinical trials; availability. *Federal Register* Vol 63, No 179:49583–49598.
5. Greenberg Report: Organization, review, and administration of cooperative studies. 1988. *Control Clin Trials* 9:137–148.
6. Ellenberg S, Fleming T, DeMets D. 2002. *Data Monitoring Committees in Clinical Trials: A Practical Perspective.* John Wiley & Sons, Ltd., West Sussex, England.
7. Friedman LM, Furberg CD, DeMets DL. 1998. *Fundamentals of Clinical Trials.* Third Edition, Springer-Verlag, New York.
8. Meinert CL. 1986. *Clinical Trials: Design, Conduct, and Analysis.* Oxford University Press, New York.
9. Pocock S. 1983. *Clinical Trials: A Practical Approach.* John Wiley & Sons, Ltd., West Sussex, England.
10. Jennison C, Turnbull BW. 1999. *Group Sequential Methods With Applications to Clinical Trials.* Chapman and Hall/CRC, Boca Raton and London.
11. Piantadosi S. 1997. *Clinical Trials: A Methodologic Perspective.* John Wiley & Sons, Inc., New York.

Contributors

Susan Anderson
Department of Biostatistics and Medical Informatics, University of Wisconsin, Madison, Wisconsin
Data Monitoring in the Prospective Randomized Milrinone Survival Evaluation: Dealing with an Agonizing Trend

Alex Bajamonde
Genentech Inc., San Francisco, California
Making Independence Work: Monitoring the Bevacizumab Colorectal Cancer Clinical Trial

Jean-Pierre Boissel
Clinical Pharmacology Department, Claude Bernard University, Lyon, France
Stopping the Randomized Aldactone Evaluation Study Early for Efficacy

Byron W. Brown, Jr.
Stanford, California
The Nocturnal Oxygen Therapy Trial Data Monitoring Experience: Problem with Reporting Lags

Julie Buring
Department of Medicine, Brigham and Women's Hospital, Harvard Medical School; Boston, Massachusetts
Stopping the Carotene and Retinol Efficacy Trial: The Viewpoint of the Safety and Endpoint Monitoring Committee

Paul L. Canner
Maryland Medical Research Institute, Baltimore, Maryland
Breaking New Ground: Data Monitoring in the Coronary Drug Project

Heidi Christ-Schmidt
Statistics Collaborative, Washington, D.C.
Making Independence Work: Monitoring the Bevacizumab Colorectal Cancer Clinical Trial

Charles Clark
Departments of Medicine, Pharmacology and Toxicology, School of Medicine, Indiana University, Bloomington, Indiana
Early Termination of the Diabetes Control and Complications Trial

Patricia Cleary
The Biostatistics Center, The George Washington University, Rockville, Maryland
Early Termination of the Diabetes Control and Complications Trial

Robert Cody
Department of Internal Medicine, Division of Cardiology, University of Michigan, Ann Arbor, Michigan
Data Monitoring in the Prospective Randomized Milrinone Survival Evaluation: Dealing with an Agonizing Trend

Theodore Colton
Department of Epidemiology, Boston University School of Public Health, Boston, Massachusetts
Challenges in Monitoring the Breast Cancer Prevention Trial

Joseph P. Costantino
Department of Biostatistics, Graduate School of Public Health, University of Pittsburgh, Pittsburgh, Pennsylvania
Challenges in Monitoring the Breast Cancer Prevention Trial

Oscar Crofford
Department of Medicine, Vanderbilt University, Nashville, Tennessee
Early Termination of the Diabetes Control and Complications Trial

Jeffrey A. Cutler
National Heart, Lung, and Blood Institute, Division of Epidemiology and Clinical Applications, National Institutes of Health, Bethesda, Maryland
Data Monitoring in the Antihypertensive and Lipid-Lowering Treatment to Prevent Heart Attack Trial: Early Termination of the Doxazosin Treatment Arm

Barry R. Davis
The University of Texas Health Science Center at Houston, School of Public Health, Houston, Texas
Data Monitoring in the Antihypertensive and Lipid-Lowering Treatment to Prevent Heart Attack Trial: Early Termination of the Doxazosin Treatment Arm

David L. DeMets
Department of Biostatistics and Medical Informatics, University of Wisconsin, Madison, Wisconsin
Data and Safety Monitoring in the Beta-Blocker Heart Attack Trial: Early Experience in Formal Monitoring Methods
Data Monitoring for the Aspirin Component of the Physicians' Health Study: Issues in Early Termination for a Major Secondary Endpoint
The Data Monitoring Experience in the Cardiac Arrhythmia Suppression Trial: The Need To Be Prepared Early
The Nocturnal Oxygen Therapy Trial Data Monitoring Experience: Problem with Reporting Lags

Kenneth Dickstein
Cardiology Division, Stavanger University Hospital, Stavanger, Norway
Data Monitoring Experience in the Moxonidine Congestive Heart Failure Trial

Fred Ederer
Bethesda, Maryland
Assessing Possible Late Treatment Effects Early: The Diabetic Retinopathy Study Experience

Susan S. Ellenberg
University of Pennsylvania School of Medicine, Center for Clinical Epidemiology and Biostatistics, Philadelphia, Pennsylvania
FDA and Clinical Trial Data Monitoring Committees

Frederick Ferris
Division of Epidemiology and Clinical Research, National Eye Institute, National Institutes of Health, Bethesda, Maryland
Early Termination of the Diabetes Control and Complications Trial

Jan Feyzi
Department of Biostatistics and Medical Informatics, University of Wisconsin, Madison, Wisconsin
Data Monitoring Experience in the Metoprolol CR/XL Randomized Intervention Trial in Chronic Heart Failure: Potentially High Risk Treatment in High Risk Patients

Dianne M. Finkelstein
Biostatistics Center, Massachusetts General Hospital; Harvard Medical School, Boston, Massachusetts

Data Monitoring Experience in the AIDS Clinical Trials Group Study #981: Conflicting Interim Results

Norman Fost
Departments of Pediatrics and Medical History and Bioethics, University of Wisconsin, Madison, Wisconsin
Monitoring a Clinical Trial with Waiver of Informed Consent: Diaspirin Cross-Linked Hemoglobin for Emergency Treatment of Post-Traumatic Shock

Gary Francis
Department of Cardiology, Cleveland Clinic Foundation, Cleveland, Ohio
Data Monitoring Experience in the Moxonidine Congestive Heart Failure Trial

Lawrence M. Friedman
Bethesda, Maryland
Data and Safety Monitoring in the Beta-Blocker Heart Attack Trial: Early Experience in Formal Monitoring Methods
The Data Monitoring Experience in the Cardiac Arrhythmia Suppression Trial: The Need To Be Prepared Early

Curt D. Furberg
Department of Public Health Sciences, Wake Forest University School of Medicine, Winston-Salem, North Carolina
Stopping the Randomized Aldactone Evaluation Study Early for Efficacy
Stopping a Trial for Futility: The Cooperative New Scandinavian Enalapril Survival Study II Trial
Lessons from Warfarin Trials in Atrial Fibrillation: Missing the Window of Opportunity

Saul Genuth
Division of Clinical and Molecular Endocrinology, Department of Medicine, University Hospitals of Cleveland, Case Western Reserve University, Cleveland, Ohio
Early Termination of the Diabetes Control and Complications Trial

Stephen L. George
Department of Biostatistics and Bioinformatics, Director, Cancer Center Biostatistics, Duke University Medical Center, Durham, North Carolina
Controversies in the Early Reporting of a Clinical Trial in Early Breast Cancer

Deborah Grady
Department of Epidemiology and Biostatistics, University of California, San Francisco, California
Consideration of Early Stopping and Other Challenges in Monitoring the Heart and Estrogen/progestin Replacement Study

Mark R. Green
Department of Hematology/Oncology, Medical University of South Carolina, Charleston, South Carolina
Controversies in the Early Reporting of a Clinical Trial in Early Breast Cancer

Robert J. Hardy
Division of Biostatistics, The University of Texas Health Sciences Center at Houston, School of Public Health, Houston, Texas
Data and Safety Monitoring in the Beta-Blocker Heart Attack Trial: Early Experience in Formal Monitoring Methods

David Harrington
Department of Biostatistics and Computational Biology, Dana-Farber Cancer Institute and Department of Biostatistics, Harvard School of Public Health, Boston, Massachusetts
Data Monitoring of a Placebo-Controlled Trial of Daclizumab in Acute Graft-Versus-Host Disease

Robert G. Hart
Department of Medicine (Neurology), University of Texas Health Science Center, San Antonio, Texas
Early Termination of the Stroke Prevention in Atrial Fibrillation I Trial: Protecting Participant Interests in the Face of Scientific Uncertainties and the Cruel Play of Chance

Charles H. Hennekens
University of Miami School of Medicine and Florida Atlantic University, Boca Raton, Florida
Data Monitoring for the Aspirin Component of the Physicians' Health Study: Issues in Early Termination for a Major Secondary Endpoint
The Data Monitoring Experience in the Candesartan in Heart Failure Assessment of Reduction in Mortality and Morbidity Program

Eric Holmgren
Genentech Inc., South San Francisco, California

Making Independence Work: Monitoring the Bevacizumab Colorectal Cancer Clinical Trial

Stephen B. Hulley
Department of Epidemiology & Biostatistics, University of California, San Francisco, California
Consideration of Early Stopping and Other Challenges in Monitoring the Heart and Estrogen/progestin Replacement Study

Mark A. Jacobson
Positive Health Program, Department of Medicine, University of California, San Francisco, California
Data Monitoring Experience in the AIDS Toxoplasmic Encephalitis Study

Desmond G. Julian
Emeritus Professor of Cardiology, University of Newcastle-upon-Tyne, London, England
Data Monitoring Experience in the Metoprolol CR/XL Randomized Intervention Trial in Chronic Heart Failure: Potentially High Risk Treatment in High Risk Patients
Stopping the Randomized Aldactone Evaluation Study Early for Efficacy
The Data Monitoring Experience in the Carvedilol Post-Infarct Survival Control in Left Ventricular Dysfunction Study: Hazards of Changing Primary Outcomes

Richard A. Kronmal
Department of Biostatistics, University of Washington, Seattle, Washington
Early Termination of the Stroke Prevention in Atrial Fibrillation I Trial: Protecting Participant Interests in the Face of Scientific Uncertainties and the Cruel Play of Chance

Henri Kulbertus
Cardiology Department, Centre Hospitalier Universitaire, Liege, Belgium
Stopping the Randomized Aldactone Evaluation Study Early for Efficacy

John M. Lachin
The Biostatistics Center, The George Washington University, Rockville, Maryland
Early Termination of the Diabetes Control and Complications Trial

Stephanie J. Lee
Department of Medical Oncology, Dana-Farber Cancer Institute, Boston, Massachusetts
Data Monitoring of a Placebo-Controlled Trial of Daclizumab in Acute Graft-Versus-Host Disease

Roger J. Lewis
Department of Emergency Medicine, Harbor-UCLA Medical Center, Torrance, California, UCLA School of Medicine, Los Angeles, California and the Los Angeles Biomedical Research Institute, Torrance, Califormia
Monitoring a Clinical Trial with Waiver of Informed Consent: Diaspirin Cross-Linked Hemoglobin for Emergency Treatment of Post-Traumatic Shock

Ruth McBride
Axio Research Corporation, Seattle, Washington
Early Termination of the Stroke Prevention in Atrial Fibrillation I Trial: Protecting Participant Interests in the Face of Scientific Uncertainties and the Cruel Play of Chance

Anthony B. Miller
Ontario, Canada
Stopping the Carotene and Retinol Efficacy Trial: The Viewpoint of the Safety and Endpoint Monitoring Committee

David Nathan
Department of Medicine, Harvard University, Boston, Massachusetts
Early Termination of the Diabetes Control and Complications Trial

James D. Neaton
Division of Biostatistics, School of Public Health, University of Minnesota, Minneapolis, Minnesota
Data Monitoring Experience in the AIDS Toxoplasmic Encephalitis Study

Milton Packer
Center for Biostatistics and Clinical Science, University of Texas Southwestern Medical Center, Dallas, Texas
Data Monitoring in the Prospective Randomized Milrinone Survival Evaluation: Dealing with an Agonizing Trend

Lesly A. Pearce
Biostatistical Consultant, Minot, North Dakota
Early Termination of the Stroke Prevention in Atrial Fibrillation I Trial: Protecting Participant Interests in the Face of Scientific Uncertainties and the Cruel Play of Chance

Stuart Pocock
Medical Statistics Unit, London School of Hygiene and Tropical Medicine, London, United Kingdom

Stopping the Randomized Aldactone Evaluation Study Early for Efficacy
The Data Monitoring Experience in the Candesartan in Heart Failure
Assessment of Reduction in Mortality and Morbidity Program
Data Monitoring Experience in the Moxonidine Congestive Heart Failure
Trial

Janice Pogue
Department of Medicine and Population Health Research Institute, Hamilton
Health Sciences and McMaster University, Hamilton, Ontario, Canada
Data Monitoring in the Heart Outcomes Prevention Evaluation and the
Clopidogrel in Unstable Angina to Prevent Recurrent Ischemic Events
Trials: Avoiding Important Information Loss
Data Monitoring in the Randomized Evaluation of Strategies for Left
Ventricular Dysfunction Pilot Study: When Reasonable People Disagree

Carol K. Redmond
Department of Biostatistics, Graduate School of Public Health, University of
Pittsburgh, Pittsburgh, Pennsylvania
Challenges in Monitoring the Breast Cancer Prevention Trial

David Sackett
Trout Research and Education Centre at Irish Lake, Markdale, Ontario, Canada
Data Monitoring in the Heart Outcomes Prevention Evaluation and the
Clopidogrel in Unstable Angina to Prevent Recurrent Ischemic Events
Trials: Avoiding Important Information Loss

Richard Schwarz
CV Ventures, LLC, Blue Bell, Pennsylvania
Data Monitoring in the Prospective Randomized Milrinone Survival
Evaluation: Dealing with an Agonizing Trend

Carolyn Siebert
Scotland, Maryland
Early Termination of the Diabetes Control and Complications Trial

Jay P. Siegel
Centocor Research and Development, Inc., Malvern, Pennsylvania
FDA and Clinical Trial Data Monitoring Committees

Steven Snapinn
Amgen Inc., Thousand Oaks, California
Stopping a Trial for Futility: The Cooperative New Scandinavian Enalapril
Survival Study II

Charles H. Tegeler
Department of Neurology, Wake Forest University School of Medicine, Winston-Salem, North Carolina
Lessons from Warfarin Trials in Atrial Fibrillation: Missing the Window of Opportunity

Eric Vittinghoff
Department of Epidemiology and Biostatistics, University of California, San Francisco, California
Consideration of Early Stopping and Other Challenges in Monitoring the Heart and Estrogen/progestin Replacement Study

Duolao Wang
Medical Statistics Unit, London School of Hygiene and Tropical Medicine, London, United Kingdom
The Data Monitoring Experience in the Candesartan in Heart Failure Assessment of Reduction in Mortality and Morbidity Program

Hans Wedel
Epidemiology and Biostatistics, Nordic School of Public Health, Göteborg, Sweden
Data Monitoring Experience in the Metoprolol CR/XL Randomized Intervention Trial in Chronic Heart Failure: Potentially High Risk Treatment in High Risk Patients

Deborah N. Wentworth
Division of Biostatistics, School of Public Health, University of Minnesota, Minneapolis, Minnesota
Data Monitoring Experience in the AIDS Toxoplasmic Encephalitis Study

Richard J. Whitley
Pediatrics, Microbiology, Medicine and Neurosurgery, University of Alabama at Birmingham, Alabama
Clinical Trials of Herpes Simplex Encephalitis: The Role of the Data Monitoring Committee

John Wikstrand
Wallenberg Laboratory for Cardiovascular Research, Sahlgrenska University Hospital, Göteborg; and Clinical Science, Astra Zeneca R&D, Mölndal, Sweden
Data Monitoring Experience in the Metoprolol CR/XL Randomized Intervention Trial in Chronic Heart Failure: Potentially High Risk Treatment in High Risk Patients

Lars Wilhelmsen

Section of Cardiology, The Cardiovascular Institute, Göteborg University, Sweden

The Data Monitoring Experience in the Candesartan in Heart Failure Assessment of Reduction in Mortality and Morbidity Program

Data Monitoring Experience in the Moxonidine Congestive Heart Failure Trial

George W. Williams

Amgen Inc., Thousand Oaks, California

The Nocturnal Oxygen Therapy Trial Data Monitoring Experience: Problem with Reporting Lags

O. Dale Williams

Division of Preventive Medicine, Department of Medicine, University of Alabama, Birmingham, Alabama

Stopping the Carotene and Retinol Efficacy Trial: The Viewpoint of the Safety and Endpoint Monitoring Committee

Consideration of Early Stopping and Other Challenges in Monitoring the Heart and Estrogen/progestin Replacement Study

Janet Wittes

Statistics Collaborative, Washington, D.C.

Stopping the Randomized Aldactone Evaluation Study Early for Efficacy

Data Monitoring Experience in the Moxonidine Congestive Heart Failure Trial

Making Independence Work: Monitoring the Bevacizumab Colorectal Cancer Clinical Trial

D.G. Wyse

Libin Cardiovascular Institute of Alberta, Calgary, Alberta, Canada

Data Monitoring in the Heart Outcomes Prevention Evaluation and the Clopidogrel in Unstable Angina to Prevent Recurrent Ischemic Events Trials: Avoiding Important Information Loss

Salim Yusuf

Department of Medicine and Population Health Research Institute, Hamilton Health Sciences and McMaster University, Hamilton, Ontario, Canada

Data Monitoring in the Heart Outcomes Prevention Evaluation and the Clopidogrel in Unstable Angina to Prevent Recurrent Ischemic Events Trials: Avoiding Important Information Loss

Data Monitoring in the Randomized Evaluation of Strategies for Left Ventricular Dysfunction Pilot Study: When Reasonable People Disagree

David Zahrieh
Department of Biostatistics and Computational Biology, Dana-Farber Cancer Institute, Boston, Massachusetts
Data Monitoring of a Placebo-Controlled Trial of Daclizumab in Acute Graft-Versus-Host Disease

Contents

SECTION 1

Introduction/Overview

CHAPTER 1

Monitoring Committees: Why and How

David L. DeMets
Curt D. Furberg
Lawrence M. Friedman

INTRODUCTION

Monitoring of clinical trials encompasses many concepts. Among these concepts are oversight of trials to ensure that the protocol meets high standards, is feasible, ethical, and is being adhered to; that participant enrollment is satisfactory; that study procedures are being done properly; and that the data are of high quality and complete. Most importantly, however, monitoring is done to make certain, to the extent possible, that participants are not being unduly harmed, either directly by the intervention or indirectly by not receiving the current standard of care. Investigators cannot wait until the end of a clinical trial to examine the data and discover that a particular intervention was beneficial, when they could have made that discovery earlier, and taken appropriate action to help people receive the better treatment. Perhaps even more importantly, investigators cannot wait until the end of a trial to discover that a new treatment that was thought to be beneficial was, in fact, harmful. They must make those decisions as early as possible in order to save lives and preserve the health of the volunteer participants. This is a moral obligation of all who are involved in clinical trials. Once a decision to stop a study has been made, study participants expect, and have a right, to be informed of that decision in a timely manner.

The kind and amount of monitoring depend on the phase of the trial (early or late), organizational structure (single or multi-center), nature of the intervention (how safe it is known to be), whether the trial is open or blinded (sometimes termed "masked"), duration of the trial, and the types of participants being studied (how vulnerable they are thought to be). Many small, single-institution trials can be adequately monitored by Institutional Review Boards (IRBs) that rely on day-to-day oversight by investigators or other individuals tasked with the responsibility. Other trials, however, are best monitored by formally established committees, which provide input to IRBs. These committees go by a variety of names, including Data and Safety Monitoring

Boards, Safety and Monitoring Efficacy Committees, and Data Monitoring Committees. These committees are commonly used for late-phase clinical outcome trials, which are typically multi-center; early-phase trials involving invasive or potentially dangerous interventions; and trials that enroll participants who are particularly vulnerable, such as children, extremely sick patients, and others incapable of providing true informed consent.

HISTORY

The concept of having committees monitor clinical trials goes back at least to the mid-1960s. Among the first trials using such a group was the Coronary Drug Project, or CDP[1] (also see Case 12). The CDP, which began enrolling participants in 1965, was a clinical trial comparing five lipid-modifying drugs against placebo in 8,341 participants who had had a myocardial infarction. The trial included 53 clinical sites, a data coordinating center, and central laboratories, plus an administrative office at the then National Heart Institute of the National Institutes of Health (NIH). Because of the large size and many participating units, the CDP had a formal committee structure, which included a Steering Committee of selected investigators, to help manage the trial. Importantly, there was a Policy Board that oversaw the trial and advised the National Heart Institute. This group was composed of nationally respected scientists representing different fields of expertise who were not involved in the actual trial. As stated in the CDP protocol (see reference 1 for a summary of the protocol), the "Policy Board is to act in a senior advisory capacity to the Technical Group [the committee of all the investigators] in regard to policy questions on design, drug selection, ancillary studies, potential investigators and possible dropping of investigators whose performance is unsatisfactory."

Because of uncertainty as to the best way of organizing and overseeing the CDP, the National Heart Institute, in 1967, commissioned a report, entitled, "Organization, Review, and Administration of Cooperative Studies."[2] This report is also known as the Greenberg Report, after the chairman of the committee that developed it, Bernard Greenberg. This report contained many recommendations, including several that are relevant to trial oversight and data monitoring:

> A Policy Board or Advisory Committee of senior scientists, experts in the field of the study but not data-contributing participants in it, is almost essential.

> A mechanism must be developed for early termination if unusual circumstances dictate that a cooperative study should not be continued.

> Such action might be contemplated if the accumulated data answer the original question sooner than anticipated, if it is apparent that the study will not or cannot

achieve its stated aims, or if scientific advances since initiation render continuation superfluous. This is obviously a difficult decision that must be based on careful analysis of past progress and future expectation. If the National Heart Institute must initiate such action, it must do so only with the advice and on the recommendation of consultants.

Until 1968, CDP investigators were informed of accumulating outcome data. But in April of that year, the Policy Board recommended that such data not be made available to the investigators. Consistent with recommendations from the Greenberg Report, it further recommended that a Safety Monitoring Committee be formed to review those data on a regular basis. If safety issues arose, they were to be referred to the Policy Board, which considered them and made recommendations to the National Heart Institute. Initially, the members of the Safety Monitoring Committee were staff of the National Heart Institute, data coordinating center staff, the chairman of the study Steering Committee, the director of the electrocardiogram reading center, and a statistician from outside the study. Others with relevant expertise from outside the study were added subsequently. Both the Safety Monitoring Committee and the Policy Board met regularly to review study progress and accumulating data, but the Safety Monitoring Committee performed a more in-depth review of the data. It made recommendations to the Policy Board with regard to protocol changes or safety concerns.[3]

The Greenberg Report was extremely influential, in that, essentially, all future cooperative clinical trials funded by the National Heart Institute and its successor incarnations incorporated the idea of a separate committee that reviewed outcome data and made recommendations with regard to trial continuation or modification.

Although the details varied among institutes, other NIH institutes then developed monitoring systems over the years. Indeed, the concept of having an external, independent data-monitoring committee spread to clinical trials supported by industry and internationally. The NIH and the U.S. Food and Drug Administration have also developed guidelines for use of such committees.[4,5]

STRUCTURE AND OPERATIONS OF MONITORING COMMITTEES

Usually, voting members of monitoring committees are independent of the study investigators and sponsor. That is, no one who is involved with either the conduct of the trial or its funding and management should serve as a voting member on the committee. The committee may need to make recommendations that go against the interests of investigators and sponsors. These recommendations may range from dropping poor-performing centers, to alerting participants about safety concerns, to stopping the trial because of adverse events. Investigators and sponsors who have financial or intellectual interests in particular outcomes have a potential conflict of interest and should not make such recommendations or be involved in the deliberations. How uninvolved a member needs to be is a matter of judgment. Can a member be from the same academic department as an investigator? Can they be from the same university? Is it appropriate for a member to be from the same organization as the sponsor, but in a different office or division from the one managing the trial? As a general rule, the more distant and independent, the better. But complete independence should not come at the expense of needed expertise. If the best person to serve on the committee is from the same university as one of the investigators, then that could outweigh concerns over potential or perceived conflicts of interest. In such cases, there needs to be sufficient care to ensure there are no real and important conflicts of interest on the part of the member and to minimize perceived conflicts.

The issue of conflict of interest applies to more than just the organization to which the committee member belongs; it also applies to financial holdings of the member and to future potential profits through holding of patents. All prospective members must be willing to disclose publicly, on an ongoing basis, their financial holdings and consulting or other relationships with companies that manufacture the drug, device, or biological being tested or with companies that manufacture direct competitor products. Having such holdings or relationships would not automatically exclude someone from serving on a monitoring committee, but there needs to be an open assessment of these potential conflicts and their magnitude. If conflicts do exist, it would be inappropriate for the member to vote on issues that relate specifically to that conflict.

What sorts of people should serve on a monitoring committee? The needed expertise is of several kinds. First, one or more experts in the scientific field of inquiry, including knowledge about the intervention, are necessary. Also essential are one or two experts in clinical trial design and biostatistics. Beyond that, monitoring committees often have bioethicists and/or patient advocates, especially for NIH-sponsored trials. Above all, at least some of the members should have served before on a monitoring committee. Experience in that activity is invaluable.

Others who may attend portions of meetings of the monitoring committee, but who are not formal, voting members, include senior investigators, representatives of the sponsor, and, although uncommon, someone from a drug (and device) regulatory agency. Attendance by someone from a regulatory agency can become complicated when the trial is multinational.

Monitoring committee meetings are typically divided into open, closed, and executive sessions. During the open session, no blinded outcome data are disclosed or discussed (even if the trial itself is open, or unblinded). Rather, administrative issues, study progress, problems in participant enrollment, baseline data, participant adherence, and other similar matters are discussed, with a study investigator present to answer any questions. Unblinded outcome data, by study group, are presented and discussed during the closed session. Usually, attendance at this session is restricted to committee members and a study biostatistician who presents the data. It is generally accepted that if the sponsor is a drug or device company, attendance by that representative at the closed session is not a good idea. An exception would be if the study biostatistician is an employee of the company. In this case, however, rules as to what the statistician is and is not allowed to communicate to the sponsor must be established in advance. If the sponsor is a government agency with no commercial interests in the trial outcome, such as the National Institutes or Health or the Department of Veterans Affairs in the United States, some have argued that attendance is permissible, whereas others think that the same rules as apply to industry-sponsored studies should pertain. There is also disagreement as to whether the biostatistician presenting the data should be part of the investigator group, part of the study data analysis group but separate from the daily study management activities, or completely independent of the investigators. This chapter will not review the reasons for these differing views, but simply recognize that they exist.[6]

Finally, there may be an executive session, where only the voting members of the committee and perhaps an executive secretary are present. This session allows the members to discuss issues more freely. If there are no contentious problems, however, the executive session may be unnecessary. The committee members can decide that at the time of the meeting.

There are two general models for monitoring committees. In the first, a committee is specifically established to monitor an individual trial. This is usually done when the trial is large and likely to go on for several years. In the second, a committee will monitor more than one trial. This is common in the case of networks of investigators that develop and conduct several or even many related protocols, such as for cancer and AIDS trials, and for IRB-appointed institution-wide monitoring committees. The advantages of the former are that the monitoring committee members have expertise in precisely the area of study and they can devote sufficient time to monitoring that single study. The primary advantage of the latter is that it is more efficient to have one committee monitor multiple protocols.

The frequency with which monitoring committees meet is determined by what is necessary to ensure the safety of the participants. The nature of the condition being studied, the kind of intervention, and how rapidly new data accumulate all influence that frequency. Typically, committees that monitor long-term trials meet every six to twelve months or when a specified percentage of participants have been accrued or a specified number of events have occurred. In addition, the option to review safety data in between, either in person or through telephone conference calls, should exist. Often, ongoing reports of individual adverse events are provided to the chairperson of the committee, who can decide whether or not to convene the full committee.

MONITORING PROCESS

It is not possible to foresee and prevent all harm. But the main purpose of monitoring is to make sure that no avoidable harm comes to the study participants as a result of being in the study. No study is risk free, but any potential harm must be counterbalanced or outweighed by potential benefits. To that end, the monitoring committee must be satisfied that the study is designed in as optimal a fashion as possible, with all reasonable safety precautions. After the study is underway, the committee regularly looks at accumulating data. In particular, it monitors study outcomes—both primary and secondary endpoints—and potential adverse events, including laboratory data, as appropriate. The committee must expect that unforeseen adverse events can and will occur, and must be prepared to modify its procedures to prevent or minimize the consequences of unexpected events.

In addition, because a study that is not well conducted cannot justifiably put participants at risk, the monitoring committee reviews study progress, in order to ensure the integrity of the trial. For example, is accrual of participants proceeding on schedule, and if not, how long will it take and will enough participants be entered eventually to address adequately the study hypotheses? Are study forms being completed and are the data of high quality? Are study procedures being done in a timely fashion? Are the analyses up-to-date? Are the participants taking the study medications as prescribed?

Monitoring committees must consider several principles. Various textbooks cover these in some detail,[7-10] so we will only summarize them here.

First, of course, are ethical standards. The trial must begin in a position of clinical equipoise.[11] That is, the informed scientific and medical communities do not know which of the approaches being tested in the trial is preferable. As the data begin to accumulate, the monitoring committee may decide that the trends in the primary outcome are so strong in one direction or another (i.e., in favor of or against the new intervention) that clinical equipoise is no longer tenable and the study must be stopped before its scheduled end. The study has achieved its goal of providing an answer. The sections that follow discuss many examples. Judgment, as well as science and statistics, enter into the decision. Connected with that is a balance of benefits and harms. Even though the primary outcome may not be clear, secondary outcomes or other clinical measures may strongly trend positively or negatively. The committee must decide if adverse events are such that continuing the study cannot be justified. This is often less a statistical decision than a medical and ethical judgment. Another important ethical issue concerns the tension between responsibilities to the study participants, to those yet to enter the study, and to the public. The data from a trial may not be sufficiently persuasive to change entrenched medical practice, but because of adverse trends, the monitoring committee has concerns about the safety of the participants already in the study and may be reluctant to allow enrollment of additional participants. If the study is stopped too early, medical practice may not be altered, and the study participants will have been put at risk to no purpose. If the study is not stopped early, additional harm may come to the study participants. The World Medical Association Declaration of Helsinki[12] clearly states that the well-being of trial participants takes precedence over societal interests. Often, however, the decisions are not clear-cut, and monitoring committees often must wrestle with these difficult issues.

A second principle, and one that drives much of data monitoring, is the concept of repeated looks at the data. Ethically, investigators and sponsors, by means of the monitoring committees, are bound to examine trends in the data during a trial. Unfortunately, the more we look at accumulating data, the greater the possibility of observing a nominally significant result by chance. Therefore, we increase the false-positive rate above that with which the study was designed (e.g., 0.05 or 0.01). For example, if a study is designed with at a 5% level of significance, and the data are looked at twice, the true false-positive, or type 1 error rate is not 5%, but about 8%; if the data are examined five times, the false-positive error rate would be about 14%.[13] Various statistical approaches to this problem have been developed, some of which will be used in the examples in the book. We will not go into detailed statistical issues here. The key point, however, is that because repeated testing of the data can affect statistical interpretation, the issue must be part of data monitoring.

Similarly, monitoring committees look at many outcomes, not just the primary one, and they usually look at different subgroups of participants. As with looking many times at a single outcome, when multiple outcomes, or multiple comparisons, are considered, the standard level of significance does not apply. Care and judgment must therefore be used in making decisions based on nominally significant results from these outcomes. As noted before, however, the safety of the participants is paramount. Therefore, the monitoring committee needs to pay serious attention to adverse events, even if they are of questionable statistical significance or have not been prespecified as outcomes of interest.

Investigators usually want to be very sure when they make claims about the benefits of a new drug or device, but they generally are not interested in proving something is harmful, using the usual level of statistical significance. Therefore, monitoring may be "asymmetric," in the sense that a different level of assurance is used for benefit than for harm.[7]

No clinical trial is done in isolation. Clinical trials are only started after there is considerable basic research, animal studies, and epidemiologic work. And of course, other clinical trials may be addressing the same or similar questions. The monitoring committee needs to be alert, not only to research done in the past that may have led to the clinical trial it is monitoring, but to ongoing research elsewhere that may affect the conduct and feasibility of, or indeed the ethical justification for, the trial. Information from other studies can necessitate modifying the protocol, revising the consent form, or even stopping the study. An example of this last situation is given in Case 24.

Finally, there are a variety of factors that affect the interpretation that the monitoring committee brings to the data it is reviewing. Among these are baseline characteristics of the study participants, including balance between the study groups, use of concomitant therapy by the participants, adherence to medication or procedures, and timeliness of the data that are being monitored. Monitoring committees need to consider these factors when making recommendations to change the protocol or discontinue the study.[3,7]

As noted, monitoring committees can make various recommendations in the course of the study. If the study is progressing reasonably well, with no clear evidence of major toxicity or overwhelming benefit, the committee would recommend continuing the trial without any changes to the protocol. Some circumstances may lead to a recommendation to continue, but with a protocol modification. For example, participant entry criteria may be restricted if it is noticed that certain subgroups of participants seem to be unduly harmed (see Case 23). Or additional measures of possible toxicity could be added. Or if an adverse event not mentioned in the protocol or consent form is observed and thought to be related to the intervention, the investigators and IRBs would be notified and the consent forms appropriately changed (see Case 17).

The monitoring committee could recommend stopping the study (or, in the case of a multi-armed study, dropping one arm) for any of several reasons. These include such overwhelming evidence of benefit from the intervention that the study hypothesis was answered earlier than expected or sufficient evidence of unexpected serious harm. Several examples of these are provided in this book. The committee may also recommend stopping early because there is little or no chance that the hypothesis can be adequately addressed. This may happen because participant recruitment is extremely slow, because compliance with the intervention is poor or there are a great many "cross-overs," or because the control group event rate is much lower than expected. It may also happen because even if the study were to continue to its scheduled end, no clinically useful information would be derived. In all these cases, if the usefulness of what will be learned is so limited that it does not outweigh the discomfort and possible harm to which the participants are being subjected, it is inappropriate to continue the study. Finally, the monitoring committee may recommend early stopping because other research studies have answered the question being posed, and the trial is no longer important or continuation would be unethical (e.g., proven therapy is being withheld).

In rare circumstances, the monitoring committee might recommend extension of the trial beyond its scheduled duration. Typically, this happens when the control group event rate is lower than planned, and a relatively short extension would yield enough outcome events to answer the question. An alternative to this is to design a trial that continues until a pre-specified number of events occurs. This alternative is preferable from a study-design perspective, and has been successfully used in some trials (see Case 8 and the REMATCH study[14]), but for fiscal and management reasons, the uncertainty of duration may be difficult for a sponsor to accept.

INTERACTIONS BETWEEN THE MONITORING COMMITTEE AND OTHERS

Because of its central role in ensuring safety and the integrity of the trial, the monitoring committee has direct or indirect interactions with several other groups. It may be appointed by, and report to, the sponsor of the trial. This is the case with most NIH funded trials. It may also be appointed by and/or make recommendations to an executive committee of the investigators.

If the monitoring committee advises the sponsor, rather than the investigators, the relationship between the monitoring committee and the investigators is indirect. The sponsor of the trial, after receiving the committee recommendations, would communicate with the investigators, informing them either that the study is proceeding well, or that certain changes need to be made. The study investigators, in turn, would inform the study participants of any recommendations, including, potentially, providing them with a revised consent form.

The IRB at each clinic has the legal responsibility to oversee the protocol at that clinic, and to ensure local participant safety. In multi-center trials, this responsibility is generally ceded to the monitoring committee, which is the only group that knows the outcome data across the entire study. When initially reviewing trial protocols, the IRBs should be informed about the plans for monitoring, so that they are comfortable that it will be done in an appropriate manner. In return for the authority to conduct the monitoring, the monitoring committee must keep all IRBs informed of its recommendations, and of any unexpected adverse events or protocol changes. For studies sponsored by the NIH, a policy requires that reports of the recommendations and any safety concerns of the monitoring committee be sent to all involved IRBs after each monitoring committee meeting.[15] We recommend that a similar policy be adopted for all industry-sponsored trials.

When the clinical trial is being conducted under the auspices of drug and device regulatory agencies, those agencies must also be kept informed of serious adverse events. Reports summarizing the committee recommendations and any protocol modifications must be communicated to the regulatory agencies, typically through the study sponsor.

Finally, it should be emphasized that except for these communications, all members of monitoring committees are expected to maintain confidentiality. Discussions of data or study issues outside of the meetings or with anyone else are completely inappropriate.

SUMMARY

This chapter reviews several key issues with regard to monitoring committees, so that the examples and discussions in the rest of this book may be better understood. The primary purpose of independent monitoring committees is to ensure, to the extent possible, that participants in clinical trials are not unduly harmed. A secondary purpose is to enhance study quality and integrity. The use of monitoring committees in late-phase and selected early-phase clinical trials has become commonplace. The compositions of these committees and the monitoring process they follow have also become more standardized, although some differences remain. Principles underlying data and safety monitoring, namely, maintenance of ethical and biostatistical standards and of public trust, and the need for considerable judgment and interpretation, are essential in the committee process. The monitoring committee also operates in the context of a larger research and participant safety environment. Therefore, recommendations from the committee must be implemented in that context.

REFERENCES

1. The Coronary Drug Project Research Group. 1973. The Coronary Drug Project: Design, methods, and baseline results. *Circulation* 47 (Suppl I): I-1–I-79.
2. Organization, review and administration of cooperative studies (Greenberg Report): A report from the Heart Special Project Committee to the National Advisory Heart Council, May 1967. 1988. *Control Clin Trials* 9:137–148.

3. Canner PL. 1983. Monitoring of the data for evidence of adverse or beneficial effects. In, (Canner PL, ed.): *The Coronary Drug Project. Methods and Lessons of a Multicenter Clinical Trial. Control Clin Trials* 4:467–483.

4. FDA Draft Guidance on Data Monitoring Committees: http://www.fda.gov/OHRMS/DOCKETS/98fr/010489gd.pdf

5. NIH Policy for Data and Safety Monitoring: http://grants.nih.gov/grants/guide/notice-files/not98-084.html

6. Ellenberg S, Fleming TR, DeMets DL. Data Monitoring Committees in Clinical Trials: A Practical Perspective. 2002. John Wiley & Sons, New York.

7. Friedman LM, Furberg CD, DeMets DL. Fundamentals of Clinical Trials, third edition. 1998. Springer-Verlag, New York.

8. Meinert CL. Clinical Trials: Design, Conduct and Analysis. 1986. Oxford University Press, New York.

9. Piantadosi S. Clinical Trials: A Methodologic Perspective. 1997. John Wiley & Sons, New York.

10. Pocock SJ. Clinical Trials: A Practical Approach. 1983, John Wiley & Sons, New York.

11. Freedman B. 1987. Equipoise and the ethics of clinical research. *N Engl J Med* 317:141–145.

12. The World Medical Association. World Medical Association Declaration of Helsinki: Ethical principals for medical research involving human subjects. October 2000 amended version, with 2002 clarification. http://www.wma.net/e/policy/b3.htm.

13. Canner PL. Monitoring clinical trial data for evidence of adverse or beneficial treatment effects. 1979. In Boissel JP, Klimt CR (eds.): *Multicenter Controlled Trials: Principles and Problems.* INSERM, Paris.

14. Rose EA, Moskowitz AJ, Packer M, Sollano JA, Williams DL, Tierney AR, Heitjan DF, Meier P, Ascheim DD, Levitan RG, Weinberg AD, Stevenson LW, Shapiro PA, Lazar RM, Watson JT, Goldstein DJ, Gelijns AC, for the REMATCH Investigators. 1999. The REMATCH trial: rationale, design, and end points. *Ann Thorac Surg* 67:723–730.

15. NIH Guidance on Reporting Adverse Events to Institutional Review Boards: http://grants.nih.gov/grants/guide/notice-files/not99-107.html

CHAPTER 2

Lessons Learned

David L. DeMets
Curt D. Furberg
Lawrence M. Friedman

In the sections that follow, the authors of the case studies identify many "lessons learned." These examples of issues faced during the monitoring of clinical trials illustrate both how the issues were addressed and how they might have been handled better. Many of these lessons learned have common themes, whereas others are specific to the particular trial. Even the latter, though, provide important guidance and warnings to others, because they are unlikely to be unique. This chapter summarizes the more common lessons in eleven major areas. The division into the eleven areas is somewhat arbitrary; there are clear overlaps among them, and many of the lessons fall into more than one area. Nevertheless, it was a useful way to categorize the many lessons learned.

MONITORING COMMITTEE COMPOSITION AND RESPONSIBILITIES

As described in Chapter 1, the monitoring committee advises both the trial sponsor and the trial investigators but also has a responsibility to the trial participants. The composition of the monitoring committee is extremely important. First, the members collectively must have experience and expertise in the area of research being studied, clinical trials, biostatistics, epidemiology, and medical ethics. Monitoring for safety and efficacy is a complex process and requires a combination of talent and knowledge. Second, members must be free of conflicts in order to make independent, unbiased recommendations. These conflicts include financial interests related to a commercial sponsor and any competitor, intellectual conflicts with the research and the trial, and ethical conflicts with respect to patient care and rights. This means that monitoring committee members should not be employees of the sponsoring company or a competitor, or of the sponsoring institute, and should not be involved in recruiting or interacting with trial participants, or be part of the data management team. Monitoring committees should have at least three members in order to achieve the necessary expertise and balance, and rarely more than seven in order to keep the logistics of arranging meetings manageable. While committee members must be quite familiar with the protocol and trial design, they must remain sufficiently independent that their discussion is not influenced by any intellectual investment in the protocol. If a monitoring committee has proper and adequate composition, it should be able to fulfill its responsibilities.

All of the monitoring committees for the trials presented later had expertise in multiple areas and were independent of the sponsor, regardless of the kind of sponsor. For example, the Antihypertensive and Lipid-Lowering Treatment to prevent Heart Attack Trial (ALLHAT) (Case 18), the Carotene and Retinol Efficacy Trial (CARET) (Case 15), and the toxoplasmic encephalitis study (Case 25) were sponsored by the National Institutes of Health, a U.S. Federal agency, while the bevacizumab colorectal cancer trial (Case 29), the Carvedilol Post-Infarct Survival Control in Left Ventricular Dysfunction Study (CAPRICORN) (Case 27), and the Cooperative New Scandinavian Enalapril Survival Study II (CONSENSUS II) (Case 23) were industry sponsored.

The example of the clinical trials of herpes simplex encephalitis (Case 21) is instructive. Until that study, it had been uncommon for monitoring committees to be established for trials in the infectious disease area. The benefit to the trial shown by this case was a key factor in the spread of the use of monitoring committees in this medical discipline.

The role of the monitoring committee should be clearly defined, preferably in a written document or charter. Although most monitoring committees currently have a charter or other written document defining their responsibilities, how they will function, what variables are to be considered for efficacy, and the statistical methods for monitoring accumulating data, these are considered at best guidelines. No current statistical methods, for example, can adequately capture the complexity of, or balance, the multiple efficacy and safety outcomes to produce a simple algorithm. When such attempts have been made, they have often failed because issues that arose were not usually included in the pre-specified methods. The complexity of the decision process has been described as early as the Coronary Drug Project (CDP)[1] and discussed in more detail by others.[2-4] Rather than rely totally on statistical methods, monitoring committees must use their collective wisdom and judgment. In addition, monitoring committees often have to react quickly to issues that were not anticipated.

Difficulties associated with lack of clear responsibilities are shown in the Randomized Evaluation of Strategies for Left Ventricular Dysfunction (RESOLVD) (Case 26), a seven-armed, two-stage pilot study in 769 patients with left ventricular dysfunction. No formal charter was agreed upon by the monitoring committee, and the investigators and no statistical monitoring boundaries were pre-specified. During the course of the trial, it became apparent that the monitoring committee and the trial investigators "had different ideas as to the roles and the function" of the committee. This led to major problems in communication. When the monitoring committee unanimously recommended trial termination due to safety concerns, the executives of the Steering Committee disagreed. An expert panel was convened to help resolve the disagreement and it concluded that there was no clear evidence of harm, but at the same time recommended that "the unanimous vote of any data monitoring board should not be overturned lightly" and found no reason to do so in this case.

Monitoring committees can unintentionally get involved in protocol modifications that later become awkward and controversial. In CAPRICORN (Case 27), the monitoring committee pointed out to the trial sponsor and steering committee early in the trial that the primary endpoint, mortality, appeared to have a lower than expected event rate and that this situation should be addressed. In addition, enrollment of study participants lagged. The steering committee responded by modifying the protocol. As discussed later in this chapter, this created awkwardness in the analysis and interpretation of the results.

With the exception, of course, of design changes necessary to ensure participant safety, it is easiest, and most rigorous, not to allow any major design changes. Many studies, however, have lower event rates than projected. One option in such cases is to make no changes. This runs the real risk of coming up with an unclear answer at the end of the trial, and, therefore, of putting participants at risk for little purpose. A second option is to change the primary endpoint. As shown in CAPRICORN (Case 27), though at times unavoidable, this is generally undesirable. If done at all, it should be implemented early in the trial and by those not aware of the comparison group findings. The second example in chapter 3 points to the problems that can arise when those who know the trends in the data make such decisions. A third option is to extend recruitment or follow-up in order to achieve the projected number of events. As with changing the primary outcome, this should be done by investigators or sponsors who do not know how the data are trending. A fourth option is to design the trial as event driven which allows the investigators to continue recruitment until the target events have been observed, increase follow up, or a combination. Since the target number of required events is pre-specified, these changes do not result in a design change. Because it is not possible even to consider whether or not to make such changes in either the third or fourth option unless one knows something about the event rate, these options imply that the investigators are informed of either the overall (all study groups combined) event rate or the event rate in the control group. If the overall event rate is lower than expected, based on the assumed control arm event rates, investigators and others may speculate that the intervention is indeed effective. However, as illustrated by several examples, such a benefit may not be the case. Investigators who want to speculate may sometimes be able to calculate the overall event rate. Providing them with the control group event rate can thus disclose the comparative numbers. In our experience, therefore, sharing the overall event rate is preferable.

On occasion, a monitoring committee is not able to come to a clear recommendation or arrive at a consensus, and a second committee may be appointed. In CARET (Case 15), which evaluated beta carotene as a cancer prevention agent, the monitoring committee recommended termination due to a negative, but not statistically significant, trend which was consistent with findings from a similar completed trial conducted in Finland (the Alpha-Tocopherol, Beta Carotene, or ATBC, cancer prevention trial).[5] When the recommendation was presented to the CARET sponsor, the National Cancer Institute, an *ad hoc* committee was formed to review the CARET monitoring committee recommendations. The *ad hoc* committee endorsed the recommendations of the monitoring committee and the sponsor, the National Cancer Institute, terminated CARET. In ALLHAT (Case 18), a trial of blood-pressure and lipid-lowering medications, the monitoring committee was narrowly divided in its recommendation to continue doxazosine, one of the interventions in this four-arm study. Because of the closeness of the vote, the sponsor, the National Heart, Lung, and Blood Institute, convened an *ad hoc* group to review the data. This group unanimously recommended early termination, which is what happened.

Though the use of second committees is sometimes necessary, it conveys a lack of confidence in the primary monitoring committee and is generally not desirable.

This situation is different from that in the CDP (Case 12) and the Diabetes Complications and Control Trial (DCCT) (Case 5), where two committees were instituted early in the trials. A policy advisory group reviewed the recommendations from the monitoring committee and advised the sponsor whether or not to accept the recommendation. Because only occasionally has the need for a second advisory committee arisen, most current trials have only a single monitoring group.

EARLY PREPARATION

The first order of business for any monitoring committee, after its roles and responsibilities are made clear, is the review and acceptance of the trial protocol and the establishment of the monitoring plan. The processes for the timely flow of data, especially outcome data, are part of the monitoring plan and should also be in place from the beginning. This includes the classification of events. Finally, the monitoring committee should be given an opportunity to comment on the layout of future data reports, for example, in the form of "table shells" or graphical displays. These items should be addressed at the first meeting of any monitoring committee. It is essential to be fully prepared before the first participant is randomized.

Trends requiring action by the monitoring committee may emerge early. In CONSENSUS II (Case 23), the angiotensin-converting enzyme inhibitor enalapril was given to patients with acute myocardial infarction. The first dose in the coronary care unit was an intravenous formulation. The infusion was given slowly due to a concern that the first dose could cause severe hypotension. At the initial meeting of the monitoring committee, 71 (7%) of the projected 1,000 deaths had accrued. A most striking finding was that 11 of 60 enalapril patients with first-dose hypotension had died compared to none of 16 placebo patients. This observation led to protocol changes, which included exclusion from enrollment of patients with low entry blood pressure, reduction in the rate of infusion, and specific criteria for termination of infusion if the blood pressure dropped below a certain level. A monitoring committee needs to be prepared to take action early.

Two other trials illustrate the same point. The Moxonidine Congestive Heart Failure (MOXCON) trial (Case 19) was terminated after accrual of only 71 (10%) of the projected 724 deaths. When the monitoring committee recommended termination, there were 46 deaths among the moxonidine and 25 deaths among the placebo patients ($p = 0.01$).

The Cardiac Arrhythmia Suppression Trial (CAST) (Case 13) evaluated arrhythmia-suppressing drugs compared to a placebo in people with heart disease. The theory was that since arrhythmias are associated with sudden cardiac death, suppressing these arrhythmias would reduce the incidence of sudden death. At the first interim analysis, with less than 10% of the participants enrolled and only about 5% of the expected number of events, the monitoring committee observed a trend in both sudden death and total mortality, but was blinded as to treatment assignment. The monitoring committee was not alarmed by the trend since there was some reason or theory to believe the active drugs would be effective and there were only small numbers of events at the time of that analysis. A few months later, the statistical center alerted the monitoring committee that these trends were getting stronger, even approaching pre-specified statistical boundaries, and that the trend was going in the opposite direction—that is, not a beneficial but a harmful direction. The monitoring committee quickly held a conference call, and agreed that a full meeting needed to be held as soon as possible with a detailed interim analysis based on as complete mortality data as possible. This detailed analysis verified that there was a harmful treatment effect, and the monitoring committee recommended that two of the three antiarrythmic drugs used in CAST be stopped. The investigators and drug regulatory agencies were immediately notified and the trial results were rapidly disseminated.

In the trial of diaspirin cross-linked hemoglobin (Case 16), a blood substitute product was being tested for use in emergency situations for trauma patients. Very early in the trial, adverse events were observed. The monitoring committee held emergency conference calls during a holiday season to review updated analyses. After careful review, the committee recommended that the trial be terminated. In this trial, the committee members had to adjust their individual schedules and be flexible to the needs of the trial, despite holiday seasons and other commitments. Another aspect of this trial was the need to waive informed consent in order to conduct emergency research. To meet U.S. federal guidelines for consent waiver, additional steps had to be taken as described in the case study, but clearly the monitoring committee carried even greater responsibility than is typical.

One approach to dealing with lagging reports of outcome data is a so-called "sweep." Each investigator is requested to contact every participant at a certain time point. In the Randomized Aldactone Evaluation Study (RALES) (Case 9), two sweeps were conducted due to the suspicion of underreporting of deaths, the primary outcome. Although the yield from the sweeps could not be precisely determined, computer simulations indicated that this effort led to an 8% increase in the number of reported deaths. In the Nocturnal Oxygen Treatment Trial (NOTT) (Case 22), a lag in reporting deaths from two centers created a nominally significant, but artificial, trend in a high-risk subgroup. A sweep of the clinical centers for mortality updates resulted in the trend largely disappearing.

Monitoring committees also need to consider the "pipeline effect" when they think about early stopping. As noted in RALES (Case 9), even with sweeps, 46 deaths were unreported at the time of the recommendation to stop the trial. These were not all identified until some time later. A recommendation to stop a study must include an estimate of the number of these unreported events, and whether the conclusions might change once all the data are known. In general, procedures need to be put in place to assure that critically important data, such as mortality and serious adverse events, are on a "fast track" in the data flow system.

ETHICS

Not surprisingly, given the reason that monitoring committees were developed, all of the case studies in this book deal with one or another aspect of ethics. In most, if not all trials, the monitoring committee faces a conflict between its responsibility to the study participants and responsibility to society, to people in general who have or may develop the disease or condition being studied. Research is useful if it leads to knowledge that can be generalized, to information that can be helpful to a broader population than just those participants in the trial. Therefore, monitoring committees resist stopping a study before it provides a clear and persuasive answer to an important question. The time, effort, expense, and risks to which participants have already been exposed would be wasted. But the primary duty of the monitoring committee is to safeguard those enrolled in the trial. If they are being unduly harmed, without likely opportunity to benefit, then the monitoring committees must recommend whatever changes are necessary, even if it means learning less than they might want. As noted in the World Medical Association's Declaration of Helsinki, "In medical research on human subjects, considerations related to the well-being of the human subject should take precedence over the interests of science and society."[6] There are no easy answers to the conflict between the need to protect the trial participants and the imperative to accrue essential, perhaps lifesaving knowledge. Statistics can help, but in the end, it comes down to the collective judgment of the committee members, using whatever data, experience, and personal perspectives they can. The Stroke Prevention in Atrial Fibrillation I (SPAF I) trial (Case 4) illustrates this tension.

Another commonly discussed issue is how long a trial should be continued once trends emerge, particularly when these trends are nominally statistically significant. As discussed later in this chapter, early results may be unreliable. Therefore, stopping a study or changing a protocol too soon may lead to false conclusions. But the responsibility of the monitoring committee to the study participants, particularly if the trend is in the direction of harm from the intervention is a major point of consideration. Examples in this book of studies that stopped arms early because of adverse trends are the CDP (Case 12) low-dose estrogen intervention, the trial of diaspirin cross-linked hemoglobin for emergency treatment of post-traumatic shock (Case 16), CAST (Case 13), and ALLHAT (Case 18). In ALLHAT, doxazosin was less effective than chlorthalidone with regard to secondary, but still clinically important, outcomes. It also had an extremely small likelihood of being shown to be superior for the primary outcome. Therefore, even though in this study where the control group was on an active intervention, and it could not be claimed that doxazosin was harmful when compared with no treatment, it was stopped ahead of schedule. In a breast cancer study (Case 28) after recruitment and treatment were completed, early emerging trends that were unexpected proved to be a challenge for the monitoring committee. Issues considered were whether early release would impact on the follow-up, affect the integrity of the trial, and interfere with long-term assessment. To complicate matters, no pre-planned interim analyses had been incorporated in the protocol. Clearly, some pre-planned but flexible interim analysis plans would be beneficial.

A related topic is the use of asymmetric monitoring guidelines. Generally, investigators are interested in proving that an intervention is beneficial, not that it is harmful. Similarly, the evidence required to take action as a results of adverse events is typically less demanding than the evidence to act on the basis of positive findings. This is because the primary responsibility is to ensure, to the extent possible, the safety of the participants. As seen above in the case study from CAST (Case 13), the first part of the trial was stopped because the advisory boundary for harm was crossed for two of the three drugs. This boundary was symmetric with the boundary for benefit. In the second part of CAST, after having seen the adverse consequences of two of the drugs, the monitoring committee established an advisory boundary for harm for the third drug that was less extreme than the boundary for benefit. Monitoring boundaries for MOXCON (Case 19) were asymmetric from the beginning. Although the nominal p-values for stopping early for benefit were two-sided 0.0001 after 25% of the data and 0.001 after 50% and 75% of the data were observed, the boundary for all-cause mortality in the harmful direction used a one-sided $p < 0.05$. The monitoring committee, in fact, recommended stopping because of increased mortality with a $p = 0.02$.

The Breast Cancer Prevention Trial (BCPT) (Case 7) illustrates the tension between accumulating evidence of the benefit of the intervention on the primary outcome (breast cancer) and adverse events, both expected (endometrial cancer, thromboembolic events) and unexpected (cataracts). The expected adverse events were addressed, at least partly, by means of a global index. But the unexpected appearance of an increased incidence of cataracts required the study to re-consent the participants. Similar disclosure of interim data because of the occurrence of adverse events took place in the Heart and Estrogen/progestin Replacement Study (HERS) (Case 17). During that trial, the participants were informed of an increased risk of pulmonary embolism and deep vein thrombosis. Despite the disclosure of the information to the participants, the vast majority continued in the studies, and the trials were successfully completed.

In the examples where interim data about adverse events were shared with participants, it was because the adverse events were either more common or more serious than had been expected, or not previously known and therefore not disclosed in the study protocol and consent form. Not only is it required that such information be provided both to the participants and the institutional ethics review committees, and, usually, to the regulatory agencies, it is an ethical obligation. An ethical obligation may also arise if the study changes course, changes the primary outcome, or needs to go longer than originally planned. The consent form that was signed by the participants is, in a sense, a contract between the investigator and the participant.

Clinical trials, indeed all clinical research, are only ethical if there is a reasonable expectation that important information will result, i.e., that clinically meaningful questions can be answered. If, during the course of a trial, it becomes clear that no such outcome is likely, the study may be stopped for what has been termed "futility." The Physicians' Health Study (PHS) (Case 3) was a factorial design study. It had as one of its primary outcomes, the effect of aspirin on cardiovascular disease mortality. However, it became apparent that the event rate for this outcome was so low that only a long (over 10-year) extension of the trial would yield a sufficient number of events to have adequate power. At the same time, a leading secondary outcome of fatal plus non-fatal myocardial infarction was becoming increasingly more significant with each review of the data. Ultimately, the monitoring committee recommended termination based on the overwhelming significance of the secondary outcome and the low probability of achieving definitive results on the primary outcome. The monitoring committee discussions show the need for flexibility, as the expected did not occur.

The AIDS Clinical Trial Group study #981 (Case 6) shows a different kind of tension between the primary endpoint and another important outcome. The monitoring committee observed a statistically significant benefit in a primary outcome related to AIDS progression but noted an adverse trend in mortality. The committee recommended continuation of the trial in order to resolve the conflicting trends. Ultimately, there was no difference in mortality.

The trial of daclizumab for treatment of acute graft-versus-host disease in allogeneic stem cell transplantation (Case 20) provides another example where a secondary endpoint led to a recommendation from the monitoring committee. In this trial, the predefined stopping guidelines for the primary outcome were not crossed. However, there was a significant increase in mortality in the daclizumab group, compared to standard treatment, while the difference in the primary outcome persisted.

The reverse happened in the Clopidogrel in Unstable Angina to Prevent Recurrent Ischemic Events (CURE) trial (Case 10). There, the monitoring committee had to balance clear benefit for the two primary outcomes (composite of cardiovascular death, myocardial infarction, and stroke; time to first outcome of any of the previous or refractory ischemia) against hemorrhagic stroke and bleeding. Even though the monitoring boundary for benefit for the primary outcomes was crossed, the committee thought that the need to obtain further information about safety, especially intracerebral hemorrhage, was important enough to justify continuing the trial until its scheduled end.

A final ethics-related issue, though one only briefly mentioned in the case studies (see Case 19), involves the monitoring committee's role in publications. Traditionally, it is the responsibility of the investigators, with or without the sponsor, to perform the final analysis and interpretation of the data, and to publish the results. Unfortunately, publication bias, where "positive" results (i.e., those studies where the intervention is shown to be better than the control) are more likely to be published than are "negative" results (i.e., no significant difference or control better than intervention) has been seen with clinical trials.[7] On average, trials with positive results are published sooner after the end of a study than are trials with negative or neutral results.[8] As an example, the results of the Prospective Randomized Amlodipine Survival Evaluation-2 (PRAISE-2) were presented at the American College of Cardiology meeting in March 2000 and have been referred to elsewhere.[9] A full report, however, has not appeared as of the publication of this book. Investigators may lose interest in publishing negative results, moving on to the next study. Despite commitments to publish negative studies, journals may have less interest in publishing the results of such trials. Sponsors of a trial may exert pressure to alter, delay, or prevent publication. A trial of a drug designed to enhance immunologic response in patients with human immunodeficiency virus (HIV) was eventually published with only incomplete data due to such pressures from the sponsor.[10,11]

There have also been occasions when individual members of the monitoring committee have disagreed with the interpretation expressed by the investigators.[12-15] Because the monitoring committee has been heavily involved in ongoing analyses, it may have as good or perhaps even a better understanding of the data than investigators, who may have seen the data only briefly before quickly submitting a paper for publication. In addition, the monitoring committee members are more likely to be independent, and to have less of a vested interest in interpreting the data in a certain way. In many studies, even though the primary responsibility for publication rests with the investigators, the monitoring committee is given the opportunity to review and comment on the draft manuscript for the main results and other major papers. The monitoring committee should especially review any aspects of the manuscripts that describe the monitoring process or reasons for early termination. Usually comments are appreciated and strongly considered. However, if there are differences of opinion, or if the publications are not timely, the responsibilities of the monitoring committee in these circumstances are not entirely clear, and further discussion is warranted.

DATA ISSUES

The responsibility of the monitoring committee to review accumulating data for early evidence of safety and effectiveness depends on the timeliness and completeness of the data. As discussed for the RALES (Case 9) example in the section on Early Preparation, interim committee reports which are based on data several months old are not helpful, especially with emerging trends. The committee reports must also be based on data that are reasonably complete and accurate. This tension between currency and completeness and accuracy is unavoidable but must be addressed. Commonly, requirements are stratified in terms of priority. The highest priority must be for the primary outcome, mortality, and other key trial-specific safety measures. Mortality, for example, should be very current, perhaps only several days old. Serious adverse events generally have regulatory reporting requirements which mandate timely data. Primary outcome data other than mortality may require more detail and a central adjudication process, which can take several months or longer. In these cases, monitoring committees may rely on preliminary reports until the adjudication process catches up. Thus, the committee will review a mix of adjudicated data and preliminary or unadjudicated data. In general, key data should not be more than two months old. Other kinds of data, such as baseline characteristics, should also not be more than two months old since they are important for checking comparability of intervention arms and also for evaluating key predefined subgroups. However, laboratory data and use of concomitant medications, for example, may not require as high a priority for timeliness.

If interim data do not meet these criteria, the monitoring committee may make an inappropriate recommendation. The Nocturnal Oxygen Therapy Trial (NOTT) (Case 22) evaluated 12 versus 24 hours of oxygen supplementation in people with chronic obstructive pulmonary disease. Early in the trial, the monitoring committee observed an emerging mortality trend favoring the group being treated with 24 hours of oxygen. This was seen overall (18 versus 9 deaths; p = 0.07) but most prominently in the highest risk subgroup (12 versus 5 deaths; p = 0.01). The committee strongly considered terminating this subgroup. However, the statistical center suspected that the data were not current for all participating clinical centers. The monitoring committee wisely suggested that further discussion be tabled until a sweep of all centers could be accomplished. With an analysis of the updated data, the subgroup trend disappeared. Indeed, two centers had been tardy in reporting mortality data. The apparent trend was an artifact of the data flow. In this case, the monitoring committee was fortunate to have uncovered this possible data issue and avoided making an inappropriate recommendation.

As discussed previously, CAST (Case 13) had unexpected early adverse mortality. It was therefore essential that the mortality data be complete and current from the beginning of the trial. The CAST monitoring committee was originally blinded as to treatment assignment. Even though it noted an emerging trend at the first interim analysis, the committee chose to remain blinded. Whether the committee would have reacted more quickly than it did had it been unblinded is only speculation. Most monitoring committees have the option of unblinding themselves at any time. Some may choose to unblind at the first interim analysis; others may choose to wait until a trend emerges. There are no regulatory requirements for a monitoring committee to remain blinded during its review of interim analyses. Most committees do not act the same way when there is an adverse trend as they do when there is a trend favorable to the intervention. Therefore, it is recommended that at the latest, when a trend emerges with any meaningful number of events, the committee be made aware of the identity of the group treatment assignments.

Monitoring committee members are usually extremely busy people. Meetings must be kept as short as possible, while allowing the committee responsibilities to be met by a careful and detailed review of the interim data. Many meetings must fit into a period of four to six hours. For example, in the Metoprolol CR/XL Randomized Intervention Trial in Chronic Heart Failure (MERIT-HF) (Case 8), the committee had a one-hour conference call each month to review safety data. Only on two occasions, when both outcomes and safety data were assessed, did the monitoring committee meet face-to-face for a longer meeting. Thus, it is paramount that monitoring reports be carefully constructed, containing both pre-specified analyses and analyses to answer anticipated committee questions, and be well presented. On occasion, a report may be so inadequate that the meeting must be deferred until a proper report can be prepared. These situations can and must be avoided with proper planning. The data center can often achieve this by preparing a mock report at the organizational or first meeting of the monitoring committee, giving an opportunity for feedback.

REACTION TO EARLY DATA

Many monitoring committees struggle with how much confidence to place in early data. Early data, by definition, consist of small numbers, which are highly variable. The observed point estimates have large confidence intervals. The lack of certainty is one reason that some monitoring boundaries require very extreme differences early in a trial. In addition, as seen in several of the case studies, early trends, even though real, might be reversed by longer follow-up. The short-term effects of interventions might not be sustained in the long-term. But monitoring committees need to be sensitive to putting study participants at risk longer than they need to. If a treatment is truly believed to be beneficial, even in the short-term, those in the control group deserve to have access to it.

Several of the case studies illustrate the hazards of reacting too soon. In the CDP (Case 12), the results from the clofibrate group exceeded the boundary p-value for benefit for the primary outcome of mortality three times in the first 30 months of the trial. Yet at the end of the study, no difference was seen. The Candesartan in Heart Failure Assessment of Reduction in Mortality and morbidity (CHARM) (Case 11) provides an example of large early differences in mortality that attenuated over time. By the end of the trial, the difference was not nearly as impressive, and failed to reach statistical significance.

It is even more difficult to continue to monitor a trial if the short-term results are in the harmful direction. Unless it is clear that the short-term results are expected to be harmful, but it is hoped that the long-term results will turn around (as might be the case with surgical procedures), short-term harm must be taken seriously. When there are early adverse trends, several options are available. If the results are clear and serious, then, of course, stopping the trial is an option. Other approaches are to wait it out, to convene an interim meeting or conference call of the monitoring committee, to request special analyses that might inform a recommendation, and to ask for additional tests to be performed.

Early in HERS (Case 17), which evaluated hormone replacement therapy for post-menopausal women, an increase in death due to coronary heart disease, one of the components of the primary outcome (non-fatal MI plus coronary heart disease death) was noted in the hormone therapy group (nominal $p = 0.02$) and seemed likely to cross the monitoring boundary. For a variety of good reasons, the monitoring committee voted to continue the trial. Later, this trend reversed and the relative hazard at the end of the trial was 0.99. In the middle years of the study, the risk of one of the pre-specified secondary outcomes, venous thromboembolic events, crossed the monitoring boundary. Instead of recommending trial termination, the monitoring committee advised the investigator leadership to inform all study participants of this risk, to modify the protocol to reduce future risk of thromboembolic complications, and to publish the venous thromboembolic data. In HERS, the continued follow-up was extremely helpful in evaluating the balance of benefit and harm.

COMPOSITE OUTCOMES

An increasing number of clinical trials today use composite outcomes. When investigators combine multiple clinical outcomes that may be affected in the same way by the study intervention, the statistical power of that trial is likely to increase. Alternatively, the sample size might be reduced. If the components are thought to be part of the same overall disease process, it can make sense to combine them. If the components of a composite outcome respond differently to an intervention, however, the interpretation of the overall findings can represent a challenge. The different components may also have very different clinical importance, and the question of "weighting" may arise. Currently, there is no generally accepted way of deciding on and interpreting composite outcomes, both overall and for individual components.

In the Heart Outcomes Prevention Evaluation (HOPE) (Case 10), the primary outcome was the combined incidence of cardiovascular death, myocardial infarction and stroke. The investigators and the monitoring committee shared the view that the individual components by themselves were sufficiently important to warrant answers as to the effect of treatment. The trial continued until the treatment benefit became clear for each of the components.

Two other recent trials not included as examples in this book, Losartan Intervention For End Point Reduction (LIFE)[16,17] and Pravastatin Or Atorvastatin Evaluation and Infection Therapy (PROVE IT)[18] relied on composite outcomes. In LIFE, losartan, compared with atenolol, reduced the combined incidence of death, myocardial infarction, and stroke in people with hypertension and left ventricular hypertrophy. Only one of the three components of the endpoint, stroke, was individually statistically significant. Myocardial infarction trended in the wrong direction. In PROVE IT, 80 mg of atorvastatin was more effective than 40 mg of pravastatin in reducing the composite outcome of death, myocardial infarction, stroke, documented unstable angina requiring hospitalization, and revascularization. The data for stroke trended in the direction opposite to other components. Questions have been raised by these findings. First, is the proper interpretation that the two interventions in LIFE and PROVE IT reduce the risk of the composite outcomes, or should the claim of benefit be limited to only individual components that are significant on their own? Requiring such a strong result, of course, would eliminate a rationale for using a composite outcome. Second, for the component analyses, should the significance level be adjusted for multiple comparisons? This is generally not done if the overall composite outcome shows a significant difference, though some would find it particularly persuasive. Third, is it fair, during the design of the trial, to exclude from a composite outcome individual outcomes that are highly likely to trend in the wrong direction? Even if such an outcome is not officially part of the original composite outcome, monitoring committees should look at the data from all relevant outcomes, and may combine them with the composite to obtain a clearer picture of the overall benefit/harm balance.

Some have proposed that if a composite outcome is used as the primary endpoint, the trial should be stopped ahead of schedule for benefit only if the clinically important components of the composite outcome cross a predefined monitoring boundary.[19] For example, if the composite endpoint is cardiovascular death plus non-fatal myocardial infarction plus angina pectoris, angina would not count in a decision to stop early. This approach would be acceptable only if the study participants have been fully informed in advance and understand the basis for stopping decisions. Clearly, this would not apply to harm, because adverse events of various sorts might reasonably lead to early stopping.

The investigators of BCPT (Case 7) and the Women's Health Initiative estrogen trials[20,21] chose another approach by creating global indices that were summary measures of the balance of benefits and harm.[22] In BCPT, the global index consisted of eleven conditions; in the Women's Health Initiative it had seven. These global indices were not the primary outcomes of the studies but were used as supporting evidence. Unlike the practice with most combined outcomes, BCPT created two global indices: one unweighted and one weighted for expected survival after development of the individual component.

In CAPRICORN (Case 27), the number of deaths (primary outcome) accrued slowly for a variety of reasons. Faced with some unattractive solutions, the monitoring committee reluctantly agreed to add a co-primary endpoint of all-cause mortality and cardiovascular hospitalization. The required sample size decreased accordingly. The pre-specified significant p-value was set at 0.005 for all-cause mortality and 0.045 for the combined endpoint. The irony in CAPRICORN was that at the end the hazard ratio for all-cause mortality was 0.77 (nominal p-value of 0.031) and for the combined outcome 0.92 (p = 0.296). CAPRICORN did not achieve its own revised criteria to demonstrate a beneficial effect. The use of a combined outcome turned out to be costly. This turn of events became awkward not only for investigators and the sponsor, but also for the monitoring committee. In retrospect, it would have been better for the monitoring committee not to have been involved at all in these design modifications, even in a limited way.

A different sense of "combined endpoints" occurred in the CHARM program (Case 11). The CHARM program was designed as three parallel but independent clinical trials of candesartan in patients with symptomatic heart failure. All three trials were conducted at the same sites. The stopping rules were trial-specific p-value criteria and statistical evidence of heterogeneity among the three trials. Monitoring included a comparison of the combined mortality experience across the three trials. The monitoring committee paid attention to the three trials in parallel and overall.

SUBGROUPS

Monitoring committees, as well as investigators, are always interested in subgroup analyses. From a monitoring perspective, if there is evidence of harm from the intervention, but that harm can be isolated to a subset of the participants, the whole study need not be stopped. The participants being harmed can be dropped from the trial, and no new participants with the identifying characteristics are enrolled. In some cases, this has worked. The National Emphysema Treatment Trial (NETT)[23,24] is an example of successfully dropping a particular subgroup. This trial compared lung-volume-reduction surgery against medical therapy in patients with severe emphysema. Partway through the trial, the monitoring committee noted that in a high-risk subgroup, 30-day mortality was 16% (11 deaths) in the 69 patients assigned to surgery and 0% in the 70 patients treated medically. Enrollment of patients meeting the identified criteria was stopped. Interestingly, the surgical group had better improvement in exercise capacity, compared with the medical group. Overall, for the participants in the remaining subgroups, the surgical treatment was eventually seen to be favorable.[25]

More often, however, subgroup findings have been less clear. The CDP example (Case 12) with high-dose estrogen and dextrothyroxine shows the hazards of relying on subgroup findings. The monitoring committee tried to identify subgroups of participants who were at particular risk from the interventions, in order to avoid discontinuing the entire arms of the trial. For the high-dose estrogen arm, the monitoring committee separated the participants into two levels of risk. It was clear that in the higher-risk group, estrogen treatment was harmful, causing increased mortality and non-fatal myocardial infarction. In the lower-risk group, there was again an increase in non-fatal myocardial infarction, as well as thromboembolic events. But mortality, the primary endpoint, trended slightly in the positive direction. The monitoring committee narrowly voted to continue this subgroup. The CDP, however, had an oversight Policy Board. This group rejected the monitoring committee's recommendation and voted to discontinue the entire high-dose estrogen arm. As seen in Case 12, the subgroup discussion for the dextrothyroxine treatment was even more complicated. Canner emphasizes that a major reason for the difficulty was the lack of *a priori* specifications of the subgroups of interest.

Although not used as examples in this book, the two Prospective Randomized Amlodipine Survival Evaluation studies (PRAISE and PRAISE-2)[9,26] are good examples of being misled by subgroup findings. These two trials were designed to evaluate the calcium channel blocker, amlodipine, for the treatment of moderate to severe heart failure. In PRAISE, the participants were stratified by etiology: ischemic and non-ischemic cause of heart failure. Mortality plus heart failure hospitalization was the composite primary outcome, with mortality alone as the leading secondary outcome. PRAISE showed a borderline overall result for the primary outcome ($p = 0.06$) but a nominally statistically significant interaction between etiology and treatment. In fact, contrary to expectations, all of the treatment effect for the composite primary outcome and for mortality was seen in the non-ischemic subgroup. Despite the internal consistency and the substantial treatment effect, the steering committee, with the concurrence of the monitoring committee, recommended that a second confirmatory trial be conducted in and limited to the non-ischemic heart failure patient population. In PRAISE-2, the previously observed treatment benefit could not be reproduced. Whether PRAISE or PRAISE-2 results were due to chance, or to changes in medical practice between the two trials, can only be the subject of speculation. No explanation was found in searching for differences in the participant characteristics or concomitant treatment.

SURROGATE OUTCOME MEASURES

Surrogate outcome measures are defined as laboratory or biological markers that may substitute for clinical outcomes in evaluating a new treatment or prevention strategy. To be a valid surrogate, the surrogate not only must correlate with the clinical outcome but also capture the full effect of the treatment.[27] The latter criterion is often challenging to verify and has led to many problems in using a proposed surrogate as a final evaluation of an intervention.[28] Nevertheless, surrogates have been useful, and even necessary, in the early evaluation of a new drug or device. The first example in Chapter 3 shows how use of interim biomarker data was used to allow accelerated approval of AIDS drugs. Monitoring committees must be aware of the strengths and limitations of proposed surrogates as they evaluate interim data.

In the previously described CAST (Case 13), enrollment was limited to participants who had their arrhythmias suppressed in the run-in part of the trial prior to randomization. Participants were randomly assigned to the drug most effective in suppressing the ventricular arrhythmia or to placebo. Despite extensive use in the cardiology community of two of the three anti-arrhythmic drugs studied in CAST, all three were found to be harmful. If a surrogate, such as arrhythmia suppression, had been the primary outcome, CAST, if even done, would have terminated very early for success. Relying on arrhythmia suppression as a valid surrogate would have been a tragedy for coronary disease patients who have ventricular arrhythmias.

In HERS (Case 17), the women assigned to hormone therapy had a net 17% decrease in LDL cholesterol and a net 10% increase in HDL cholesterol, compared with the women assigned to placebo. Based on observational studies, these favorable changes in biomarkers would be expected to lead to at least a 25% reduction in coronary events. HERS, however, showed no reduction in these events in the hormone group.

A parallel situation occurred with the Prospective Randomized Milrinone Survival Evaluation (PROMISE) (Case 14), which compared milrinone, an inotropic drug that was known to increase cardiac function in patients with heart failure, with placebo. The primary outcome in PROMISE was mortality. The investigators hypothesized that improvement in cardiac function would translate to improvement in mortality. As the trial progressed, the monitoring committee noted an increase, rather than a decrease, in mortality among the milrinone-treated patients. The trial was ended early, showing a harmful mortality effect of milrinone in moderate to severe heart failure patients.

Monitoring committees must be careful not to react quickly to trends in supposed surrogate measures. In DCCT (Case 5), the value of tight control of glucose levels was compared with the standard of care for patients with type 1 diabetes. The study included two trials; one of primary prevention (no evidence of either retinopathy or renal disease at baseline) and one of secondary prevention (evidence of minimal retinopathy and perhaps early nephropathy), each with about 700 participants. Possible outcome measures considered during protocol design ranged from microaneurysms in the retina to blindness, tracking the progression of diabetic retinopathy from very mild to severe. After some initial discussion, the DCCT investigators chose as the primary endpoint a persistent level of retinopathy using a standardized scale based on reading fundus photographs. It was not thought that there was adequate power to look at clinical events within each trial individually. Clinical events, however, would be used in any decision to end the study early. At the beginning, the monitoring committee observed a worsening of microaneurysms in the patients on the tight control regime in the secondary prevention trial. This soon turned around, and clear beneficial trends for tight control were seen in both trials. Because many clinicians believed that early worsening of microaneurysms was the beginning of a visual acuity decline, this might have been reason to terminate the DCCT early for harm. However, the monitoring committee waited to see if the changes in primary outcome of retinopathy and other more clinically apparent effects would emerge. The evidence for these outcomes later became so convincing of a treatment benefit that the DCCT ended early. If the monitoring committee had responded to the early negative trends in microaneurysms, diabetic patients would have been deprived of a very beneficial treatment strategy. Even though the occurrence of microaneurysms trended in a negative direction early in the trial, the study investigators and monitoring committee realized that the addition of clinical outcomes would be needed to persuade the medical community to change practice.

EXTERNAL INFORMATION

A classical illustration of the importance of external information is the series of trials of warfarin in people with atrial fibrillation (Case 24). Five randomized clinical trials were initiated during a 21-month period between

September 1985 and June 1987. After three of them were terminated early and published showing a clinical benefit, completion of the remaining two trials became an ethical issue. Due to the very favorable benefit of warfarin for prevention of stroke, it was considered unethical to withhold anticoagulants from patients in the placebo groups. The case illustrates that the time frame to find answers to scientific questions often has a defined window of opportunity.

Relevant external information also emerged during the conduct of the Beta-blocker Heart Attack Trial (BHAT) (Case 2). A Norwegian trial of the beta-blocker timolol[29] in the secondary prevention of acute myocardial infarction was published while BHAT was in its follow-up phase. The timolol results were very favorable, showing a marked survival improvement. Both trials recruited patients prior to hospital discharge following an acute myocardial infarction. However, recruitment of the last participant in BHAT had been completed six months earlier. The monitoring committee concluded that the benefit of early initiation of beta-blocker treatment after an acute event may be very different from initiation post-discharge. Because the results from the timolol trial were not necessarily applicable to the control group participants in BHAT, all of whom were well beyond the acute myocardial infarction phase, there was no ethical reason to stop BHAT and put those participants on a beta-blocker. Thus, no change in the BHAT protocol was recommended. When the mortality results from BHAT finally exceeded the statistical monitoring criteria, the monitoring committee took into account not only the internal consistency of the data but the consistency of the results with the other recently competed beta-blocker trials when making its recommendation to stop.

External information had a greater impact on CARET (Case 15). A Finnish trial of alpha-tocopherol and beta carotene (ATBC)[5] showed an unexpected increase in the incidence of lung cancer. These findings were communicated to the CARET investigators. Although the active interventions differed, both evaluated beta-carotene and the trials had the same pre-specified primary outcome, lung cancer incidence. The communication between the trials was facilitated by the National Cancer Institute (NCI), the sponsor of both trials. The excess of lung cancer in CARET was similar to that observed in the Finnish trial. Almost 1.5 years after the CARET investigators had been made aware of the ATBC results, the monitoring committee recommended termination of the trial regimen. The weighted log-rank test for confirmed lung cancer yielded a p-value of 0.053 (RR = 1.24) and for all-cause mortality 0.014 (RR = 1.18). An NCI-appointed *ad hoc* group concurred with the recommendation by the CARET monitoring committee to stop the trial, taking into account the ATBC, as well as CARET, results.

While CAPRICORN (Case 27) was still recruiting post-infarction patients with poor left ventricular function, two other clinical trials of beta-blockers, the Cardiac Insufficiency Bisoprolol Study II (CIBIS II)[30] and MERIT-HF (Case 8), reported survival benefits. Faced with lagging recruitment and increasing non-trial use of beta-blockers, the monitoring committee recommended, although reluctantly, to add a second primary endpoint of all-cause mortality or hospitalization for a cardiovascular reason to the original primary endpoint of all-cause mortality. The recruitment goal of 2,600 patients was reduced to 1,850 patients.

The unexpected development in MOXCON (Case 19) of excess all-cause mortality, the primary endpoint, in the moxonidine group led the monitoring committee to look for any other evidence that might help in the recommendation. Limited, though supportive, information was found in a dose-response phase II trial which had 10 deaths among 230 patients on moxonidine (five different dose groups) versus no deaths among 38 placebo patients.

POST-TRIAL FOLLOW-UP

Usually, when a trial ends, the responsibility of the monitoring committee also ends. At the end of most trials, the participants and their physicians are informed of the study findings and recommendations. There is generally little expectation that there will be any follow-up of the participants. However, for some studies, primarily when clinical trials are stopped ahead of schedule, but even when they continue to their planned end, there may be reasons for longer-term, or post-trial, follow-up. For interventions that are intended to last for years, or even life-long, the relatively short span of a trial does not provide sufficient information about later experience. Does the benefit persist? Do adverse consequences appear? Are adverse events that were noted during the trial reversed once an intervention is stopped? Do biochemical or physiological measures observed during the trial translate into subsequent clinical events? Sometimes, answers to these sorts of questions can be obtained during the trial itself. The Diabetic Retinopathy Study (DRS) (Case 1) saw very early benefit from photocoagulation, but the monitoring committee members and the study sponsors were concerned that late harmful effects of the procedure might reduce or eliminate the benefit. They did not continue the trial beyond the point when the benefit became clear and persuasive. However, they performed analyses using assumptions for late harm. These analyses showed that the early benefit was extremely unlikely to be reversed by any late harm. After benefit was seen, the investigators stopped enrollment of additional participants and implemented appropriate treatment of those reaching high risk status. The observed early benefit persisted with the group differences continuing, even during the extended follow-up. Late harmful effects were not noted.

The CDP (Case 12) did conduct long-term follow-up after the end of the study, which, for two of the interventions, was on schedule. One of those interventions, niacin, was not shown at the end of the trial to lead to a reduction in mortality, the primary outcome. There was, however, a significant reduction in both non-fatal myocardial infarction and the combination of death from coronary heart disease or non-fatal myocardial infarction. Nine years after the end of the trial, mortality was assessed. At that time, a significant reduction in mortality in the niacin group was seen, compared with the group assigned to placebo and the other intervention groups. Although not shown as a case study in this book, a similar result was noted for the Multiple Risk Factor Intervention Trial. In that study, a difference in clinical outcome did not occur until several years after the official end of the trial.[31] In both of these cases, the investigators, not the monitoring committee, made the decision to conduct post-trial follow-up.

Post hoc analysis in HERS (Case 17) showed a statistically significant time trend. An early adverse trend with more coronary events in the hormone group reversed, with fewer events occurring in years 3 to 5 of the study. An unblinded follow-up for 2.7 years (HERS II) was conducted to determine whether the risk reduction seen in the later years persisted. This extended follow-up demonstrated no group difference in the rates of coronary events.[32]

It is not an example in this book, but the two estrogen components of the interventions in the Women's Health Initiative (WHI) were stopped ahead of schedule because of concerns about harm. Surprisingly, and contrary to the data from observational studies, the estrogen-alone intervention showed a trend toward lower incidence of breast cancer. Whether this finding is real, a result of biased assessment, or a play of chance, is unclear. Here, the monitoring committee strongly recommended that mammography examinations be conducted on the women subsequent to the trial's end.[21]

Although post-trial follow-up is uncommon, if may be important in selected situations. Usually, it will be the investigators who make the decision for follow-up. But the monitoring committee may help to identify particular instances, as with the WHI.

EARLY TERMINATION FOR REASONS OTHER THAN SCIENCE OR ETHICS

There are exceptions to the rule that trials are terminated early only for ethical and scientific reasons. Trials have been aborted for failure to enroll an adequate number of study subjects. A more troubling reason is termination early by the sponsor for commercial reasons. A recent such case is the Controlled Onset Verapamil Investigation of Cardiovascular End Points (CONVINCE) Trial.[33] CONVINCE was designed to compare a new formulation of verapamil to a physician's choice of atenolol or hydrochlorothiazide as first-line treatment of hypertension. The planned average follow-up was 5 years, the revised sample size was 16,600, and the revised target number of primary endpoints was 2,246. Recruitment of 16,602 participants was completed in December 1998. Two years later and two years earlier than initially planned, the sponsor stopped the trial "for commercial reasons." In this case, the original sponsor had been acquired by another sponsor, so there were substantial management changes in the trial. The aborted trial had accrued 729 (32%) of the 2,246 primary events. It did not demonstrate the hypothesized equivalence between verapamil and hydrochlorothiazide/atenolol, perhaps due to the shortened follow-up. The accompanying editorial[34] was sharply critical of the sponsor's decision to terminate the trial and referred to it as "a broken pact with researchers and patients." The termination of any trial for purely commercial reasons violates multiple ethical principles.

First, participant rights were violated. Participants who willingly volunteer for clinical trials expose themselves to risk. By enrolling, they expect that important information will accrue and that they will contribute to science and to improved health for others. Inconclusive findings from prematurely terminated trials do not meet these objectives.

Second, the principles of the Declaration of Helsinki which state that "considerations related to the well-being of the human subject should take precedence over the interests of science and society" were violated.[6,35]

Third, the Institutional Review Boards at the institutions participating in CONVINCE were misled. No IRB would approve an important long-term prevention trial with a mortality/morbidity outcome that was intentionally underpowered. If a sponsor reserves the right to terminate a trial prematurely for purely administrative or commercial reasons, this should be clearly stated, perhaps even in the informed consent.

Fourth, the independence of the monitoring committee was undermined. In CONVINCE, the monitoring committee "specifically recommended against stopping the trial since none of the traditional criteria for stopping applied."

Fifth, the premature termination violated U.S. Food and Drug Administration and perhaps other regulatory agency guidelines. According to the Guidance on Statistical Principles for Clinical Trials from the International Conference of Harmonization,[36] "trials should only be stopped early for ethical reasons or if the power is no longer acceptable."

The editorial on CONVINCE[34] discusses six other cases of commercial interruption. They include two trials of iron-chelation therapy and one each of amino-guanidine, liposomal doxorubicin, diltiazem, intravenous immunoglobulin, and fluvastatin. In at least one case, the sponsoring company also issued legal warnings to the trial investigators to prevent publication of the results and dissemination of them to participants.

The experience of the second Sibrafiban Versus Aspirin to Yield Maximum Protection from Ischemic Heart Events Post-Acute Coronary Syndromes (2nd SYMPHONY) trial illustrates a somewhat more positive outcome.[37] Even though the corporate sponsor stopped the study for commercial reasons, the monitoring committee and investigator group were able to work constructively with the sponsor to complete data analysis and assure orderly termination of the trial.

SUMMARY

As the case studies in this series demonstrate, monitoring of a clinical trial is a complex process. No simple algorithm can capture all of the variations and issues. Rather, flexibility and wisdom of a properly constituted monitoring committee are essential. Interpretation of interim analyses depends on the direction of a trend, internal and external consistency, kind and clinical importance of the primary and secondary outcomes and adverse events, and the completeness and timeliness of the accumulating data.

We believe, based on the 29 case studies and the other examples, and on our collective experience, that monitoring committees, along with appropriate statistical methodology, have served investigators, sponsors, regulatory agencies, study participants, and the public extremely well. Additional experience will undoubtedly make the process even better. Sharing those experiences, the "lessons learned," is essential to that process.

REFERENCES

1. Canner PL. 1983. Monitoring of the data for evidence of adverse or beneficial treatment effects in the Coronary Drug Project. *Control Clin Trials* 4:467–483.
2. DeMets D. 1984. Stopping guidelines vs. stopping rules: A practitioner's point of view. *Commun Statist-Theor Meth A* 13:2395–2417.
3. Fleming T, DeMets DL. 1993. Monitoring of clinical trials: issues and recommendations. *Control Clin Trials* 14:183–197.
4. Pocock SJ. 1992. When to stop a clinical trial. *BMJ* 305:235–240.
5. The Alpha-Tocopherol Beta Carotene Cancer Prevention Study Group. 1994. The effect of vitamin E and beta carotene on the incidence of lung cancer and other cancers in male smokers. *N Engl J Med* 330:1029–1035.
6. The World Medical Association. World Medical Association Declaration of Helsinki: Ethical principals for medical research involving human subjects. October 2000 amended version, with 2002 clarification. http://www.wma.net/e/policy/b3.htm.
7. Dickersin K, Chan S, Chalmers TC, Sacks HS, Smith H Jr. 1987. Publication bias and clinical trials. *Control Clin Trials* 8:343–353.
8. Ioannidis JPA. 1998. Effect of the statistical significance of results on the time to completion and publication of randomized efficacy trials. *JAMA* 279:281–286.

9. Thackray S, Witte K, Clark AL, Cleland JGF. 2000. Clinical trials update: OPTIME-CHF, PRAISE-2, ALL-HAT. *Eur J Heart Fail* 2:209-212.

10. Kahn JO, Cherng DW, Mayer K, Murray H, Lagakos S for the 806 Investigator Team. 2000. Evaluation of HIV-1 Immunogen, an immunologic modifier, administered to patients infected with HIV having 300 to 549 × 10^6/L CD4 cell counts: a randomized controlled trial. *JAMA* 284:2193-2202.

11. DeAngelis CD. 2000. Conflict of Interest and the Public Trust (editorial). *JAMA* 284:2237-2238.

12. Berson EL, Rosner B, Sandberg MA, Hayes KC, Nicholson BW, Weigel-DiFranco C, Willett W. 1993. A randomized trial of vitamin A and vitamin E supplementation for retinitis pigmentosa. *Arch Ophthalmol* 111:761-772.

13. Norton EWD. 1993. Letter to the editor. *Arch Ophthalmol* 111:1460.

14. Marmor MF. 1993. Letter to the editor. *Arch Ophthalmol* 111:1460-1461.

15. Berson EL, Rosner B, Sandberg MA, Hayes KC, Nicholson BW, Weigel-DiFranco C, Willett C. 1993. Letter to the editor. *Arch Ophthalmol* 11:1463-1465.

16. Dahlof B, Devereux R, de Faire U, Fyhrquist F, Hedner T, et al. 1997. The Losartan Intervention For Endpoint reduction (LIFE) in hypertension study: rationale, design, and methods. The LIFE Study Group. *Am J Hypertens* 10:705-713.

17. Dahlof B, Devereux RB, Kjeldsen SE, Julius S, Beevers G, de Faire U, et al. 2002. Cardiovascular morbidity and mortality in the Losartan Intervention For Endpoint reduction in hypertension study (LIFE): A randomised trial against atenolol. *Lancet* 359:995-1003.

18. Cannon CP, Braunwald E, McCabe CH, Rader DJ, Rouleau JL, et al. 2004. Intensive versus moderate lipid lowering with statins after acute coronary syndromes. *N Engl J Med* 350:1495-1504.

19. Chen YHJ, DeMets DL, Lan KKG. 2003. Monitoring mortality at interim analyses while testing a composite endpoint at the final analysis. *Control Clin Trials* 24:16-27.

20. Writing Group for the Women's Health Initiative Randomized Controlled Trial. 2002. Risks and benefits of estrogen plus progestin in healthy postmenopausal women. *JAMA* 288:321-333.

21. The Women's Health Initiative Steering Committee. 2004. Effects of conjugated equine estrogen in postmenopausal women with hysterectomy. The Women's Health Initiative Randomized Controlled Trial. *JAMA* 291:1701-1712.

22. Freedman L, Anderson G, Kipnis V, Prentice R, Wang CY, Rossouw J, Wittes J, DeMets D. 1996. Approaches to monitoring the results of long-term disease prevention trials: Examples from the Women's Health Initiative. *Control Clin Trials* 17:509-525.

23. National Emphysema Treatment Trial Research Group. 2001. Patients at high risk of death after lung-volume-reduction surgery. *N Engl J Med* 345:1075-1083.

24. Lee SM, Wise R, Sternberg AL, Tonascia J, Piantadosi S, for the National Emphysema Treatment Trial Research Group. 2004. Methodologic isssues in terminating enrollment of a subgroup of patients in a multicenter randomized trial. *Clin Trials* 1:326-338.

25. National Emphysema Treatment Trial Research Group. 2003. A randomized trial comparing lung-volume-reduction surgery with medical therapy for severe emphysema. *N Engl J Med* 348:2059-2073.

26. Packer M, O'Connor CM, Ghali JK, Pressler ML, Carson PE, et al. 1996. Effect of amlodipine on morbidity and mortality in severe chronic heart failure. Prospective Randomized Amlodipine Survival Evaluation Study Group. *N Engl J Med* 335:1107-1114.

27. Prentice RL. 1989. Surrogate endpoints in clinical trials: Definition and operational criteria. *Stat Med* 8:431-440.

28. Fleming TR, DeMets DL. 1996. Surrogate end points in clinical trials: are we being misled? *Ann Intern Med* 125:605-613.

29. Norwegian Multicenter Study Group. 1981. Timolol induced reduction in mortality and reinfarction in patients surviving acute myocardial infarction. *N Engl J Med* 304:801-807.

30. CIBIS II Investigators and Committees. 1999. The Cardiac Insufficiency Bisoprolol Study II (CIBIS II): A randomised trial. *Lancet* 353:9-13.

31. The Multiple Risk Factor Intervention Trial Research Group. 1990. Mortality rates after 10.5 years for participants in the Multiple Risk Factor Intervention Trial. Findings related to *a priori* hypotheses of the trial. *JAMA* 263:1795-1801.

32. Grady D, Herrington D, Bittner V, Blumenthal R, Davidson M, et al. 2002. Cardiovascular disease outcomes during 6.8 years of hormone therapy: Heart and Estrogen/progestin Replacement Study follow-up (HERS II). *JAMA* 288:49-57.

33. Black HR, Elliott WJ, Grandits G, Grambsch P, Lucente T, White WB, et al. 2003. Principal results of the Controlled Onset Verapamil Investigation of Cardiovascular End Points (CONVINCE) trial. *JAMA* 289:2073-2082.

34. Psaty BM, Rennie D. 2003. Stopping medical research to save money. A broken pact with researchers and patients. *JAMA* 289:2128-2131.

35. Boyd K. 2001. Commentary: Early discontinuation violates Helsinki principles. *BMJ* 322:605-606.

36. Food and Drug Administration, Department of Health and Human Services. 1998. International Conference on Harmonisation: Guidance on statistical principles for clinical trials; availability. *Federal Register* Vol 63, No 179:49583-98. http://www.fda.gov/cber/gdlns/ichclinical.pdf.

37. Armstrong PW, Newby LK, Granger CB, Lee KL, Simes J, Van de Werf F, White HD, Califf RM for the Virtual Coordinating Centre for Global Collaborative Cardiovascular Research (VIGOUR) Group. 2004. Lessons learned from a clinical trial. *Circulation* 110:3610-3614.

CHAPTER 3

FDA and Clinical Trial Data Monitoring Committees

Susan S. Ellenberg*

Jay P. Siegel*

Data Monitoring Committees (DMCs) or Data and Safety Monitoring Boards (DSMBs) have long been components of clinical trials of investigational treatments in a limited number of clinical areas, such as cardiovascular disease, ophthalmologic diseases and conditions, and AIDS. The Food and Drug Administration (FDA) has never required such committees (except for certain trials in emergency research as described below), however; and FDA reviewers have therefore not routinely evaluated the planned operation of DMCs in their assessment of trial protocols. As DMCs have come into increasing use in a wider range of applications, and as DMC decisions have increasingly had significant implications for the regulatory process, the FDA is increasing its focus on their role in the conduct of clinical trials.

The first regulatory document to include mention of monitoring committees was the Guideline for the Format and Content of the Clinical and Statistical Sections of New Drug Applications,[1] issued by the FDA in 1988. This document noted that any plans for interim monitoring and/or the use of a DMC and the operational procedures for such monitoring should be described. The document also notes that minutes of any meetings of a data monitoring group may be requested by the FDA division reviewing the application.

The emergence of human immunodeficiency virus (HIV) in the early 1980s and the urgency of identifying effective treatments led the investigative community and the FDA to a new focus on the interim monitoring process, which offered the opportunity for closing trials sooner than had been anticipated should interim analysis demonstrate a high level of efficacy. Such a possibility raised some concerns at the FDA. First, it was essential that trials not be stopped unless the results were truly definitive. The FDA recognized that, especially when studying unmet medical needs in serious dis-

---

* Based on authors' work at the Center for Biologics Evaluation and Research, Food and Drug Administration.

eases, it was critical to avoid a situation in which a trial was stopped early with positive results widely publicized, followed later by a revelation that, with further follow-up and analysis, the results were actually inconclusive or negative. Second, the FDA recognized that the potential benefits of early demonstration of efficacy could be lost or even turn into liabilities if manufacturers were not yet prepared to meet the resulting demand. FDA leadership participated in a National Institutes of Health-organized international workshop held in 1992 in which many aspects of the data monitoring process were debated[2,3] and held its own workshop the following year that concentrated on interim monitoring of trials conducted by industry.[4]

Other exigencies in the 1990s led to further attention to interim data monitoring in regulatory documents. In 1996, the FDA developed regulations on waiver of informed consent in emergency research, including a requirement for an independent data monitoring committee among a series of additional protections to be established in trials conducted in settings in which informed consent of subjects or legally authorized representatives is not feasible.[5,6] The International Conference on Harmonization, a consortium of regulatory authorities and pharmaceutical manufacturers in the United States, Europe and Japan, issued several guidance documents mentioning DMCs; the most detail was provided in a document on statistical issues in clinical trials, issued in 1999.[7,8]

In 1998, the Office of the Inspector General of the U.S. Department of Health and Human Services issued a report on institutional review boards (IRBs). In this report, some attention was given to the role of DMCs; the FDA and NIH were urged to establish standards and requirements relating to the use of such committees in clinical research. In 1999 and 2000, growing concerns about protection of subjects' rights and welfare in gene therapy research further fueled the call to strengthen and standardize the role of DMCs in human subjects protection. In response, the FDA developed a draft guidance focused entirely on DMCs and the processes of monitoring interim data from clinical trials.[9] This guidance represents by far the most extensive commentary FDA has issued on this topic.

The FDA has reason to be concerned with the process of clinical trial data monitoring. The knowledge of interim data could potentially influence aspects of the trial conduct in ways that could lead to biased or uninterpretable results, inability to complete a trial, or other problems. Thus, the FDA generally expects trial sponsors and investigators to keep themselves blinded to the accumulating results as the trial progresses. The need to develop interim reports at regular intervals during the trial, and present these reports to an oversight committee, raises the possibility that those interim results may become known to sponsors and/or investigators. Any evidence that interim results may have influenced the conduct of the trial will reduce or even destroy the credibility of the trial results.

For similar reasons, FDA reviewers generally remain blinded to accumulating trial results. Sponsors may request changes to trial protocols after the trial is initiated for a variety of defensible reasons; FDA must consider such requests and cannot do so objectively if they know the potential impact of the proposed change on the final results. For example, if the sponsor proposes to switch the primary and secondary endpoints, and the FDA reviewer knows that the interim results for the current secondary endpoint are more favorable than for the current primary endpoint, the reviewer will not be able to evaluate the proposed change on its merits, even under the assumption that the sponsor does not know the interim results and so the proposed change could not have been motivated by those data.

While knowledge of interim data by those managing a trial raises scientific and regulatory concerns, inadequate monitoring of data can subject participants to excess risk, and lead to improper trial management and to participant's receiving treatments already demonstrated to be inferior. FDA shares with investigators, sponsors, IRBs, and DMCs responsibility for protection of human subjects, and has the responsibility to provide regulations and or guidance to other parties in order to promote practices that optimize patient protection.

The FDA has had a variety of experiences with DMCs, many of which have identified potential problems and have informed and influenced development of regulatory policy and practices. A few of these are summarized below.

DIDANOSINE FOR TREATMENT OF AIDS: USE OF INTERIM DATA FOR EARLY DRUG APPROVAL

In 1990, when the only antiviral drug available to treat HIV/AIDS was AZT, the FDA was developing new policies that permitted "accelerated approval" of potentially life-saving new drugs on the basis of early "surrogate" endpoints that were thought likely to predict clinical benefit. A new antiviral drug, didanosine, had shown promise in early trials, demonstrating improvements in markers, in particular, CD4 + cell counts. Large trials of didanosine, being conducted by the NIH-funded AIDS Clinical Trials Group, were evaluating the effect of didanosine on survival but were also collecting the early marker endpoints. The FDA, having data only on approximately 100 patients from the early trials, was interested in reviewing the interim data on markers from the larger ongoing trials; if those data were supportive of the smaller data set already available, the FDA would be more comfortable moving ahead with a rapid approval based on the larger set of marker data.

When the FDA requested this interim data from the NIH, however, concerns arose regarding the potential impact on the ongoing trials from the release of the interim marker data, which would inevitably be made public if they were to be the basis of an FDA approval. Because of the urgency felt by the FDA and the NIH, and the shared understanding of the importance of ultimately completing the ongoing studies and evaluating the treatment's effect on the clinical endpoints, the Director of FDA's Center for Drug Evaluation and Research took the unprecedented step of meeting with the DMC for these trials to try to work out an optimal way to proceed. It was jointly decided that interim marker data from only one of the three ongoing trials would be provided. That trial was close to completion, so that the early release of interim marker data was very unlikely to endanger its ability to provide valid conclusions; and it included sufficient data on markers to satisfactorily enhance the existing database.

The accelerated approval regulations issued in 1992[10] note that for drugs approved under this mechanism, data verifying and describing the ultimate clinical benefit must be made available following initial approval, and that trials to produce such endpoints would normally be ongoing at the time of approval on the basis of surrogate endpoints. In the area of HIV/AIDS, this regulation has been used to approve drugs based on interim marker data from ongoing trials designed to provide definitive clinical evidence of safety and efficacy, as was done for didanosine. (Currently, early data on viral load is used as a surrogate, with longer-term data on viral load considered the definitive endpoint.) For the most part, these trials have been successfully completed despite the release of the interim marker data.[11]

HA-1A FOR TREATMENT OF SEPSIS: IMPACT OF SPONSOR UNBLINDING

HA-1A, a monoclonal antibody against the lipopolysacharide of gram-negative bacteria, was developed for treatment of severe sepsis. In 1990, a randomized controlled study was underway to assess the benefits and risks of this new treatment. The trial was monitored by a DMC that was independent of the sponsors and study investigators, who were to remain blinded to interim data throughout the study. While the study was ongoing, the sponsor proposed, and the FDA accepted, a new analytic plan that changed several aspects of the study that were critical to its ability to support approval of the treatment. These included changing the primary endpoint from survival at 14 days to survival over 28 days, changing the primary analysis subgroup from sepsis patients with gram-negative bacteremia to those with pure gram-negative infection (regardless of bacteremia but excluding mixed infections), and clarifying how the analysis would deal with patients lost-to-follow-up, covariates, and non-septic deaths. The study's results were reported as showing a favorable impact on 28-day survival in patients with gram-negative bacteremia.[12]

During the review of the licensing application, the FDA became aware that prior to submission of the new analytic plan, two executives of the sponsor had met with the DMC and had seen an interim analysis based on outcomes in approximately two-thirds of the patients to be entered. The interim analysis presented at that meeting showed not only outcomes of the existing primary analyses (based on the original primary endpoint and primary analysis group) but outcomes of several alternative analyses as well. Subsequent to this meeting, at least one of the two executives who had seen the interim data signed off on the new analytic plan before it was submitted to the FDA. The analytic plan was also reviewed and approved for submission to the FDA by a statistician in the contract research organization (CRO) managing the trial, who also had seen the interim data. None of this involvement of unblinded individuals in the decision to change the primary analyses of the trial was mentioned in the FDA submission proposing these changes, or in the application ultimately submitted to the FDA. Indeed, the application included wording denying knowledge of interim data by sponsor employees involved in changing the analytic plan.

The sponsor and the CRO maintained that the proposal to change the analytic plan arose entirely independently of, and was not influenced by, knowledge of the interim data; the FDA found no evidence that this was untrue. Nonetheless, the FDA felt that even well-intentioned sponsor and CRO experts, knowing the interim outcomes on various endpoints, could not make a decision to change those endpoints without raising concern that such change was influenced by knowledge of the endpoints. As noted earlier, FDA personnel recognize that, when they themselves know interim data, they cannot ensure that such knowledge will not impact decisions about trial amendments while the trial is ongoing.

FDA analysis, whether based on the protocol-defined analytic plan or problematic amended analytic plan, determined that this study did not show statistical significance on its primary endpoints and did not demonstrate efficacy. A larger, confirmatory trial focusing on the patient subset with the greatest observed treatment different in the first trial (i.e., those in gram-negative septic shock) failed to confirm efficacy (see discussion of the CHESS trial in next case study). (For additional discussion of this case, see Siegel.[13])

HA-1A FOR TREATMENT OF SEPTIC SHOCK AND MENINGOCOCCEMIA: AVOIDING UNBLINDING AT FDA

In 1992-3, HA-1A was under further study for two indications: pediatric meningococcemia, a type of gram-negative sepsis thought to be particularly likely to respond to this drug;[14] and septic shock, being evaluated in the CHESS trial (Confirming HA-1A Efficacy in Septic Shock).[14] In January 1993, the independent DMC for the pediatric meningococcemia trial met and recommended continuation as designed. On the next day, however, the DMC of the CHESS trial recommended stopping based both on observed excess mortality (p = 0.07, one-tailed) for the subset of patients with gram-negative bacteremia, and on the futility of continuing the attempt to demonstrate efficacy in the total population. Upon receiving this recommendation, the sponsor, still blinded to the meningococcemia data, halted enrollment in both trials, began withdrawing the product from Europe, where the drug had already been approved for the treatment of sepsis based on data from the study discussed in the previous example, and approached regulatory authorities to discuss the conditions under which the meningococcemia trial might be reopened. Some European authorities indicated they would need to review the interim data from the meningococcemia trial. The FDA preferred to remain blinded so as not to compromise its role and requested that advice be sought from the meningococcemia trial DMC, who would be reconvened and provided with the interim data from the CHESS trial. The committee met, reviewed the CHESS data, and recommended continuation of the meningococcemia trial. The FDA remained blinded, relied on the DMC's recommendation, and allowed the trial to continue.

A few years later the sponsor approached FDA with a request to terminate enrollment of the meningococcemia trial somewhat short of reaching the target sample size because the meningococcemia season had ended for that year and supplies were not readily available to continue into the next season. The FDA was able to consider this request on its merits, without any potential influence of the interim data to which it had remained blinded, and determined the proposal to be acceptable.

ACTIVASE ((T-PA) IN STROKE: POSSIBLE INFLUENCE OF INTERIM DATA ON PROTOCOL CHANGE

The NIH was funding a phase 2 trial in which the primary endpoint was a measure of neurological function at 24 hours (the NIH Stroke Scale). This endpoint was intended to determine if the treatment was promising enough to warrant a definitive phase 3 trial with clinical endpoints (e.g., survival and functional status after 90 days), which were defined as secondary endpoints in the phase 2 trial. However, the steering committee and sponsor grew increasingly concerned that a successful phase 2 trial might make it difficult to mount a definitive phase 3 efficacy trial; since the drug was already available as an approved treatment of acute MI, physicians might be impressed enough with promising phase 2 data to adopt this treatment for stroke even without the FDA-approved indication. The study steering committee therefore proposed switching the primary and secondary endpoints in the ongoing trial so that the primary endpoint would be the longer-term functional outcome needed for regulatory approval and clinical acceptance, and also proposed increasing study size to provide adequate power for the new endpoint.

The proposal was brought to the FDA following DMC review of interim analyses examining primary and secondary endpoint data on the majority of patients to be enrolled. Study steering committee members met with FDA to discuss the proposal, which was presented by the study statistician, a member of the steering committee who also served as study coordinator. This statistician was responsible for conducting the interim analyses and presenting them to the DMC, and was therefore aware of the interim data. At the meeting, the statistician explained that the proposal to modify the endpoints had arisen from the blinded members of the steering committee and that the interim data were not revealed and did not influence the discussion.

The FDA felt that the unblinded statistician's knowledge of interim data could well have inadvertently influenced the proposal, especially as the statistician had played a prominent role in discussing and presenting the proposal. Therefore, the FDA was not comfortable accepting the proposal and indicated that if the primary analysis were to change, the population for the new analysis would need to include only those entered following the change. In order to facilitate efficient completion of the trial, the portion of the trial that had been completed up to that point was termed "Part A," and the subsequent portion, containing data collected after the change in primary analysis, was termed "Part B."

Ultimately, Parts A and B gave very similar results—both showing clinical efficacy. The Part A data, both at interim and final analysis, showed a larger treatment effect on the clinically relevant endpoint at 90 days than on the 24-hour stroke score endpoint, despite the fact that the power had been thought to be lower for the clinical endpoint.[16] Due to the controversies in this treatment area (this class of drugs can increase the risk of hemorrhagic conversion of stroke and had not provided net benefit in other trials under somewhat different conditions), the fact that there were two trials (Part A and Part B) with consistent and confirmatory results was quite valuable in establishing the benefit of this therapy.

BETASERON (INTERFERON BETA) IN SECONDARY PROGRESSIVE MULTIPLE SCLEROSIS: RESOLVING INCONSISTENCIES IN ONGOING TRIALS

Betaseron had been approved for reducing relapses in patients with relapsing, remitting multiple sclerosis (MS) and was under study for the additional indication of secondary progressive MS. Two trials of similar design, one in Europe and one, initiated about two years later, in the United States, were exploring efficacy using a measure of progression of disability in this patient population. The European trial was completed in 1998, and the results, showing a statistically significant difference in progression of disability favoring patients on Betaseron, were published with an accompanying editorial recommending use of the drug.[17,18]

In serious diseases such as MS, a single efficacy study has often been deemed sufficient for approval by the FDA. In this case, the new indication was closely related to one in which efficacy had already been established (primary, progressive MS), so the data from the related indication could be considered confirmatory, as per FDA guidance on evidence of effectiveness.[19] The data from the European trial were submitted to the FDA in support of the new indication.

While reviewing the application containing data from the European study, FDA reviewers learned that in spite of, and with full awareness of, the positive data from Europe, the DMC for the U.S. study nonetheless recommended continuation of the U.S. study. These circumstances raised concern at the FDA that the results of the two studies might be substantially divergent for, had the U.S. study been trending favorably, it seemed likely that the DMC would have stopped it given the already definitive data from the European study showing delay in progression of disability. The FDA was also concerned that an approval of the new indication in the United States at that time would endanger the completion of the U.S. study, which its own DMC had clearly indicated should be continued even in the face of the European results.

As discussed above, FDA is reluctant to view interim data because of the concern that knowledge of interim results may leave the FDA unable to render unbiased judgments about future proposals to alter the trial. This concern was somewhat lessened in this case by the fact that the U.S. trial had already been fully enrolled and had a detailed analytic plan. More importantly, however, FDA felt there were compelling reasons to pursue access to the interim data of the U.S. trial and to discuss them with the DMC. Specific concerns included the following:

- Were the interim data such that they would likely influence the decision to approve the expanded indication?
- Did the interim data contain information that would affect the labeling for the expanded indication in important ways (e.g., absence of efficacy in certain populations or settings, emerging safety concerns)?
- Might FDA approval inadvertently interfere with the investigators' ability to answer critical questions about the safety and effectiveness of this therapy?

FDA reviewers requested interim data reports and learned that the U.S. study was showing no difference at all between treatment groups.

Preliminary analyses could not identify differences between the studies that appeared to account for the different outcomes. With the sponsor's and DMC chair's permission, FDA reviewers met with the DMC to brainstorm about the data and to ensure that neither group inadvertently and unnecessarily compromised the objectives of the other. Based upon analysis of all data available, the FDA notified the sponsor of its determination that approval would not be further considered until the U.S. study was completed and data submitted.

DRUG X IN SERIOUS DISEASE Y: ADDRESSING A POTENTIAL SAFETY ISSUE

The investigational drug in this example was never approved, so neither the drug nor manufacturer will be identified. As in the previous example, Drug X was being evaluated in multiple trials simultaneously. They were being managed by different coordinating centers and were being overseen by different DMCs. The director of one of the statistical centers became concerned about a potentially emerging safety issue and elected to alert the manufacturer to the problem, despite the fact that the manufacturer had indicated a preference to remain blinded to interim results. Once the manufacturer had received the information, he contacted the FDA for advice as to how to proceed. In order to minimize further release of interim data to parties whose knowledge of interim data could jeopardize the integrity of the ongoing trials, the FDA advised the manufacturer to ask the study DMCs to share interim data among themselves and jointly discuss them. If the other trials provided data supportive of the existence of a safety concern, such data sharing would provide mutual confirmation of the concern and all the studies would likely be halted. If the other studies showed no evidence of a safety concern, the DMC for the "index" study might be reassured that the data they were observing more likely represented a random temporal imbalance in outcomes than a true problem. The manufacturer asked the DMCs to proceed in this way. The joint review revealed that only the "index" study data suggested the safety concern. No further action was taken at that time. At a later meeting of the DMC for the "index" study, however, the DMC recommended termination of the study on the basis of futility; the announcement of the study termination also noted the safety concern, the observed evidence of which had diminished but had not disappeared. The termination of this study did not affect one of the remaining two studies, which had virtually completed its enrollment by that time, but did create an obstacle to enrollment in the other study despite any evidence of any safety concern in that trial; ultimately that study was terminated due to an inability to continue enrollment.

The experiences described above have elevated awareness of DMC procedures and their implications for regulatory decision-making at the FDA, and informed the development of the draft guidance document on DMCs that was issued in 2001.[9] In particular, the issues surrounding availability of interim data to those who manage and/or conduct the trial have received substantial attention. Clinical trials are highly resource intensive, with major investment on the part of the sponsor, investigators, and individuals who voluntarily participate in them; it is in no one's interest to find, at the time a trial has been completed, that the results may be unreliable due to inappropriate awareness of interim results by those directing and/or carrying out the trial. The FDA has tried to highlight problematic issues in this regard in its draft DMC guidance document.

Because FDA reviewers prefer to remain blinded to interim results, for the reasons described earlier, the FDA relies on DMCs to identify emerging serious safety issues in trials in which such issues require comparison of frequencies among two or more study arms. Thus, in order to ensure that trial conduct will comply with regulatory requirements in terms of protecting the safety of participants, the FDA is increasingly interested in evaluating whether DMCs are appropriately constituted and operate under a clear and satisfactory set of procedures. Clinical trial sponsors may note more frequent FDA requests for details on plans for DMCs, such as their membership, approaches to ensuring absence of conflicts of interest, and the standard operating procedures (often referred to as a charter) under which the DMC will operate.

We would like to acknowledge helpful comments and suggestions from Drs. Robert O'Neill and Robert Temple from the Center for Drug Evaluation and Research, U.S. Food and Drug Administration.

REFERENCES

1. U.S. Food and Drug Administration. 1988. *Guideline for the Format and Content of the Clinical and Statistical Sections of an Application.* Rockville, MD: FDA. http://www.fda.gov/cder/guidance/statnda.pdf.
2. Ellenberg SS, Geller N, Simon R, Yusuf S (eds.). 1993. Proceedings of "Practical Issues in Data Monitoring of Clinical Trials," Bethesda, Maryland, USA, 27–28 January 1992. *Stat Med* 12:415–616.
3. O'Neill RT. 1993. Some FDA perspectives on data monitoring in clinical trials in drug development. *Stat Med* 12:601–608.
4. O'Neill RT. 1993. A regulatory perspective on data monitoring and interim analysis. In Buncher CR, Tsay JY (eds.): *Statistics in the Pharmaceutical Industry.* Marcel Dekker, New York.
5. Title 21, US Code of Federal Regulations. Part 50.24
6. Ellenberg SS. 1997. Informed consent: Protection or obstacle? Some emerging issues. *Control Clin Trials* 18:628–636.
7. US Food and Drug Administration. 1998. International Conference on Harmonisation: Guidance on Statistical Principles for Clinical Trials. http://www.fda.gov/cber/gdlns/ichclinical.pdf.

8. ICH E9 Expert Working Group 1999. ICH Harmonised Tripartite Guideline: Statistical principles for clinical trials. *Stat Med* 18:1905–1942.
9. US Food and Drug Administration. 2001. Guidance for Clinical Trial Sponsors on the Establishment and Operation of Clinical Trial Data Monitoring Committees. FDA, Rockville, MD. http://www.fda.gov/cber/gdlns/clindatmon.htm.
10. Title 21, US Code of Federal Regulations, Parts 314.500–314.560. http://straylight.law. cornell.edu/cfr/cfr.php?title=21&type=part&value=314
11. Murray JM, Elashoff MR, Iacono-Connors LC, Cvetkovich TA, Struble KA. 1999. The use of plasma HIV RNA as a study endpoint in efficacy trials of antiretroviral drugs. *AIDS* 13:797–804.
12. Ziegler EJ, Fisher CJ Jr, Sprung CL, et al. 1991. Treatment of gram-negative bacteremia and septic shock with HA-1A human monoclonal antibody against endotoxin. A randomized, double-blind, placebo-controlled trial. The HA-1A Sepsis Study Group. *N Engl J Med* 324:429–436.
13. Siegel JP. 2002. Biotechnology and clinical trials. *J Infect Dis* 185:S52–S57.
14. Derkx B, Wittes J, McCloskey R. 1999. Randomized, placebo-controlled trial of HA-1A, a human monoclonal antibody to endotoxin, in children with meningococcal septic shock. European Pediatric Meningococcal Septic Shock Trial Study Group. *Clin Infect Dis* 28:770–777.
15. McCloskey RV, Straube RC, Sanders C, Smith SM, Smith CR. 1994. Treatment of septic shock with human monoclonal antibody HA-1A. A randomized, double-blind, placebo-controlled trial. CHESS Trial Study Group. *Ann Intern Med* 121:1–5.
16. The National Institute of Neurological Disorders and Stroke rt-PA Stroke Study Group. 1995. Tissue plasminogen activator for acute ischemic stroke. *N Engl J Med* 333:1581–1588.
17. PRISMS Study Group. 1998. Randomised double-blind placebo-controlled study of interferon beta-1a in relapsing/remitting multiple sclerosis. *Lancet* 352:1498–1504.
18. Goodkin DE. 1998. Interferon β therapy for multiple sclerosis. *Lancet* 352:1486–1500.
19. U.S. Food and Drug Administration. 1998. Guidance for Industry: Providing Clinical Evidence of Effectiveness for Human Drug and Biological Products. http://www.fda.gov/cder/guidance/1397fnl.pdf

SECTION 2

General Benefit

Introduction to Case Studies Showing Benefit from the Intervention

David L. DeMets
Curt D. Furberg
Lawrence M. Friedman

This section contains examples of clinical trials that showed benefit from the intervention being tested. Most of the examples are of trials that stopped earlier than scheduled because the benefit was overwhelmingly clear, but a few continued to their planned end. The specific issues and the kinds of discussions that took place are diverse. And rarely was the decision an easy one.

A common problem faced by the monitoring committees was how to balance short-term results against the desire for long-term information. The Metoprolol CR/XL Randomized Intervention Trial in Chronic Heart Failure (MERIT-HF—Case 8), Diabetic Retinopathy Study (DRS—Case 1), Diabetes Control and Complications Trial (DCCT—Case 5), Candesartan in Heart Failure Assessment of Reduction in Mortality and Morbidity (CHARM—Case 11), and the AIDS Clinical Trials Group (ACTG) study of fluconazole versus clotrimazole (Case 6) all discuss the difficulties in deciding how long to continue after early benefit was clearly seen. With treatments that will be used for months or years, knowledge of long-term effects (possible toxicity as well as benefit) is clearly important. Yet keeping participants in the control groups off interventions shown to be beneficial (at least in the short-term) has serious ethical implications that the monitoring committees wrestled with.

The Stroke Prevention in Atrial Fibrillation I (SPAF I) trial (Case 4) addresses the issue of having large early differences, but with small numbers of events. The monitoring committee needed to consider how much of the difference might have been due to chance, and whether longer follow-up was justifiable.

Some studies, such as the Beta-blocker Heart Attack Trial (BHAT—Case 2), the Physicians Health Study (PHS—Case 3), and MERIT-HF (Case 8) were faced with interpreting and dealing with results (both published and unpublished) from other trials. How these external data are factored into monitoring committee recommendations is discussed.

CHARM (Case 11) had the issue of monitoring more than one trial of similar or even identical interventions. In CHARM, there were three trials of the same intervention in patients with somewhat different baseline characteristics. All three trials were combined in the final analysis.

Not all clinical outcomes trend in the same direction in a trial. The PHS trial of aspirin (Case 3) had cardiovascular mortality as its primary outcome. However, it soon became apparent that a very low event rate made arriving at a conclusion for this outcome infeasible. Yet there were extremely strong positive results for myocardial infarction and negative trends for stroke. How the monitoring committee assessed these outcomes provides important lessons. The ACTG trial of fluconazole (Case 6) showed significant benefit for the primary outcome of fungal infections, but a non-significant adverse trend for death. Balancing these was not easy.

Monitoring committees often need to consider not just other outcomes, but also individual components of combined outcomes and subgroup findings, as in the paper discussing the Heart Outcomes Prevention Evaluation (HOPE) and Clopidogrel in Unstable Angina to Prevent Recurrent Ischemic Events (CURE) trials (Case 10). Here, the monitoring committees balanced the clear overall findings against the desire to obtain important information on subgroups and components of the composite outcome.

Toxicity, both expected and unexpected, can raise difficult issues. The Breast Cancer Prevention Trial of tamoxifen (Case 7) had both of these. In this study, the use of a "global index" for an intervention that had effects on multiple organ systems helped the monitoring committee to interpret the data and make recommendations.

An important issue in some of the cases is the currency of the data being reviewed. Long lag times can yield misleading information and incorrect recommendations to stop or not stop a trial. The Randomized Aldactone Evaluation Study (RALES—Case 9) showed the need for current data and, at times, "data sweeps."

Some of the case studies (e.g., BHAT, DCCT, RALES, MERIT-HF) discuss mechanics of data monitoring committees. Blinding or masking of monitoring committee members; use of group sequential monitoring and conditional power; interactions with investigators, sponsors, and regulatory agencies; and whether more than one review committee is needed are addressed.

Finally, despite clear benefit, two of the studies (CURE—Case 10) and ACTG fluconazole—Case 6) continued to the scheduled end. And some of those that stopped early continued past the time when they showed statistical significance, even when adjusted for repeated looks at the data. The reasons for the different decisions vary. Probably most important are persuasiveness of the results and the need to obtain sufficient information to evaluate fully the balance between observed benefits and harm.

CASE **1** _____

Assessing Possible Late Treatment Effects Early: The Diabetic Retinopathy Study Experience

Fred Ederer

ABSTRACT

The Diabetic Retinopathy Study (DRS)[1] assessed the ability of photoco-agulation to delay or prevent severe visual loss in people with proliferative diabetic retinopathy. Benefit was detected early, but there were concerns about the possibility of late adverse effects. Calculations using projected blindness and death rates reassured the data monitoring committee that even large late adverse effects would not offset the early benefit already observed.

INTRODUCTION AND BACKGROUND

Treatments for diseases, whether they be medical or surgical, can have separate early and late effects, effects that need not be concordant. The early effects could be harmful (i.e., "complications") and the late effects benefi-cial; or conversely, the early effects could be beneficial and the late effects harmful.

This chapter presents a case history from the DRS of a perplexing problem in the early stopping of a fixed-sample clinical trial in a disease with a long response time. The following problem confronted the data monitor-ing committee: In a surgical study with a projected follow-up of five years, a substantial, statistically significant treatment benefit came to light three years after initiation of the study, when only 350 of the 1732 enrolled patients had been followed for at least two years. Although it seemed obvious to some that the trial should be stopped so that the benefits of the finding could be made available to untreated eyes not only of patients enrolled in the study, but also of those outside the study, to others the course of action was not so clear-cut. Only 11 patients had been followed for as long as three years, and it was possible that the treatment could also produce a late-developing adverse effect. What should be the course of action? Should the trial be

55

stopped and a beneficial treatment effect be proclaimed? Or should the trial be continued to find out if there is indeed a late-developing adverse effect? The first alternative would be wrong and costly if there was in fact a late adverse effect that outweighed the beneficial effect already observed. The second choice would be wrong and costly if no late adverse effect turned out to exist, because then the better treatment would be withheld from patients in and outside the study for several years.

PROTOCOL DESIGN

Proliferative diabetic retinopathy is a chronic complication of diabetes that, after a long asymptomatic period, can progress to severe visual loss. It is a leading cause of blindness in the United States. The Diabetic Retinopathy Study, a randomized, controlled clinical trial, was sponsored by the National Eye Institute in the early 1970s to assess the ability of photocoagulation to delay or prevent severe visual loss in patients with proliferative diabetic retinopathy. Although the treatment had been widely used, its benefit in preserving vision had not been established. In five small (fewer than 100 patients), controlled (but not randomized) studies the published results conflicted.[2]

More than 1,700 diabetic patients were enrolled in the 15 medical centers participating in the DRS. One eye was randomly selected for photocoagulation, while the other eye remained untreated. A five-year follow-up was planned for each patient, and the principal response for gauging the efficacy of the treatment was the occurrence of severe visual loss ("blindness"). This was defined as visual acuity less than 5/200 at two or more consecutive follow-up visits scheduled at four-month intervals.[3] At the time it was launched, the study was widely publicized in medical journals and in direct mailings to some 12,000 physicians specializing in ophthalmology or diabetes whose cooperation with the study was sought. Patient enrollment began in 1972 and ended in 1975.

In 1975, after an average of only 15 months of follow-up (range 0–38 months), a highly statistically significant finding emerged: the two-year cumulative incidence of blindness was 16.3% in untreated eyes, but only 6.4% in treated eyes (Figure 1). Photocoagulation treatment had reduced the two-year risk of blindness by about 60%.[4] Losses to follow-up, but not deaths, had been negligible in number.

Because of the large size of the study, its public health importance, and the national and international attention it had already received, those who had to decide what to do in the face of these findings were acutely aware that any recommendations they might make could have a considerable influence on medical practice.

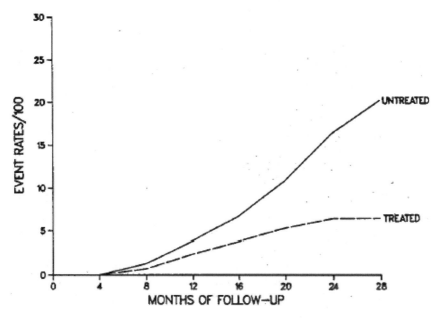

Figure 1 Cumulative event rate of severe visual loss ("blindness") as of September 30, 1975. Reprinted from DRS (1976) from Amer J Ophthal.

THE DATA MONITORING EXPERIENCE

In December 1975, members of the DRS Data Monitoring Committee and some members of the DRS Policy Advisory Group, a body that was charged with scientific oversight of the study, proposed to the director of the National Eye Institute, who would eventually make the final decision, that the treatment protocol be changed promptly—more than three years before the planned termination of the study—to allow treatment of untreated (control) fellow eyes at high risk of blindness. This change would allow study patients to benefit from the favorable treatment effect. The protocol change would be accompanied by a recommendation to treat similar eyes outside the study.

A major obstacle to deciding on an early protocol change was the possibility, suggested by findings from another study published in February 1975,[5] that severe late complications of photocoagulation might reverse the initial beneficial effect. Some members of the Policy Advisory Group believed that these complications could become manifest as new cases of blindness and proposed that the study be continued to its planned conclusion to allow evaluation of this possibility.

In summary, an early protocol change would give untreated eligible eyes both in and outside the study an immediate substantial reduction in risk of blindness, but it might also subject them to a possible risk, of unknown magnitude, of late-developing complications. Continuing the trial without change, on the other hand, although protecting untreated eyes against exposure to the possible harmful late effects, would deprive them of the known immediate benefit. These, then, were the horns of the dilemma facing the decision-makers.

A step toward the resolution of this problem was to develop quantitative estimates of the consequences of a postulated late harmful effect. The general objective was to determine whether such an effect was likely to vitiate or possibly even reverse the known early beneficial effects of photocoagulation. The specific objective was to obtain, assuming long-term follow-up of all study patients and no change in treatment protocol, estimates of the percentage of treated and untreated eyes retaining vision (i.e., not going blind).

Because the mortality of patients with proliferative diabetic retinopathy is not negligible,[6] the calculations had to take projected mortality as well as blindness into account. The general format of the estimating procedure was to project long-term annual rates of incidence of blindness in treated and untreated eyes, and of mortality from all causes, and to cumulate these rates in a double-decrement life table[8,9] so as to obtain estimates of percentage of treated and untreated eyes retaining vision over the lifetime of the patients.[10] For simplicity, risks of death were assumed to be independent of risks of blindness.[9]

For the first 32 months of follow-up, the annual blindness incidence rates were based on observed study data. For subsequent years of follow-up, for which results were not yet available, changes in blindness incidence were postulated that were adverse to the hypothesis of a long-term benefit of treatment: the annual blindness rates were assumed to increase progressively in treated eyes and decrease progressively in untreated eyes. The magnitude of these assumed changes was greater than believed probable by the experienced ophthalmologists involved in the decision. Specifically, the annual blindness rate in treated eyes was assumed to increase from 0.04 in the second and third years of follow-up to 0.07 in the fourth year, and to *increase* exponentially at 10% per year thereafter. A rate that increases 10% per year doubles every $7^{1}/_{4}$ years. In untreated eyes, the rate for the fourth year was assumed to be 0.107, the rate that was observed for the last two years for which data were available; and this rate was assumed to *decrease* exponentially at 10% per year thereafter. An annual death rate of 0.05 was assumed for the 32–48-month follow-up interval, a rate that was similar to that for the second year of follow-up, and for subsequent years this rate was assumed to increase exponentially at 10% per year.

The foregoing annual blindness and death rates are illustrated in Figure 2 and the consequent cumulative life table results in Figure 3. The projected

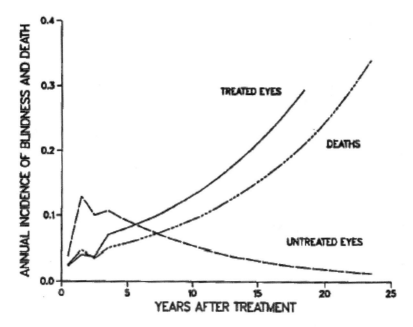

Figure 2 Annual incidence (expressed as a proportion) of blindness and death under the assumption of a delayed harmful effect of treatment. Reprinted with permission from *Control Clin Trials*.[1]

annual blindness rates for treated and untreated eyes in Figure 2 converge rapidly during the first five years of follow-up, cross during the sixth year, and then diverge rapidly. The areas under the curves of Figure 3 are proportional to the years of sight remaining after treatment. The percentage of eyes retaining sight is greater for treated eyes during the first eleven years of follow-up and greater for untreated eyes after the twelfth year. However, the gain from treatment in the early years exceeds the subsequent loss, and this is indicated by the fact that the average years of sight remaining at time of treatment is greater for treated (6.9) than for untreated (6.5) eyes.[10] According to this model, virtually all surviving patients would be bilaterally blind after 25 years (Figure 3).

The obvious implication of these calculations is that the substantial early benefit of treatment is not likely to be vitiated by subsequent combined effects of severe complications in treated eyes and a considerably improved prognosis in untreated eyes.

All groups involved in the decision process were reassured by the foregoing calculations. In particular, the director of the National Eye Institute believed that these results constituted the turning point in deciding what to do. As a result, the following decisions were made:[4]

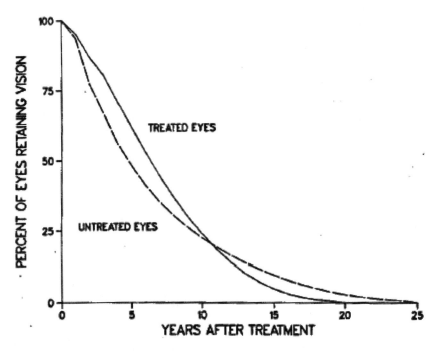

Figure 3 Percentage of eyes retaining vision since treatment-under the assumption of a delayed harmful effect of treatment.[10]

- The study protocol was changed so as to allow treatment of control eyes at high risk of blindness (control eyes at lesser risk would generally not be treated until they developed high risk characteristics); the untreated eyes of all patients would be screened at a special recall visit to identify those at high risk.
- Patient follow-up was continued so as to make possible the detection of a possible severe late-developing adverse effect.
- The results were announced to study physicians and patients, and to the scientific and general public.

Patient follow-up was terminated in 1979.

The projections had overestimated longevity: the actual five-year cumulative mortality rate was 22.6%[12] rather than 19.6%, as had been projected.[10] Therefore, fewer patients than projected would be alive to sustain the hypothetical adverse effect. Had the mortality projections been correct, the arguments for early stopping would have been even more compelling.

The protocol change in 1976[4] and an additional change in 1977[13] served to "contaminate" the control group: A number of hitherto untreated control

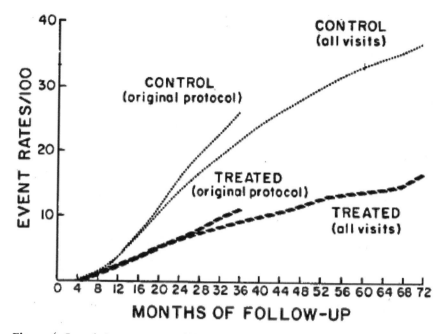

Figure 4 Cumulative event rate of blindness as of June 30, 1979. Reprinted with permission from *Ophthalmology*.[14]

eyes that during follow-up developed high-risk characteristics received photocoagulation treatment consequent to the protocol changes; the percentage of control eyes treated was 12 after two years, 24 after three years, and 40 after five years.[14]

The observed long-term cumulative incidence rates of blindness in treated and control eyes, plotted in Figure 4, provide no evidence for a delayed severe adverse effect of treatment. Such an effect might manifest itself, in Figure 4, by (a) an increase in the slope of the "treated" line, or (b) a decrease in the proportionate difference between cumulative rates represented by the "treated" and "untreated" lines:

1. No increase in the slope of the "treated" line is observable.

2. After two years of follow-up, the proportionate difference between the "treated" and "untreated" lines (original protocol) was 60%; i.e., treatment had reduced the risk of blindness by 60%. Before we address the question of a possible delayed deleterious effect on the proportionate difference, we need to deal with the effect of the aforementioned contamination of the control group. The expected effect of this contamination is in the direction of diminishing the proportionate difference. Additionally, the expected effect of the hypothetical delayed severe complications of treatment is also in the

direction of diminishing the difference, with the magnitude of the diminution depending on the severity of the complications. The hypothetical adverse complications quantified in the projections, which were stipulated to commence in the fourth year after treatment, would have had the effect of diminishing the proportionate difference by two-fifths within two years, and by nearly three-fourths within four years. No diminution even approaching this magnitude is evident in Figure 4: the proportionate difference diminished only modestly from 60% after two years to 59%, 58%, and 58% after three, four, and five years, respectively.

Although the protocol changes in 1976 and 1977, allowing treatment of some control eyes and thereby contaminating the control group, limited the capacity of the study to detect a delayed deleterious treatment effect, the study maintained the capacity to detect an effect as severe as that projected. After six years of follow-up, there was no hint of such a severe change.

LESSONS LEARNED

1. The crucial step in resolving the dilemma facing the DRS was the decision to develop quantitative estimates of the consequences of a postulated harmful effect. This was similar to a step taken by the Coronary Drug Project when faced by an analogous problem. In that study, after an average follow-up of about five years, mortality (the major response variable) was found to be somewhat higher in patients assigned to low-dose estrogen than those assigned to placebo.[11] Projections showed that this trend was unlikely to reverse itself before the end of the study. Based on this information, the decision was made to stop administering low-dose estrogen.

2. The projections in the DRS showed that late severe complications in treated eyes accompanied by a considerably improved prognosis in untreated eyes would not outweigh the substantial early benefit of treatment. The availability of this information made the decision to allow treatment of control eyes easy. Whereas in the Coronary Drug Project the projections were made for the length of the study, in the Diabetic Retinopathy Study they were made for the life of the study population.

3. The mere possibility of a late effect of treatment that is opposite to an early observed effect is not sufficient reason to keep a clinical trial going without change. Quantitative estimates may show that even large late effects will not offset the early beneficial effects already observed.

REFERENCES

1. Ederer F, Podgor MJ, and The Diabetic Retinopathy Study Research Group. 1984. Assessing possible late effects of in stopping a clinical trial early: A case study. Diabetic Retinopathy Study Report No. 9. *Control Clin Trials* 5:373–381.

2. Ederer F, Hiller R. 1975. Clinical trials, diabetic retinopathy, and photocoagulation: A reanalysis of five studies. *Surv Ophthalmol* 19:267–286.

3. The Diabetic Retinopathy Study Research Group. 1981. Diabetic Retinopathy Study Report Number 6: Design, methods, and baseline results. *Invest Ophthalmol Vis Sci* 21:149–209.

4. The Diabetic Retinopathy Study Research Group. 1976. Preliminary report on effects of photocoagulation therapy. *Am J Ophthalmol* 81:383–396.

5. Francois J, DeLaey JJ, Cambie E, Hanssens M, Victoria-Troncoso V. 1975. Neovascularization after argon laser photocoagulation of macular lesions. *Am J Ophthalmol* 79:206–210.

6. Davis MD, Hiller, R, Magli YL, Podgor MJ, Ederer F, Harris W A, et al. 1979. Prognosis for life in patients with diabetes: Relation to severity of retinopathy. *Trans Am Ophthalmol Soc* LXXVII:144–170.

7. Cutler SJ, Ederer F. 1958. Maximum utilization of the life table method in analyzing survival. *J Chronic Dis* 8:699–712.

8. Bayo F. United States Life Tables by Causes of Death: 1959–61, Vol 1, No. 6, National Center for Health Statistics, Public Health Service Publication No. 1252, U.S. Dept. HEW, Washington, DC, May 1968.

9. Berg JW. 1964. Disease-oriented end results. A tool for pathological clinical analysis. *Cancer* 17:693–707.

10. Ederer F, Podgor MJ. 1978. Estimates of a hypothetical delayed deleterious effect of photocoagulation treatment for diabetic retinopathy. *Office of Biometry and Epidemiology. National Eye Institute. Biometrics Note* No. 6, February.

11. The Coronary Drug Project Research Group. 1981. Practical aspects of decision making in clinical trials: The Coronary Drug Project as a case study. *Control Clin Trials* 1:367–376.

12. The Diabetic Retinopathy Study Research Group. Unpublished data

13. The Diabetic Retinopathy Study Research Group. 1978. Photocoagulation treatment of proliferative diabetic retinopathy. The second report of the Diabetic Retinopathy Study. *Ophthalmology* 85:82–106.

14. The Diabetic Retinopathy Study Research Group. 1981. Photocoagulation treatment of proliferative diabetic retinopathy. Clinical application of Diabetic Retinopathy Study (DRS) findings. DRS Report Number 8. *Ophthalmology* 88:583–600.

CASE **2** _____

Data and Safety Monitoring in the Beta-Blocker Heart Attack Trial: Early Experience in Formal Monitoring Methods

Lawrence M. Friedman
David L. DeMets
Robert Hardy

ABSTRACT

The Beta-Blocker Heart Attack Trial (BHAT) compared the beta-blocker propranolol against placebo in 3,837 people who had recently had a myocardial infarction. The primary outcome was total mortality. The trial ended nine months ahead of schedule because of clear benefit from propranolol. The independent monitoring committee considered several newly developed statistical approaches in recommending early stopping, as well as other factors, including what had been communicated in the consent form to the participants.

INTRODUCTION AND BACKGROUND

In the 1970s, it was thought that blockade of the beta-adrenergic receptors might be beneficial for patients with myocardial infarction. This led to the conduct of several clinical trials. Some of these trials treated patients with intravenous beta-blockers at the time of the acute MI;[1-3] others began treatment intravenously at the time of the acute event and continued with oral beta-blockers after hospital discharge;[4] still others began long-term oral treatment of patients after the acute recovery phase.[5,6,7] Relevant to the development of BHAT were concerns that the long-term trials that had been conducted were inconclusive. In particular, some were underpowered, one used a beta-blocker that had unexpected serious toxicity, and some may have used inadequate doses of medication.[8] Therefore, a workshop, conducted by the National Heart, Lung, and Blood Institute (NHLBI) recommended that another long-term trial with a sufficiently large sample size and using appro-

64

priate doses of a beta-blocker with which there was considerable experience and a known toxicity profile, such as propranolol, be conducted.[9]

PROTOCOL DESIGN

The design of BHAT, which was sponsored by the NHLBI, called for enrollment of 4,020 patients, aged 30–69 years, who had had a myocardial infarction 5–21 days prior to randomization. The primary objective of the study was to determine if long-term administration of propranolol would result in a difference in all-cause mortality. The alpha level was set at two-tailed 0.05, with 90% power to detect a 28% relative change in mortality, from a three-year rate of 18% in the control (placebo) group to 12.96% in the intervention group. This projected benefit was derived from the earlier beta-blocker trials. It was also assumed that over the three-year average follow-up, 26% of patients assigned to propranolol would discontinue the study drug, and 21% of patients assigned to placebo would begin taking a beta-blocker.[9] Thus, after taking into account non-adherence, the adjusted estimated control group event rate was 17.46% and the adjusted estimated treatment group event rate was 13.75%. The adjusted relative benefit was 21.25%, rather than 28%.

Participants were randomly assigned to either daily propranolol or placebo. Initial dosing was propranolol, 40 mg, three times a day or matching placebo. Depending on the serum drug level at one month, the dose was changed to either 60 mg three times a day or 80 mg three times a day. Approximately 80% of the participants randomized to propranolol were on the 60-mg regimen. Participants assigned to placebo also had their dose formulation changed in order to preserve the double-blind. Participant accrual was planned for two years, with follow-up for a minimum of two years and a maximum of four years (average follow-up of three years).

Participant enrollment began in 1978; a total of 3,837 participants were enrolled, instead of the planned 4,020. This reduced the power from the planned 90% only a small amount (to 89%), assuming all other factors remained unchanged.

As noted, several studies of beta-blockers had been conducted prior to BHAT. In addition, other studies were ongoing simultaneously. One, a trial of timolol, which was similar in many respects to BHAT, was published in April 1981.[10] This trial of 1,884 survivors of an acute myocardial infarction showed a statistically significant reduction in all-cause mortality, from 16.2% to 10.4%, during a mean follow-up of 17 months.[10] At this point, BHAT was no longer enrolling patients, but follow-up was continuing.

Six months later, in October 1981, the independent Policy and Data Monitoring Board (PDMB), which was advisory to the NHLBI, recommended

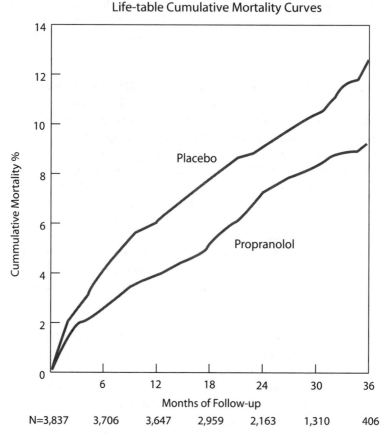

Life-table cumulative mortality curves for groups receiving propranolol hydrochloride and placebo. N indicates total number of patients followed up through each time point.

Figure 1 Life-table Cumulative Mortality Curves. Reprinted from BHAT[11] with permission from *JAMA*.

that BHAT be stopped, nine months ahead of schedule, because of a significant reduction in mortality in the propranolol group (Figure 1).[11]

DATA MONITORING EXPERIENCE

Early in the trial, the PDMB considered several monitoring boundaries. These included the ones suggested by Pocock[12] and Peto.[13] However, the PDMB selected the then recently published O'Brien–Fleming procedure for establishing monitoring boundaries.[14] The reasons for selecting this procedure were that (1) it protects the overall alpha; (2) it is quite conservative early in the study when small numbers and enrollment of participants who are perhaps not representative of the final study sample could lead to misleading conclusions; (3) the final critical value is close to the nominal critical value, so that the power and sample size are not affected and communication of the outcome to the medical community is more straightforward; and (4) the decreasing boundary over time appropriately reflects confidence in the accumulating data.

The PDMB first reviewed the BHAT data in May 1979. Subsequent data reviews were to occur approximately every six months, until the scheduled end of the trial in June 1982. The logrank z-value exceeded the conventional 1.96 critical value for a nominal p of 0.05 at the October, 1979 meeting of the PDMB. However, because of the conservative nature of the O'Brien–Fleming boundaries early in the study, this was far from significant. At the regularly scheduled meeting in April 1981, the PDMB reviewed not only the accumulating BHAT data, but the results of the timolol trial that had just been published.[10] The PDMB recommended that BHAT continue, primarily because, despite the timolol findings, the BHAT data did not show convincing evidence of benefit. Not only had the monitoring boundary not been crossed, but the long-term effect on mortality and possible adverse events was unknown. Importantly, all patients in BHAT had been in the trial for at least six months post-infarction, and there was no evidence that beta-blockers started after that time produced benefit. Thus, there was not an ethical concern about leaving the participants on placebo off treatment. The PDMB advised that the study investigators be informed of the timolol results. However, it also advised that because there had been conflicting results from other beta-blocker trials, the positive results of the timolol trial should not preclude the continuation of BHAT. Furthermore, timolol was not then available for sale in the United States, where BHAT was being conducted.

At its October 1981 data review, the PDMB noted that the upper O'Brien–Fleming boundary had been crossed.[14] The normalized logrank statistic was then 2.82, which exceeded the boundary value of 2.23. (At the prior meeting of the PDMB, in April, 1981, the logrank statistic was 2.34, which was just short of the then boundary value of 2.44.) Figure 2 shows the logrank statistics at each time, along with the upper monitoring boundary.[15]

The PDMB considered a number of factors in addition to the monitoring boundaries in its recommendation to stop early. One was conditional power; that is, the likelihood that the observed results would remain significant if BHAT were to continue to its scheduled end.[15-17] Based on prior control group data, several estimates of the number of future events were made. If there were no additional benefit from propranolol (i.e., if the null hypothesis were to hold for the next nine months), the conditional probability of seeing a significant benefit at the end of the trial was calculated for these

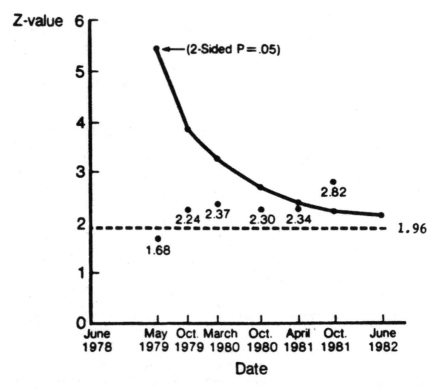

Figure 2 Beta-Blocker Heat Attack Trial Monitoring Boundary. Reprinted from DeMets et al.[15] with permission from *Control Clin Trials*.

different numbers of control group events. Under the most likely estimate, the error rate would at most be 5.5%, or only 0.5% more than the original type I error of 5%.[16,17]

The PDMB also looked at the additional precision that would derive from the added events. All participants had already been followed for one year, and only a few remained to be seen for their second annual visit. Therefore, the results for those years were complete, or essentially so. The additional precision for year 2 would have been minor. The year 3 data would have been somewhat improved by additional follow-up, as only about half of the participants had been seen for their third year visit. But even here, the increase in precision, as reflected by the narrowing of the standard error in the propranolol group from 0.0079 to 0.0068, and in the placebo group from 0.0130 to 0.0082, would have been modest. Very few participants had completed a four-year visit, so additional follow-up would have been helpful in estimating benefit at that point.[15]

The PDMB discussed whether the practicing medical community would be less likely to accept the BHAT results if the study were stopped early than if it were to continue to its scheduled end. Because the BHAT results were consistent with the recently published trial of timolol, this was not thought to be a serious problem. Ethical considerations were also raised. Although all of the control group participants were well past the time after their MI when propranolol was started, some might suffer a repeat MI. If so, it would be important for them to be aware of the BHAT results. For patients in the general public, knowledge of the BHAT outcome would be important to their medical care.

The PDMB reviewed a checklist of items to be considered when possibly recommending early termination. This checklist had been developed by one of the members of the PDMB.[18] In addition to the factors mentioned above, the list included examination of comparability of baseline variables and subsequent management of patients between the groups whether outcome ascertainment was sufficiently complete and equal in the groups consistency of subgroup results and overall benefit-to-risk, taking into account multiple outcomes and adverse events. None of these factors suggested that the observed outcome was due to anything other than the administration of propranolol or that the validity of the reported results would be seriously challenged.

A further consideration was the consent that had been signed by the study participants. The consent stated that "if propranolol proves to be beneficial for heart attack patients, the study will be stopped as soon as this is known. If, on the other hand, it proves to be harmful, the study will also be stopped, or those who have a tendency to be harmed will be removed from the study." Because the monitoring boundary had been crossed, it was argued that this "contract" with the patients required stopping the study.

In summary, the points in favor of early stopping were—

1. The pre-specified monitoring boundary had been crossed and propranolol was clearly beneficial.
2. Conditional power calculations indicated that there was little likelihood that the conclusions of the study would be changed if follow-up were to continue.
3. The gain in precision of the estimated results for the first two years would be tiny, and only modest for the third year.
4. The results were consistent with those of another beta-blocker trial.
5. There would be potential medical benefits to both study participants on placebo and to heart attack patients outside the study.
6. Other factors, such as subgroup examinations and baseline comparability, confirmed the validity of the findings.

7. The consent form clearly called for the study to end when benefit was known.

The points in favor of continuing until the scheduled end were—

1. Even though slight, there remained a chance that the conclusions could change.
2. Because therapy would be continued indefinitely, it would be important to obtain more long-term (4 year) data.
3. It would be important to obtain more data on subgroups and secondary outcomes.
4. The results of a study that stopped early would not be as persuasive to the medical community as would results from a study that went to completion, particularly given the mixed results from earlier trials.

The PDMB considered these issues and, in a closely divided vote, recommended early stopping. The NHLBI accepted this recommendation, and the investigators were informed of the decision.

As noted earlier, the sample size estimate assumed a three-year mortality rate of 18% in the control group. The mortality at one year was 5.99%. However, the two-year mortality was 9.15% and the three-year mortality (with a relatively small number of deaths) was 12.52%. At the time BHAT was stopped, the average follow-up was 25 months, with a control group mortality of 9.8%.[11] Thus, except for the first year, which included the high-risk early post-MI period, the observed mortality was considerably less than expected. However, the mortality in the propranolol group after the average follow-up of 25 months was 7.2%, an observed relative benefit of 26.5%, rather than the estimated relative benefit (after adjustment for non-adherence) of 21.25%.

LESSONS LEARNED

1. BHAT was one of the first major trials to use the O'Brien–Fleming approach to sequential boundaries. It proved particularly helpful in fostering a cautious attitude with regard to claiming significance prematurely. Even though conventional significance was seen early in the study, the use of sequential boundaries gave the study added credibility and probably helped make it persuasive to the practicing medical community.

2. The use of conditional power added to the persuasiveness of the results, by showing the extremely low likelihood that the conclusions would change if the trial were to continue to its scheduled end.

3. The decision-making process involves many factors, only some of which are statistical. Confidence that the data being observed are correct,

reasonably complete and current, and are not confounded by baseline or subsequent treatment imbalances provides assurance that the conclusions are due solely to the random assignment of the intervention. Use of a checklist of these factors helps ensure that they are adequately considered.

4. The lower than expected event rate in the control group is another demonstration of the need for randomized trials to assess treatment benefit or harm.

5. Ethical issues are paramount. If a study similar to the one being conducted presents results while the study is ongoing, the implications must be faced fully and honestly. The effect of the completed study on participant medical care and safety needs to be considered, as does the question as to whether the ongoing study remains important and ethical. The investigators need to be fully informed as to the data and relevance of the reported study, as do Institutional Review Boards. Study participants should also be informed of information pertinent to their medical care and continued involvement in the trial. During any discussion about continuation or early termination, the monitoring committee must be aware of the "contract" that was made with the subjects, namely, what was said during the informed consent process.

6. In the planning stages of a long-term trial, it is rare that all issues that might affect early termination can be anticipated. Because statistical considerations are only part of the deliberations, members of monitoring committees must always use their best judgment. The trial data themselves usually will not provide clear answers to key questions such as whether the results will be sufficiently persuasive to change practice, or the overall balance of benefits and risks. Judgment from a monitoring committee that contains members with diverse backgrounds and experience must come into play. Recommendations to stop or continue a trial are almost always accepted by the study sponsor, whose responsibility it is to implement those recommendations. Particularly when a recommendation involves a close vote, as in the case of BHAT, the study sponsor must also use judgment in its decision to accept or reject the recommendation. In BHAT, the recommendation to stop was accepted. But in situations where the recommendation is not accepted, the sponsor must fully and openly explain why it made its decision.

REFERENCES

1. Norris RM, Clarke ED, Sammel NL, et al. 1978. Protective effect of propranolol in threatened myocardial infarction, *Lancet* 2:907–909.
2. Sloman G, Stannard M. 1967. Beta-adrenergic blockade and cardiac arrhythmias. *BMJ* 4:508–512.
3. Waagstein F, Hjalmarson AC. 1976. Double-blind study of the effect of cardioselective beta-blockade on chest pain the acute myocardial infarction. *Acta Med Scand* (suppl) 587:201–208.

4. Andersen MP, Bechgaard P, Frederiksen J, et al. 1979. Effect of alprenolol on mortality among patients with definite or suspected acute myocardial infarction: Preliminary results. *Lancet* 2:865–868.

5. Ahlmark G, Saetre H, Korsgren M. 1974. Reduction of sudden deaths after myocardial infarction, *Lancet* 2:1563.

6. Multicentre International Study. 1977. Supplementary report: Reduction in mortality after myocardial infarction with long-term beta-adrenoceptor blockade. *BMJ* 2:419–421.

7. Wilhelmsson C, Vedin JA, Wilhelmsen L, et al. 1974. Reduction of sudden deaths after myocardial infarction by treatment with alprenolol. Preliminary results. *Lancet* 2:1157–1160.

8. Furberg CD, Friedewald WT. The effects of chronic administration of beta-blockade on long-term survival following myocardial infarction. 1978. In Braunwald E (ed.): *Beta-Adrenergic Blockade: A New Era in Cardiovascular Medicine*, Excerpta Medica, Amsterdam.

9. Byington RP for the Beta-Blocker Heart Attack Trial Research Group: Beta Blocker Heart Attack Trial. 1984. design, methods, and baseline results. *Control Clin Trials* 5:382–437.

10. The Norwegian Multicenter Study Group. 1981. Timolol-induced reduction in mortality and reinfarction in patients surviving acute myocardial infarction. *N Engl J Med* 304:801–807.

11. β-Blocker Heart Attack Trial Research Group. 1982. A randomized trial of propranolol in patients with acute myocardial infarction. 1. Mortality results. *JAMA* 247:1707–1714.

12. Pocock SJ. 1977. Group sequential methods in the design and analysis of clinical trials. *Biometrika* 64:191–199.

13. Peto R, Pike MC, Armitage P, et al. 1976. Design and analysis of randomized clinical trials requiring prolonged observations of each patient. I. Introduction and design, *Br J Cancer* 34:585–612.

14. O'Brien PC, Fleming TR. 1979. A multiple testing procedure for clinical trials, *Biometrics* 35:549–556.

15. DeMets DL, Hardy R, Friedman LM, Lan KKG. 1984. Statistical aspects of early termination in the Beta-Blocker Heart Attack Trial. *Control Clin Trials* 5:362–372.

16. Lan KKG, Simon R, Halperin M. 1982. Stochastically curtailed tests in long-term clinical trials. *Comm Stat* C1:207–219.

17. Halperin M, Lan KKG, Ware JH, Johnson NJ, DeMets DL. 1982. An aid to data monitoring in long-term clinical trials. *Control Clin Trials* 3:311–323.

18. Canner PL. 1983. Monitoring of the data for evidence of adverse or beneficial treatment effects. *Control Clin Trials* 4:467–483.

Data Monitoring for the Aspirin Component of the Physicians' Health Study: Issues in Early Termination for a Major Secondary Endpoint

David L. DeMets
Charles H. Hennekens

ABSTRACT

The Physicians' Health Study was a randomized, double-blind, placebo controlled, 2 × 2 factorial primary prevention trial whose primary aims were to test whether aspirin reduces risks of cardiovascular disease (CVD) mortality and beta-carotene decreases the incidence of cancer. The trial was conducted among 22,071 apparently healthy U.S. male physicians aged 40–84 years at entry. After five years of treatment and follow-up, on December 17, 1987, the independent Data and Safety Monitoring Board (DSMB) recommended unanimously the early termination of the aspirin component due principally to the emergence of a statistically extreme (p < 0.00001) 47% reduction in risk of a first myocardial infarction (MI), the major secondary endpoint, in the context of a far lower than anticipated CVD mortality as well as use of aspirin among the vast majority of individuals who experienced a non-fatal event. Several additional factors were involved, including little or no trend in either CVD mortality or stroke, although the numbers of events were too low to distinguish between small benefit, no effect, and small harm. These circumstances suggested clear evidence for aspirin in preventing a first MI, a major outcome of clinical and public health importance in the context of inadequate power to test the primary endpoint of CVD mortality.

INTRODUCTION AND BACKGROUND

Cardiovascular disease (CVD) is the leading cause of mortality in the United States, so primary prevention as well as treatment strategies are crucial. While atherosclerosis is the principal underlying cause, thrombosis is the proximate cause of virtually all occlusive vascular events. Blood platelets play a crucial role in the initiation and propagation of clinical thrombotic events. The effect of aspirin on reducing the aggrebility of blood platelets has been well established, suggesting that this over-the-counter and inexpensive, widely used drug might have clinical benefit in the treatment and prevention of CVD.[1,2]

In some senses aspirin is as old as medicine itself.[1] In the fifth century B.C., Hippocrates found that an extract from the bark of the white willow tree relieved aches and pains of his patients. This extract was later found to contain an aspirin-like compound. In 1897 aspirin was synthesized by Felix Hoffmann, a chemist working in the laboratory of Friedrich Bayer. During the 20th century aspirin became the most widely used drug in the world, but its potential to decrease risks of cardiovascular disease (CVD) only became apparent during the last 30 years. In 1971, Sir John Vane demonstrated that small amounts of aspirin irreversibly inhibit platelet aggregation. Since the proximate cause of virtually all acute coronary syndromes is thrombosis, it seemed reasonable to hypothesize that aspirin might break the chain of events leading to CVD. Some, but not all, observational epidemiological studies were compatible with the possibility of small to moderate benefits of 10–50%.[3,4] For small to moderate effects, however, the amount of uncontrolled and uncontrollable confounding inherent in all observational study designs is about as big as the effect sizes. Thus, reliable data about whether aspirin reduces risks of CVD could only derive from randomized trials of sufficient size and duration to detect the postulated benefit.[5-7] During the decades of the 1970s and 1980s randomized trials were conducted among patients who had survived a prior myocardial infarction (MI), stroke, transient ischemic attacks, or unstable angina. In meta-analysis, these trials demonstrated significant benefits on subsequent MI, stroke, and CVD death.[8] There were no data, however, from large-scale randomized trials of primary prevention of CVD.

With respect to beta-carotene, basic research and observational analytic studies were compatible with a possible reduction in cancer incidence.[9] By the late 1970s it seemed important and timely to hypothesize in apparently healthy individuals that aspirin decreased CVD mortality and that beta-carotene reduced cancer incidence. Stampfer et al.[10] determined that the most efficient design was a 2×2 factorial trial to test this hypothesis.

PROTOCOL DESIGN

The Physicians' Health Study (PHS) was a randomized, double-blind, placebo-controlled, 2×2 factorial primary prevention trial among 22,071 apparently healthy male U.S. physicians aged 40–84 years at entry.[11] The PHS was funded as an investigator-initiated grant by the U.S. National Institutes of Health with the National Heart, Lung, and Blood Institute (NHLBI) supporting the aspirin component and the National Cancer Institute(NCI) the beta-carotene component. The PHS was designed and conducted as a far larger companion trial to a primary prevention trial of British doctors. A number of pilot studies were completed which demonstrated the willingness and ability of U.S. physicians to comply with their assigned regimen as well as to provide complete follow-up data. In addition, 325 mg aspirin on alternate days was demonstrated to inhibit platelet aggregation and prolong the bleeding time so this regimen was chosen to enable the participants to take one pill each day.

For the aspirin component, the primary prespecified endpoint was CVD mortality and the major secondary objectives were to assess the impact on. Additional prespecified endpoints were MI and stroke, total mortality and cause specific mortality as well as side effects, especially bleeding. Since aspirin and beta-carotene had no known beneficial or deleterious interactions, a randomized double-blind 2×2 factorial design was used to test the two hypotheses simultaneously.[10] Based on the results of previous secondary prevention trials of aspirin,[8] the hypothesis was that aspirin would reduce CV mortality by 20%. Although it was expected that such an effect might reduce total mortality by 10%, it was not expected that this trial would have sufficient power to detect this outcome. Considering cost and feasibility, a large cohort of apparently healthy U.S. male physicians between 40 and 84 years of age, having no previous CVD, was selected as the study population. The PHS design assumed that these physicians would have a lower mortality rate than the general U.S. population. Specifically, the assumption was that the cohort would have a CV mortality rate 25% of the U.S. population for the first year, 50% for the second year of follow-up, and 75% for subsequent years of follow-up. This led to the final design of 22,000 physicians being randomized to 7.5 years of follow-up. This sample size would provide 0.95 power to detect a 20% reduction in CV mortality with a one-tailed 0.05 significance level. With recruitment to start in early 1982, follow-up was scheduled to be completed in late 1990.

An independent and multi-disciplinary Data and Safety Monitoring Board (DSMB) was established jointly by the principal investigator, NHLBI, and NCI. The primary responsibilities of the DSMB were to monitor the progress of the PHS as well as the accumulating data for cogent evidence of benefit or harm. The DSMB included clinicians with expertise in aspirin, CVD, beta-carotene, and cancer as well as epidemiologists and biostatisticians, all experienced in the design, conduct, analysis, and interpretation of randomized trials. The DSMB was scheduled to meet every six months throughout the trial. For data monitoring, the DSMB chose the method proposed by Haybittle[12] and Peto[13] to provide guidelines for early termination. This method requires that the standardized test statistic exceeds 3.0 (or three standard deviations) on any interim analysis. This corresponds to a nominal p-value of 0.0013. Since the interim analyses are conducted no more frequently than twice annually, the final p-value can be used without any further adjustment. The terms of reference for early termination included proof beyond a reasonable doubt that is likely to influence clinical practice in the context of the above-mentioned statistical guidelines.

Introductory letters and consent forms were mailed to over 261,000 U.S. male physicians aged 40–84 years. About half returned the forms and about half were willing to participate. Of these, about 33,000 were initially eligible. Interestingly, the chief exclusion criterion was regular use of aspirin. Of these, after a three-month run-in on active aspirin and beta-carotene placebo about a third were excluded because of non-compliance, leaving 22,071 willing and eligible participants who were randomized (11,037 to aspirin and 11,034 to placebo).

The DSMB recommended early termination of the aspirin arm on December 17, 1987.[14,15] The beta carotene arm continued to its completion date, which was December 31, 1995. In this report, the issues surrounding the DSMB decision to recommend early termination of the aspirin component are reviewed and implications are summarized. A more detailed discussion has been published.[14]

DATA MONITORING EXPERIENCE

As expected, with such a large number of participants randomized, the baseline risk factors were virtually identical between the aspirin and placebo arms. Compliance to the assigned trial medication was over 85% for most of the follow-up period in both the active and placebo groups. Follow-up was 100% for mortality and over 99% for major morbidity. Endpoints were classified by a separate committee blinded to the assigned intervention. These aspects were not issues in the DSMB deliberations. Bleeding problems, including bruising, gastrointestinal bleeding, and nose bleeding, were increased in the aspirin arm compared to placebo but appeared to be lower than reported in previous aspirin trials. Gastrointestinal ulcers were also higher on aspirin but not statistically significant. Thus, the DSMB did not consider these sufficient to recommend any change in the trial.

During the last 1.5 years of the PHS aspirin component, the DSMB held three formal meetings with five issues of primary concern;[14] these were—

1. Low CVD overall mortality rate resulting in reduced statistical power
2. No emerging trends in CVD mortality

3. Emerging trends in MI rate difference
4. No emerging trend in stroke rate difference
5. Placebo arm cross-over rate

Data for these key outcomes are presented in Tables 1–3, and represent a summary of what was available at each of the DSMB meetings. Relative risks (RR) are shown for each time period.

The DSMB was aware early in the trial that the mortality event rate was far lower than the already low rate assumed in the design, and that trend persisted. By the December 1987 meeting, 733 CV deaths were expected, in contrast to the 88 that were reported and confirmed. At that time, about 68% of the reported events had been confirmed or refuted. The design had assumed the PHS rate would be between 50% and 75% of the U.S. healthy male age-matched population. However, only 12% of the assumed rate was observed. The projected mortality rates for the remaining follow-up period were also examined, but even modest increases did not alter the conclusion that the overall mortality rates would be far lower than assumed. The lower rate implied a reduced power of the trial. The DSMB conducted extensive calculations[14] which suggested that power of the trial would be only 0.50 with

Table 1   Mortality Outcome in PHS

Date*	Mortality Outcome	Aspirin	Placebo	RR
6/86	CV	28	33	0.83
	Total	58	75	0.76
1/87	CV	37	42	0.86
	Total	91	102	0.88
12/87	CV	44	44	0.99
	Total	110	115	0.95

* Date of Data Monitoring Board meeting for which analysis was presented.
Modified Table 1. *Ann Epidemiol* 1:395–405, 1991.

Table 2   Confirmed Myocardial Infarctions

Date*	Outcome	Aspirin	Placebo	RR	P-value
7/86	Non-fatal	71	111	0.61	0.003
	Total	75	122	0.61	0.0007
1/87	Non-fatal	85	137	0.60	0.0004
	Total	89	154	0.56	<0.0001
12/87	Non-fatal	99	171	0.56	<0.0001
	Total	104	189	0.53	<0.0001

* Date of DMB meeting for which analysis was presented.
Modified Table 2. *Ann Epidemiol* 1:395–405, 1991.

Table 3 Confirmed Stroke*

Date*	Outcome	Aspirin	Placebo	RR	P-value
7/86	Ischemic	31	40	0.76	0.47
	Hemorrhagic**	9	4	2.45	0.17
	(Mod–fatal)	(8)	(0)		(0.0078)
1/87	Ischemic	43	52	0.82	0.35
	Hemorrhagic	12	4	3.23	0.05
	(Mod–fatal)†	(10)	(0)		(0.0020)
12/87	Ischemic	64	61	1.05	0.79
	Hemorrhagic	13	6	2.19	0.11
	(Mod–fatal)	(10)	(2)	(5.06)	(0.02)

* Date of DMB meeting for which analysis was presented.
** Excludes strokes unclassified as to ischemic, hemorrhagic.
† Mod–fatal = moderate, severe, or fatal.
Modified Table 3. *Ann Epidemiol* 1:395–405, 1991.

the mortality rate as observed and a sample size of 22,000. In order to have 0.90 power for mortality, the effect of aspirin would have to result in a 35% reduction or greater, rather than the 20% as assumed.

In addition, Table 1 indicates that the observed difference in CV mortality between aspirin and placebo was also smaller than assumed and decreasing over time. The observed relative risk for CV mortality went from 0.83 to 0.86 to 0.99. For total mortality, the RR was initially encouraging but at the December 1987 meeting was only 0.95. Thus, the smaller intervention effect further reduced the chances of a statistically significant result at the end of the scheduled follow-up. The DSMB calculated the power of detecting a significant difference at the end of follow-up, taking into consideration the already observed intervention effects and the lower mortality rates using methods of conditional power.[16] These conditional power calculations, assuming a 20% aspirin effect for the remainder of the trial, indicated only a 0.32 chance of obtaining a significant result at the scheduled termination date in 1990. In order for the conditional power to increase to just 0.80, the aspirin effect would have to be 40%, double that of the initial assumptions.

The conclusion of both the unconditional and conditional power calculations was that the PHS aspirin component was substantially underpowered for the primary outcome of CVD mortality as well as for total mortality. Based on the mortality outcome, the choices were to (1) continue as is and hope for the best, (2) increase the sample size (but recruitment had been completed five years earlier), or (3) increase the follow-up period. In order to accumulate the desired number of primary events to compensate for the lower observed event rate, the DSMB calculated that the follow-up would have to be extended an additional 16.5 years for a total of 20.5 years of follow-up.

While the primary prespecified endpoint of CV mortality did not seem encouraging to the DSMB, the major secondary outcome of MI was of considerable interest. As shown in Table 2, the results for non-fatal MI or total (fatal and non-fatal) MI became apparent within six months and statistically extreme over the last three DSMB meetings, with a nominal p-value less than 0.0001 at the December 1987 meeting. Early in the trial, the PHS study chair and the DSMB had discussed the possibility of MI's becoming statistically significant before the primary endpoint because of the larger event rate, assuming that some portion of the hypothesized effect of aspirin would carry over to fatal MI as well as non-fatal MI. The policy was that while MI would be an endpoint of major interest, it would not by itself be sufficient to terminate the trial early. The physician participants had been advised that CV mortality was the primary endpoint. However, the MI results seemed to indicate a protective effect of aspirin for this secondary but important clinical and public health outcome.

Another key secondary outcome was the effect of aspirin on stroke. The data over the same period of time is shown in Table 3. While the number of stroke events are small and thus the data are inconclusive, the results shown are consistent with the hypothesis that aspirin is possibly beneficial for ischemic stroke and possibly adverse for hemorrhagic stroke (although the beneficial effect was not seen at the December 1987 meeting). For hemorrhagic strokes classified as moderate, severe or fatal, there were ten events in the aspirin group and two in the placebo group. While nominally significant ($p = 0.02$), the number of events is very small and not conclusive, but consistent with the available evidence from trials of secondary prevention.

Finally, the DSMB also noted that by December 17 1987 over 85% of participants who suffered a non-fatal MI were prescribed aspirin. This prescribing pattern was compatible with the results from the secondary prevention trials, and, indeed, the U.S. Food and Drug Administration (FDA) had labeled aspirin for this indication. The effect of the treatment cross-over or "drop-in" phenomenon was that individuals at higher risk for having a primary outcome were now on active aspirin treatment and future intervention effects of aspirin were likely to be diminished. Thus, this situation further lowered the ability of the PHS to reach its primary objective during the funded follow-up period.

After considering all of the issues in much more detail than described here, the DSMB recommended to the study chair at its December 1987 meeting that he be unblinded and consider the options listed below.[14]

1. Extend the length of follow-up.
2. Increase the study population.

3. Continue as planned with no change.
4. Terminate the trial early and report the results.

Extension of follow-up for a considerable period was considered, assuming funding could be obtained. However, ethical issues suggested that the participants needed to be told about the MI results so they could make an informed decision whether to continue in their assigned study arm. This information might have the effect of increasing the cross-over to aspirin. The DSMB did not believe extension with immediate disclosure of the MI results was a viable option. Additional recruitment was not feasible. Continuing as planned for another three years could be achieved with little additional effort but also with very little gain at the expense of not sharing the MI and stroke results. The DSMB recommended unanimously on December 17, 1987, to the study chair that the aspirin component be terminated early.

Following the unanimous recommendation of the DSMB, the principal investigator spoke with the Steering Committee and prepared a preliminary report. A manuscript was submitted for expedited review to the *New England Journal of Medicine* (NEJM) on December 23, 1987, and accepted for publication on December 30, 1987.

Interestingly, of seven independent experts chosen by the editor of NEJM to review the manuscript, six concurred with the decision of the DSMB concerning early termination of the blinded aspirin component of the PHS. The preliminary report was published on January 25, 1988.[15]

Unblinding of PHS Participants

Letters were written, printed, and mailed to all participants to arrive on or before January 25, 1988, together with reprints of the preliminary report. Of those assigned to aspirin, over 99% elected to remain on the drug. Over the 2–3 years following termination, 74% of the physicians who were assigned to the placebo arm elected to take aspirin with an additional 15% already on aspirin. Thus, 89% of the placebo arm physicians elected to take aspirin, suggesting that these individuals accepted and endorsed the recommendations of both the DSMB and the study's advisory committee. In addition, the CV mortality rate remained low and confirmed the DSMB recommendation that this primary outcome would not likely yield definitive results.

Postscript

The results of the PHS were accompanied by the simultaneous publication of the results of the British Doctors Trial (BDT) on January 28, 1988, in the British Medical Journal. The BDT showed no significant effect of aspirin on first MI.[17] Considerable confusion occurred among health care providers and the general population, so the principal investigators of both trials along with the chairs of their DSMB's published a meta-analysis of the two trials. For non-fatal MI, the PHS showed a significant benefit of 42% ± 9% and the BDT showed a non-significant benefit of 3% ± 19%. Not surprisingly, due to the far larger sample size of the PHS the meta-analysis of the two trials showed a 33% ± 9% reduction in first MI whose p-value is less than 0.00002.[18] In the final report of the PHS, with 100% of reported events confirmed or refuted, aspirin reduced the risk of a first MI by 44% (p ≤ 0.00001).[19]

Starting in 1999, three additional randomized trials of aspirin in the primary prevention of CVD have been completed and published. The Thrombosis Prevention Trial (TPT),[20] Hypertension Optimal Treatment Trial (HOT),[21] and Primary Prevention Project (PPP)[22] all showed significant benefits of aspirin on first MI. In fact, the PPP was also terminated early based on the recommendation of its DSMB. A meta-analysis of the five trials provides conclusive evidence to corroborate the initial finding from the PHS that aspirin significantly reduces the risk of a first MI by 32% (p ≤ 0.00001).[23] Further, even after randomization of over 55,000 subjects, of which about 12,000 are women, there are non-significant effects on stroke and CVD mortality. The beta-carotene component of the PHS ended as scheduled on December 31, 1994. At that time there were an additional seven years of observational aspirin use. In the analyses of 12 years of aspirin (five randomized and seven observational) there was a significant reduction in CVD mortality of about 20% among aspirin takers.[24,25]

LESSONS LEARNED

1. The PHS DMB experience confirms what the Coronary Drug Project investigators described earlier: that the decision process is complex and hard to define in advance.[26] While statistical procedures such as the Peto-Haybittle group sequential boundary are useful in interpreting interim analyses of the primary prespecified endpoint cautiously, they provided little help to the DSMB for most of the issues under discussion in the PHS. They did, however, help interpret the "significance" of the MI finding.

2. Secondary endpoints can play a major role in the decision. The DSMB did anticipate in advance that MI (fatal and non-fatal) might become significant, using the Peto-Haybittle criteria, before the primary outcome of CVD mortality. At the beginning of the PHS, the participants were clearly informed that the primary outcome was CV mortality. However, this does not assure that those participants would not respond to the significant MI results. In fact, over 99% of those assigned to aspirin remained on the active drug, and 89% of those assigned to placebo choose to take active aspirin after the results were disseminated.

3. The role of a DSMB in addressing a non-significant primary endpoint in the context of a statistically extreme finding on the major secondary endpoint is a very challenging task. Any DSMB recommendations or comments must be based on unblinded or partially blinded interim data, and thus subject the trial to possible bias. Yet, this DSMB had to struggle with the fact that the CV mortality rate, the primary outcome, was less than half the rate assumed, which reduced the power to be far less than 0.50 at the same time that a secondary endpoint, MI, was becoming more and more significant with time. Extending or expanding the trial was considered but determined to be not feasible.

4. Conditional power methods were used to assess whether the primary outcome could ultimately be statistically significant, given the observed data, projected mortality rates, and a range of hypothesized aspirin effects for the remainder of the trial. None of the calculations with reasonable variations in the assumptions indicated that the primary mortality outcome would be significant in the next several years. This methodology was helpful.

5. The DSMB did not formulate the recommendation to terminate at the meeting on December 17, 1987. Rather, the discussions about terminating early began much earlier as the observed trends began to emerge and gained momentum at the last three meetings with the data as summarized in Tables 1–3. The DSMB was interested in observing whether the trends would become stronger, fluctuate, or weaken. The fact that the CVD mortality rate did not increase and that fatal and non-fatal MI results were apparent by six months and became statistically extreme over time helped the DSMB in their deliberations. Thus, over the last three meetings the DSMB became increasingly convinced that nothing more would be gained by continuing the aspirin component. In this case, tracking the emerging trends was important.

6. The principal investigator found the advice of external reviewers useful in dealing with the DSMB recommendations. In the PHS, the external experts came by way of the editorial process of the New England Journal of Medicine but served the useful purpose of a second opinion.

7. Despite the PHS results for fatal and non-fatal MI, the endorsement of the aspirin as a primary prevention strategy has been mixed. The physician participants in the PHS overwhelmingly accepted the results by taking aspirin themselves. Other later trials[22,23] have suggested similar results. In early 2002, the United States Preventive Services Task Force (USPSTF) issued guidelines that all apparently healthy individuals with ten-year risk of a first CHD event of greater than 6% should be considered for aspirin prophylaxis to prevent a first MI.[27] Later that year the American Heart Association (AHA) issued similar guidelines for all apparently healthy individuals whose ten-year risks are greater than 10%.[28]

Nevertheless, the Food and Drug Administration has not as yet labeled aspirin to prevent a first MI. In 1989, following the publication of the final report of the PHS as well as the BDT, the Cardio-Renal Drugs Advisory Committee (CRDAC) to the U.S. FDA voted 6-2 to label aspirin to prevent a first MI. The FDA did not act on this recommendation, citing the apparently discrepant results of the PHS and BDT. In 2003, CRDAC reviewed the evidence from all five published trials and their meta-analysis, and voted not to approve aspirin for primary prevention of a first MI. One recently completed and two ongoing trials should provide important relevant information. The recently completed Women's Health Study of about 40,000 apparently healthy female health professionals provides relevent important information.[29] The recently begun ASPREE trial in Australia among the elderly (Mark Nelson, personal communication) is evaluating the high risk primary prevention subjects for which regulatory authorities are requiring further data.

Monitoring committees should bear in mind the likely impact of the results on clinical and public health practice when considering early termination but should still give the participants in a trial the highest priority.

REFERENCES

1. Williams A, Hennekens CH. 2004. The role of aspirin in cardiovascular diseases-forgotten benefits? *Expert Opin Pharmacother* 5:109-115.
2. Vane JR. 1971. Inhibition of prostaglandin synthesis as a mechanism of action for aspirin-like drugs. *Nat. New Biol* 231:232-235.
3. Hennekens CH, Karlson LK, Rosner B. 1978. A case control study of regular aspirin use and coronary deaths. *Circulation* 58:35-38.
4. Manson JE, Stampfer MJ, Colditz GA, Willett WC, Rosner B, Speizer FE, Hennekens CH. 1991. A prospective study of aspirin use and primary prevention of cardiovascular disease in women. *JAMA* 266:521-527.
5. Friedman LM, Furberg CD, DeMets DL. 1998. *Fundamentals of Clinical Trials.* Third Edition, Springer-Verlag, New York.
6. Hennekens CH, Buring JE. 1986. *Epidemiology in Medicine.* Little, Brown & Company, Boston.
7. Hennekens CH, Buring JE, Manson J, Ridker PM. 1999. *Clinical Trials in Cardiovascular Disease: A Companion to Braunwald's Heart Disease.* W Saunders Company, Philadelphia.
8. Antiplatelet Trialists Collaboration. 1988. Secondary prevention of vascular disease by prolonged anti-platelet therapy. *BMJ* 296:320-332.
9. Peto R, Doll R, Buckley JD, Sporn M. 1981. Can dietary beta-carotene materially reduce human cancer rates? *Nature* 290:201-205.
10. Stampfer MJ, Buring JE, Willett W, Rosner B, Eberlein K, Hennekens CH. 1985. The 2 × 2 factorial design: Its application to a randomized trial of aspirin and beta-carotene in U.S. physicians. *Stat Med* 4:111-115.
11. Hennekens CH, Eberlein K for the Physicians' Health Study Research Group. 1985. A randomized trial of aspirin and beta-carotene among US physicians *Prev Med* 14:165-168.
12. Haybittle JL. 1971. Repeated assessment of results in clinical trails of cancer treatment. *Br J Radiol* 44:793-797.

13. Peto R, Pike ML, Armitage P, Breslow NE, Cox DR, Howard SV, et al. 1976. Design and analysis of randomized clinical trails requiring prolonged observations of each patient. I. Introduction and design. *Br J Ca* 34:585-612.

14. Data Monitoring Board of the Physicians' Health Study: Cairns J, Cohen L, Colton T, DeMets DL, Deykin D, Friedman L, Greenwald P, Hutchison GB, Rosner B. 1991. Issues in the early termination of the aspirin component. *Ann Epidemiol* 1:395-405.

15. Steering Committee of the Physicians' Health Study Research Group. 1988. Preliminary report: Findings from the aspirin component of the ongoing Physicians' Health Study. *N Engl J Med* 318:262-264.

16. Lan KKG, Simon R, Halperin M. 1982. Stochastically curtailed tests in long-term clinical trials. *Comm Stat* 1:207-219.

17. Peto R, Gray R, Collins R, Wheatley K, Hennekens C, Jamrozik K, et al. 1988. Randomized trial of prophylactic daily aspirin in British male doctors. *BMJ* 296:313-316.

18. Hennekens CH, Peto R, Hutchison GB, Doll R. 1988. An overview of the British and American aspirin studies. *N Engl J Med* 318:923-924.

19. Steering Committee of the Physicians' Health Study Research Group. 1989. Final report on the aspirin component of the ongoing Physicians' Health Study. *N Engl J Med* 321:129-135.

20. The Medical Research Council's General Practice Research Framework. 1998. Thrombosis prevention trials: randomized trial of low intensity oral anticoagulation with warfarin and low-dose aspirin in the primary prevention of ischemic heart disease in men at increased risk. *Lancet* 351:233-240.

21. Hansson L, Zanchetti A, Carruthers SG, Dahlof B, Elmfeldt D, Julius S, Menard J, et al. 1998. Effects of intensive blood pressure lowering and low-dose aspirin in patients with hypertension: Principal results of the Hypertension Optimal Treatment (HOT) randomized trial. *Lancet* 351:1755-1762.

22. Collaborative Group of the Primary Prevention Project. 2001. Low-dose aspirin and vitamin E in people at cardiovascular risk: a randomized trial in general practice. *Lancet* 357:89-95.

23. Eidelman RS, Hebert PR, Weisman S, Hennekens CH. 2003. An update on aspirin in the primary prevention of cardiovascular disease *Arch. Intern Med* 163:2006-2010.

24. Cook N, Hebert P, Manson J, Buring J, Hennekens CH. 2000. Self-selected post-trial aspirin use and subsequent cardiovascular disease and mortality in the Physicians' Health Study. *Arch Intern Med* 160:921-928.

25. Cole S, Cook N, Hennekens CH. 2002. Use of a marginal structural model to determine the effect of aspirin on cardiovascular mortality in the Physicians' Health Study. *Am J Epidemiol* 155:1045-1053.

26. Coronary Drug Project Research Group. 1981. Practical aspects of decision making in clinical trials: The Coronary Drug Project as a case study. *Control Clin Trials* 1:363-76.

27. United States Preventive Services Task Force. 2002. Aspirin for the primary prevention of cardiovascular events; recommendation and rationale. *Ann Intern Med* 136:157-160.

28. Pearson TA, Blair SN, Daniels SR, Eckel RH, Fair JM, Fortmann SP, et al. 2002. American Heart Association guidelines for primary prevention of cardiovascular disease and stroke: 2002 Update: Consensus panel guide to comprehensive risk reduction for adult patients without coronary or other atherosclerotic vascular diseases. *Circulation* 106:388-391.

29. Ridker PM, Cook NR, Lee IM, Gordon D, Gaziano JM, Manson JE, Hennekens CH, Buring JE. 2005. A randomized trial of low-dose aspirin in the primary prevention of cardiovascular disease in women. *N Engl J Med* 352:1293-1304.

Early Termination of the Stroke Prevention in Atrial Fibrillation I Trial: Protecting Participant Interests in the Face of Scientific Uncertainties and the Cruel Play of Chance

Robert G. Hart
Lesly A. Pearce
Ruth McBride
Richard A. Kronmal

ABSTRACT

The Stroke Prevention in Atrial Fibrillation (SPAF) I trial evaluated aspirin and warfarin for prevention of stroke and nonCNS emboli in elderly patients with nonvalvular atrial fibrillation. Participants were categorized as either warfarin-eligible or warfarin-ineligible based on contraindications to or refusal of anticoagulation, and interim efficacy monitoring examined treatment effects separately by warfarin eligibility. The planned primary analyses compared aspirin to placebo among *all* participants and warfarin to placebo among warfarin-eligible patients. The study was terminated early following the second interim analysis due to a large reduction in thromboembolic events by aspirin versus placebo among the subgroup of warfarin-eligible participants (1 vs. 18, respectively, relative risk reduction = 94%, p < 0.001). This reduction was not evident among warfarin-ineligible patients (25 vs. 28, respectively, relative risk reduction = 8%, p = 0.8). The reduction by aspirin vs. placebo for all aspirin-assigned patients (the planned primary analysis) was significant (26 vs. 46, respectively, relative risk reduction = 42%, p = 0.02), but this resulted from pooling of subgroups with dissimilar responses. While the extreme effect of aspirin in anticoagulation-eligible participants was suspected to be due to the play of chance, termination of the SPAF I trial was justified to protect the interests of warfarin-eligible participants assigned placebo. The potential implications of interim efficacy monitoring of multiple subgroups should be carefully considered when planning interim monitoring.

INTRODUCTION AND BACKGROUND

Atrial fibrillation is a strong, independent risk factor for ischemic stroke because it leads to formation and embolism of stasis-precipitated left atrial appendage thrombi. Some 60,000 strokes occur yearly among 2.3 million Americans with this dysrhythmia. Strokes in people with atrial fibrillation are especially large and disabling, and consequently prevention is paramount.

By the mid-1980s, epidemiological, case-control, and autopsy studies had demonstrated an independent association between nonvalvular atrial fibrillation and stroke. While it had been proposed that anticoagulation could prevent strokes in patients with atrial fibrillation, the advanced age of most atrial fibrillation patients (average age in the 70s) and the high intensity of anticoagulation then commonly prescribed caused clinicians to be wary due to the risk of serious hemorrhage. No antithrombotic prophylaxis was routinely prescribed for most atrial fibrillation patients. Clinical trials to assess the benefit versus risk of treatment with anticoagulants and antiplatelet agents were clearly warranted.

PROTOCOL DESIGN

In 1987, the SPAF I trial, sponsored by the National Institute of Neurological Disorders and Stroke, was launched to assess the efficacies of adjusted-dose warfarin and, separately, of aspirin for prevention of stroke and systemic embolism (primary thromboembolic events) in atrial fibrillation patients.[1] Patients with sustained or intermittent nonvalvular atrial fibrillation were entered at 15 clinical sites in the United States. Participants deemed eligible to receive anticoagulation were randomized to warfarin (open-label), aspirin 325 mg/day, or placebo (double-blind), while those not eligible for warfarin were randomly assigned to either aspirin 325 mg/day or placebo (double-blind)[2] (Figure 1).

Anticoagulation eligibility was based on the safety of anticoagulation (e.g., recent gastrointestinal hemorrhage, frequent falling) and willingness to receive it. A major reason for exclusion from anticoagulation was age >75 years, considered a relative contraindication during that era of high-intensity anticoagulation monitored in the United States by inaccurate laboratory techniques. In short, the categorization of patients as warfarin-eligible versus warfarin-ineligible was based on considerations of anticoagulation safety and not on an *a priori* hypothesized differential efficacy of aspirin. The primary comparison of the occurrence of thromboembolic events in those assigned

SPAF I Study

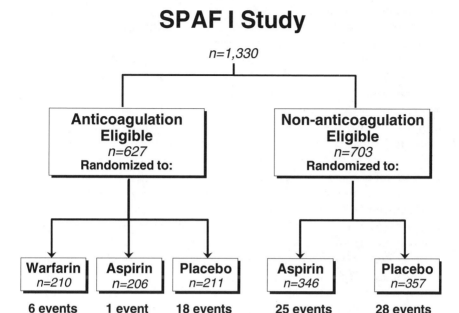

Figure 1 Design and main results of the SPAF I Study.

aspirin versus placebo was to include all patients randomized to aspirin versus placebo, both anticoagulation-eligible and anticoagulation-ineligible. This required a sample size of 1,407 participants followed for a mean of 2.5 years to detect a 33% relative risk reduction.[2] A larger 50% relative risk reduction was believed to be the minimum clinically important difference for the warfarin vs. placebo comparison and required that 472 participants be followed for a mean of 2.5 years.

DATA MONITORING EXPERIENCE

Based on a somewhat unusual design for that era (Figure 1), interim efficacy monitoring included comparison of aspirin versus placebo separately in anticoagulation-eligible and anticoagulation-ineligible patients, as well as for both groups combined, and in warfarin versus placebo and warfarin versus aspirin among warfarin-eligible participants (i.e., five separate comparisons).[2] Although the primary hypothesis of aspirin efficacy was to be tested by comparing all patients assigned to aspirin to all patients assigned to placebo, separate interim monitoring of warfarin-eligible and warfarin-ineligible seemed prudent based on the study design. Eight interim analyses were anticipated, to occur after every 25 primary events with the preset probability values for statistical significance at each interim analysis adjusted to preserve an overall alpha of 0.05 (e.g., 0.003 at the second interim analysis following accumulation of 50 primary events).

In November 1989 at the second interim analysis, the DMC recommended that the placebo arm of the anticoagulation-eligible stratification be terminated due to a striking reduction in primary thromboembolic events among those assigned to aspirin vs. placebo (1 vs. 18 primary events, respectively), a relative risk reduction of 94% (p < 0.0001). At that point, mean follow-up averaged 1.2 years per participant, and about 25% of the planned number of primary events had accrued. The DMC did not recommend that the placebo comparison among anticoagulation-ineligible patients be ended; the observed efficacy of aspirin versus placebo among these patients was quantitatively different (25 versus 28 primary events, respectively; relative risk reduction of 8%, p = 0.75) and statistically heterogeneous (p = 0.009) compared to its effect in anticoagulation-eligible patients.[3,4]

The SPAF I Executive Steering Committee was surprised by the large, unanticipated difference in aspirin efficacy between atrial fibrillation patients deemed anticoagulation-eligible versus anticoagulation-ineligible. Despite the DMC's recommendation, four scientific considerations favored continuing the placebo arm among anticoagulation-eligible patients:

1. The efficacy of aspirin among the larger group of anticoagulation-ineligible participants was modest and did not approach statistical significance. Yet, this subset was stratified based on perceived risks of anticoagulation and not response to aspirin.

2. Analysis of participant features comparing those deemed anticoagulation-eligible vs. anticoagulation ineligible did not explain the unexpected difference in aspirin efficacy; i.e., there was no obvious biologically plausible explanation.

3. In early 1989 (ten months before), the Copenhagen AFASAK randomized trial reported only a small (14%), non-statistically significant effect of aspirin 75 mg/day among anticoagulation-eligible atrial fibrillation patients[5] (Table 1).

4. Results of an influential 1988 meta-analysis of the efficacy of aspirin on vascular events in a broad range of patients with vascular disease made it unlikely that the observed 94% reduction in stroke and systemic emboli was a generalizable effect.[6]

It was the view of the SPAF I Executive Steering Committee that the very large effect of aspirin seen in SPAF I trial anticoagulation-eligible participants most likely represented an extreme play of chance. However, faced with the high statistical significance (p < 0.0001), the SPAF I Executive Steering Committee concurred that placebo treatment among anticoagulation-eligible

Table 1 Features of Atrial Fibrillation Patients Assigned to Aspirin/Placebo in Randomized Trials

	SPAF I (1991)		AFASAK I* (1989)	EAFT** (1993)
	Warfarin-eligible	Warfarin-ineligible		
Aspirin dosage	325	325	75	300
Number of patients	417	703	672	444
Mean age (yr)	65	68	73	70
Men (%)	72	69	54	56
Hypertension (%)	55	51	32	42
Diabetes (%)	18	16	9	13
Tobacco smoking (%)	14	18	36	20
Prior MI (%)[†]	17	14	7	8
Intermittent AF (%)[‡]	33	34	0	25
Prior stroke/TIA (%)[§]	8	8	6	100
Relative risk reduction by aspirin (%)	94	8	14	4

* All participants were warfarin-eligible.
** Subset of warfarin-eligible participants.
[†] MI = myocardial infarction.
[‡] AF = atrial fibrillation.
[§] TIA = transient ischemic attack.

participants should not continue, and the trial was terminated to protect the interests of these participants. When subsequent, more detailed analyses failed to identify differences in patient features between anticoagulation-eligible and anticoagulation-ineligible participants that would account for the discrepancy in aspirin efficacy,[3] the SPAF I Executive Steering Committee recommended to the DMC that the placebo arm of the anticoagulation-ineligible arm also be terminated, and this recommendation was accepted by the DMC and the NINDS. The rationale was as follows: if it is established that aspirin reduces stroke in anticoagulation-eligible patients and that differences in aspirin efficacy between anticoagulation-eligible and anticoagulation-ineligible patients could not be explained by differences in patient features, it is likely that aspirin is efficacious to some degree for all atrial fibrillation patients, making continued treatment with placebo not in the best interest of the participants. In short, while the early termination of the SPAF I trial did not permit confident estimation of the effect of aspirin on thromboembolism in atrial fibrillation patients, it was very likely that aspirin was of some benefit, precluding further placebo treatment.

Further, interim results of the warfarin versus placebo comparison (5 vs. 18 events, $p = 0.04$) coupled with the results of the recently published AFASAK trial showing a similar effect (risk reduction of 54%, $p < 0.05$)[5] established the efficacy of warfarin over placebo. Hence, the relevant clinical question evolved to a comparison of warfarin with aspirin, and this was the basis of the subsequent SPAF II randomized trial.[7] In order to facilitate SPAF II recruitment, the results of the separate effects of warfarin and aspirin versus placebo in Group I of the SPAF I trial were not initially revealed.[8] The efficacy of aspirin was reported for all randomized patients, as planned in the study design, as the overall best estimate of the effect of aspirin from the SPAF I trial[4] with the differential effect according to anticoagulation eligibility published later as an exploratory result.[3]

LESSONS LEARNED

The early termination of the SPAF I trial before the efficacy of aspirin was satisfactorily defined serves to illustrate two important aspects of DMC function:

1. The design of the plan for interim efficacy monitoring should be carefully thought through to consider the implications of all potential monitoring outcomes on the conduct of trial.
2. Protection of participant interests by the DMC should outweigh demands of clinical science.

It appeared likely during the deliberations of November 1989 that the extreme effect of aspirin among anticoagulation-eligible patients in the SPAF I trial, but not among anticoagulation-ineligible participants, was mainly due to the play of chance. The genie was let out of the bottle by a planned interim efficacy comparison that seemed logical based on the specific study design. Protection of the trial participants was paramount to the DMC and the SPAF I Executive Steering Committee. The clinical issue of aspirin's efficacy for patients with atrial fibrillation was left muddy at the termination of the SPAF I trial because the participants' interests were properly placed ahead of the need for more data.

The efficacy and safety of aspirin in atrial fibrillation was eventually sorted-out from other randomized trials. In addition to the SPAF I trial, five other randomized clinical trials have compared aspirin to placebo in patients with atrial fibrillation (Figure 2).[9] All have shown trends toward reduction in stroke by aspirin, with their pooled results showing a 22% (95% CI 3, 38) relative risk reduction.[9] Of note, the efficacy of aspirin in two other trials restricted to anticoagulation-eligible participants with atrial fibrillation have not demonstrated the large effect that prompted early termination of the SPAF I trial (Table 1). Attempts to identify atrial fibrillation patients who are "aspirin-responders" through pooled analysis of individual patients from these trials were unrevealing.[10] Aspirin is now generally accepted as offering a modest (~20%) reduction in stroke and other vascular events in patients

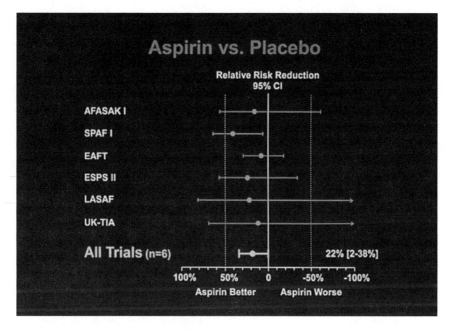

Figure 2 Metanalysis of six randomized trials testing aspirin in atrial fibrillation.[9]

with atrial fibrillation,[9,11] although it is much less efficacious than adjusted-dose warfarin.[12]

How external results from a comparably large, similar study should influence DMC deliberations continues to be debated.[13] In retrospect, perhaps the results of the Copenhagen AFASAK trial, available at the time of the SPAF I trial termination, might have been weighted more heavily to justify continued observation of the SPAF I participants assigned to aspirin. This difficult issue continues to challenge the best judgment of DMCs today.

REFERENCES

1. Hart RG, Halperin JL, Pearce LA, Anderson DC, Kronmal RA, McBride R, et al. 2003. Lessons from the Stroke Prevention in Atrial Fibrillation trials. *Ann Intern Med* 138:831–838.
2. Stroke Prevention in Atrial Fibrillation Investigators. 1990. Design of a multicenter randomized trial for the Stroke Prevention in Atrial Fibrillation Study. *Stroke* 21:538–545.
3. Stroke Prevention in Atrial Fibrillation Investigators. 1993. A differential effect of aspirin in the Stroke Prevention in Atrial Fibrillation Study. *J Stroke Cerebrovasc Dis* 3:181–188.
4. Stroke Prevention in Atrial Fibrillation Investigators. 1991. The Stroke Prevention in Atrial Fibrillation Study: Final results. *Circulation* 84:527–539.
5. Petersen P, Boysen G, Godtfredsen J, Andersen ED, Andersen B. 1989. Placebo-controlled, randomized trial of warfarin and aspirin for prevention of thromboembolic complications in chronic atrial fibrillation. The Copenhagen AFASAK study. *Lancet* 1:175–179.

6. Antiplatelet Trialists' Collaboration. 1988. Secondary prevention of vascular disease by prolonged antiplatelet treatment. Antiplatelet Trialists' Collaboration. *BMJ* 296:320-331.
7. Stroke Prevention in Atrial Fibrillation Investigators. 1994. Warfarin vs. aspirin for prevention of thromboembolism in atrial fibrillation: Stroke Prevention in Atrial Fibrillation II Study. *Lancet* 343:687-691.
8. Stroke Prevention in Atrial Fibrillation Investigators. 1990. Preliminary report of the Stroke Prevention in Atrial Fibrillation Study. *N Engl J Med* 322:863-868.
9. Hart RG, Benavente O, McBride R, Pearce LA. 1999. Antithrombotic therapy to prevent stroke in patients with atrial fibrillation: A Meta-analysis. *Ann Intern Med* 131:492-501.
10. Atrial Fibrillation Investigators. 1997. The efficacy of aspirin in patients with atrial fibrillation: Analysis of pooled data from three randomized trials. *Arch Intern Med* 157:1237-1240.
11. Antithrombotic Trialists' Collaboration. 2002. Collaborative meta-analysis of randomized trials of antiplatelet therapy for prevention of death, myocardial infarction, and stroke in high risk patients. *BMJ* 324:71-86.
12. van Walraven C, Hart RG, Singer DE, Laupacis A, Connolly S, Petersen P, et al. 2002. Oral anticoagulants vs. aspirin in nonvalvular atrial fibrillation: An individual patient metanalysis. *JAMA* 288:2441-2448.
13. Pocock SJ. The role of external evidence in data monitoring of a clinical trial. 1996. *Stat Med* 15:1285-1293.

Early Termination of the Diabetes Control and Complications Trial

John M. Lachin
Patricia Cleary
Oscar Crofford
Saul Genuth
David Nathan
Charles Clark
Frederick Ferris
Carolyn Siebert
for the DCCT Research Group

ABSTRACT

The Diabetes Control and Complications Trial (1983-1993) of 1,441 subjects followed for an average of 6.5 years assessed the effects of intensive therapy aimed at maintaining near normal levels of blood glucose versus conventional therapy on the risks of diabetes complications of the eyes, kidneys, and nerves. The study was designed to test the hypothesis that the higher than normal blood glucose levels associated with conventional insulin therapy caused these complications. The study was terminated one year ahead of schedule by the monitoring board. This paper describes the medical, ethical, and statistical challenges faced by the study group and the monitoring board.

INTRODUCTION AND BACKGROUND

The Diabetes Control and Complications Trial[1] was a multi-center, randomized, controlled clinical trial of the relative effects of a program of intensive versus conventional management of blood glucose levels on the development and/or progression of microvascular complications of type 1 diabetes mellitus (T1DM). The trial was organized and funded by the National Institute of Diabetes, Digestive, and Kidney Diseases (NIDDK) of the National

Institutes of Health (NIH). The study group was appointed in January 1982, the first subject randomized in August 1983, and the last in June 1989. The study was terminated after an average of 6.5 years of follow-up in June 1993, one year ahead of schedule.

The Director of the NIDDK appointed an external data monitoring committee, called the Data, Safety. and Quality Review Group (DSQRG), to review the accruing data from the trial periodically and to advise on the early termination of the trial or modification of the protocol based on the emerging results. Early in the trial, the DSQRG prepared a document entitled *Operating Procedures for the Data, Safety, and Quality Review Group* which delineated the roles, responsibilities, and functions of the DSQRG. That document was later described in detail by Siebert and Clark.[2] The DSQRG met approximately every six months for the duration of the trial. At the December 1992 meeting, the DSQRG recommended that the DCCT initiate closeout activities as a prelude to consideration of early termination.

The NIDDK had also appointed a second oversight committee, the Policy Advisory Group (PAG), that met periodically to review the continuing viability of the DCCT in light of other emerging evidence while masked to the DCCT results. It was also the responsibility of the PAG to offer a final recommendation on termination of the DCCT when so recommended by the DSQRG. Thus, the analyses of the updated study data were presented to a joint meeting of the DSQRG and PAG in June 1993 at which time both groups concurred that the study should be stopped. The principal results were then rapidly published,[1] followed by dozens of papers on the detailed results of the study. A complete bibliography is available from the website of the Coordinating Center at the George Washington University Biostatistics Center (www.bsc.gwu.edu). The members of the DSQRG and PAG are named in DCCT.[1]

This chapter describes the various considerations which lead to the conclusion by the DSQRG in December 1992 that a statistically significant and clinically meaningful difference between the treatment groups had been observed. Some, but far from all, considerations were statistical. We also describe lessons learned from the monitoring of this trial that may bear on the conduct of future trials.

The Glucose Hypothesis

Type 1 diabetes mellitus (T1DM) is the result of an autoimmune process that leads to ablation of the insulin secreting β-cells of the islet of Langerhans in the pancreas. Eventually the patient decompensates with rising blood glucose levels and other metabolic abnormalities and untreated, eventually dies. In 1922, Banting and Best of the University of Toronto showed that injections of insulin extracted from animals could lower glucose levels and sustain life.

Within 20 years of the introduction of insulin therapy, a variety of long-term complications of the eyes, kidneys, and nerves (retinopathy, nephropathy, and neuropathy), rarely if ever seen in the pre-insulin era, were observed that ultimately lead to blindness, end stage renal disease, and amputations, respectively. One school of thought postulated that these complications were a manifestation of the underlying course of diabetes per se, or perhaps side effects of exogenous insulin therapy. The other school advocated *The Glucose Hypothesis* that complications resulted from the elevated levels of glycemia (hyperglycemia) that persisted with conventional insulin therapy, and could be prevented by maintaining near-normal levels of glycemia.

The principal weakness of prior studies of this hypothesis was that the technology to achieve and sustain levels of glycemia close to the non-diabetic range simply did not exist. However, by 1980 advances in therapy allowed subjects to achieve near-normal day-to-day levels of glycemia. Multiple daily injections of combinations of short, intermediate and long-acting insulins, or use of a continuous subcutaneous insulin infusion device (or pump), in conjunction with hand-held blood glucose meters, allowed subjects to test their blood glucose levels frequently during the day, before and after meals, and to adjust their insulin doses accordingly. In addition, the glycosylated hemoglobin (HbA_{1c}) assay provided an objective, reliable measure of the average glucose level over the preceding 2–3 months. This provided direct feedback that allowed the clinician and patient to tailor a regimen of diet, exercise, and insulin administration to achieve long-term glucose levels as close to normal as possible. These advances made it practical to conduct a definitive clinical trial to formally test the glucose hypothesis.

PROTOCOL DESIGN

Treatments and Timeline

Since it was impractical to "clamp" a subject at a randomly assigned specific level of glucose, the chosen design assigned half the subjects to receive an intensive therapy aimed at near-normal glycemia, and half to receive conventional therapy with no glucose targets using no more than two insulin injections daily. The principal potential adverse effect of intensive therapy was an increased risk of episodes of hypoglycemia, where low levels of blood glucose cause symptoms ranging from sweating or dizziness to loss of consciousness and seizure. The objective of the study was to evaluate the effects of intensive versus conventional therapy on the risks of retinopathy principally, and also the risks of nephropathy, neuropathy, and hypoglycemia.

The design of the study has been published[3-5] and the protocol, manual of operations, and complete study data sets can be obtained from the National Technical Information Service. Briefly, the study consisted of two independent trials designated as the Primary Prevention Trial and the Secondary Intervention Trial with different eligibility criteria. The primary prevention trial consisted of 726 subjects with early duration type 1 diabetes (1–5 years), no retinopathy, and near-normal renal function (albumin excretion rate (AER) < 40 mg/24 hr). The secondary trial included 715 subjects with longer duration diabetes (1–15 years), minimal background retinopathy, and possibly some early signs of nephropathy (AER < 200 mg/24 hr).

The DCCT study group was organized in January 1982. The study began with the enrollment of 278 subjects into a preliminary trial from August 1983 to March 1984 that demonstrated feasibility.[6] Recruitment to the full-scale study was opened in February 1985 and closed in July 1988 for the secondary trial and June 1989 for the primary trial with an additional 1,163 subjects enrolled, or 1,441 total.[5] All subjects were to be followed through 1993. However, the DSQRG recommended early termination and the final subject visits were held during January–April 1993.

Primary Outcome ~ Retinopathy

The principal DCCT outcome was onset or progression of diabetic retinopathy based on centrally graded fundus photographs obtained from each subject at baseline and at six-month intervals during the trial. Photographs were graded using a 25-step scale of increasing severity of retinopathy in the two eyes (Table 1) that had been developed for the Early Treatment of Diabetic Retinopathy Study.[7] The principal outcome measure was a sustained progression of at least three steps (*sustained 3+ step progression*) from the level on entry (step 1 in the primary trial, steps 2–9 in the secondary) that was observed on two successive six-monthly visits. The principal analysis was specified to be a lifetable analysis of the cumulative

Table 1   Steps of severity of diabetic retinopathy (DR) and levels of severity of diabetic nephropathy

Step	Retinopathy Severity of DR
1	No retinopathy
2–3	Microaneurysms only
4–5	Mild non-proliferative (NPDR)
6–9	Moderate NPDR
10–11	Severe NPDR (SNPDR)
12–25	Proliferative (PDR) and worse

incidence of the onset or progression of retinopathy using a modified Kaplan-Meier estimator and the Mantel-logrank test.[8] Using the method of Lachin and Foulkes,[9] 700 subjects were required to provide 90% power to detect a 37.5% risk reduction, allowing for 10% losses to follow-up and 20% non-compliance, for the primary and secondary trials, or 1,400 total. Power was higher if the rate of loss to follow-up and non-compliance were lower.

However, a 3+ step progression within the above ranges of retinopathy severity is a surrogate outcome that is not usually associated with any lesions or overt symptoms, such as change in vision, requiring treatment. Thus, prior to the start of the full-scale trial, the study investigators recommended to the DSQRG that a treatment group difference in the cumulative incidence of 3+ step progression alone should not be used as a criterion for premature termination of the trial. Rather, they desired that a treatment effect on the incidence of more severe levels of retinopathy be used as the basis for such a decision, such as the incidence of severe non-proliferative diabetic retinopathy or the incidence of laser surgery (photocoagulation). Owing to the lower expected frequency, the protocol specified that treatment group differences for these outcomes would be assessed in the combined primary and secondary trials.

Other Outcomes—Nephropathy and Neuropathy

The DCCT was not designed to detect differences between the treatment groups in the incidence of progression of nephropathy or neuropathy, which occur less frequently than retinopathy. Nevertheless, these and other outcomes were monitored and employed in analyses of the emerging results. Nephropathy outcomes were predefined using the albumin excretion rate (AER). *Microalbuminuria* (or worse) is a value distinctly above normal (AER ≥ 40 mg/24 hr), and *albuminuria* (AER ≥ 300 mg/24 hr) is equivalent to overt proteinuria, the earliest clinical manifestation of significant diabetic renal disease. Upon entry, subjects were required to have an AER <40 or <200 mg /24 hr in the primary or secondary trial, respectively. It was pre-specified that the cumulative incidence of albuminuria would be assessed in the combined trials due to the expected low incidence.

Autonomic neuropathy was assessed every two years, and neuropathy assessed clinically and by testing of nerve conduction velocity at baseline, five years, and study end. Other outcomes included quality of life, neuro-cognitive function, mental status, macrovascular events, and risk factors such as blood pressure and serum lipids level. In addition, various adverse effects of diabetes or its treatment were monitored continuously, especially episodes of hypoglycemia. Virtually all outcome assessments were analyzed and monitored periodically by the DSQRG.

The investigators and patients were masked to progression of complications until such time as a level was reached for which treatment was clinically indicated, including severe non-proliferative treatment that could require photocoagulation, renal insufficiency, hypertension, hyperlipidemia, or macrovascular events.

Group Sequential Procedures

The DSQRG and the Coordinating Center jointly specified the statistical procedures for interim monitoring of the accumulating data at approximately six-month intervals. The group-sequential procedure of Lan and DeMets[10] was employed using the "O'Brien-Fleming-like" $\alpha_1^*(t)$ alpha-spending function where t is a measure of the fraction of study information available at a given interim analysis. No formal procedures were applied for monitoring of adverse events (e.g., hypoglycemia) or to monitor for futility (lack of effectiveness).

While these methods provide a stopping boundary, they were employed in a less rigorous way to assess the strength of evidence that a true difference had likely emerged. The DSQRG did not commit itself to terminating the trial if significance was reached for any one analysis, but rather agreed in advance to consider early termination when a body of evidence had emerged that was clinically compelling and that addressed all of the study objectives. The Operating Procedures for the DSQRG described a number of criteria other than statistical significance which should be met prior to any decision to terminate the trial prematurely (see Table 2).

In statistics, "information" has a precise meaning, but for many of the analyses employed in the DCCT, such as lifetables, the precise amount of statistical information to be observed during the entire trial could not be quantified before the end of the trial was reached. Thus, as later described by Lan and DeMets,[11] a function of the duration of the trial was used as a surrogate measure of information. The DSQRG met in November 1985 to monitor for the first time both treatment effectiveness and safety. Since close-out was scheduled to occur at the end 1993, 17 semi-annual meetings of the DSQRG were anticipated through December 1993. The fraction of DSQRG meetings held was employed, as a surrogate measure of information. Thus, at each meeting, the Lan–DeMets spending function was employed, with an increment in information of $1/17 = 0.059$.

Longitudinal analyses of repeated measurements over time were also performed using the multivariate rank test of Wei and Lachin[12] that provides a single test of the average difference between treatment groups over all repeated visits combined.[13,14] This method was employed to assess group differences in the distributions of the ordinal retinopathy severity scores over

Table 2 DSQRG Considerations for Early Termination

Excerpted from *Operating Procedures for the Data, Safety and Quality Review Group*.

a. Whether the magnitude or character of an observed difference constitutes a clinically important benefit or risk;

b. Whether the results could be explained by possible differences in baseline variables between the groups;

c. Whether the results could be due to ascertainment bias caused by differences in the treatment regimens;

d. Whether the results are consistent with those for other variables which should be associated with the variable in question;

e. Whether the results are consistent among various subgroups of subjects and across the various centers involved in the study;

f. Whether the risk which is under consideration is outweighed by assessment of the overall potential benefit of therapy;

g. Whether the results could be due to concomitant therapy not directed at blood glucose control rather than due to the different treatment regimens;

h. Whether it is likely that the current trends in the data could be reversed if the trial were to be continued unmodified;

i. Whether and how much additional precision or certainty in the results could be obtained by continuing the trial under the present Protocol; and,

j. Whether there would be significant loss in external validity or credibility of the trial by change in Protocol or discontinuation.

time, longitudinal measures of renal function with severely skewed distributions, and measures of nerve conduction for which there is a lower limit of quantification. These analyses were implemented at the 11th meeting of the DSQRG in December 1990 at an information fraction of 0.647, with subsequent increments of 0.059 in the study information as for the lifetable analyses. For each outcome variable, the correlations of successive test statistics from each DSQRG meeting were computed using the methods described in Su and Lachin.[15] The critical values then were computed by numerical multivariate integration or Monte Carlo simulation.

For more serious but less frequent outcomes such as severe nonproliferative diabetic retinopathy and albuminuria, it was decided to employ a nominal significance level of 0.05 at the end of the trial. For such outcomes, criteria for statistical significance alone were considered less important than the observation of a biologically consistent treatment group effect in conjunction with an effect on 3+ step progression that met group sequential criteria for significance.

In order to maximize the scientific gain from procedures performed infrequently (e.g., nerve conduction studies), the DCCT protocol included a "study-end" evaluation of all DCCT subjects. Thus the study adopted a *Closeout Protocol* which called for a staged termination of the trial if warranted.

The DSQRG would first decide that the trial should initiate closure activities. Thereafter, all subjects would be comprehensively evaluated over a five-month period. These data would then be analyzed and presented to a joint meeting of the DSQRG and PAG at which a decision would be reached regarding the termination of the trial.

THE DATA MONITORING EXPERIENCE

The following is a synopsis of the principal findings at the meetings of the DSQRG leading up to the decision to terminate the study ahead of schedule. A summary of the levels of significance of the principal analyses is presented in Table 3. Only the lifetable analyses of retinopathy and nephropathy progression, and the Wei-Lachin point-prevalence analyses of neuropathy at five years of follow-up are presented.

Figure 1 presents the cumulative incidence of sustained 3+ step retinopathy progression in the primary and secondary cohorts, from DCCT.[1] At the conclusion of the study in June 1993, some subjects had been followed for nine years, with an average of 6.5 years. During the early part of the study there was much discussion of the lack of evidence of benefit. In both cohorts, there was no discernible benefit of intensive therapy between groups during the first five years of follow-up. In the secondary intervention cohort, the risk of "early worsening" during the first two years was increased somewhat with intensive therapy. Nevertheless, intensive therapy continued to yield mean-

Table 3   Emergent Significant Results (P-values and Relative Risk Estimates)

	P-values				Relative risk (95% CI) 12/92
	6/91	12/91	6/92	12/92	
Lifetable analyses					
Boundary (p)	0.011	0.015	0.019	0.024	
Sustained 3+ Step change					
Primary trial	NS	0.004	<0.0001	<0.0001	3.7 (2.2, 6.2)
Secondary trial	0.005	0.0006	<0.0001	<0.0001	2.2 (1.6, 2.9)
Total	0.004	<0.0001	<0.0001	<0.0001	2.5 (1.9, 3.3)
SNPDR	NS	NS	0.048	0.044	1.6 (1.0, 2.6)
Photocoagulation	0.027	0.037	NS	0.013	2.9 (1.2, 6.8)
Albuminuria	NS	NS	0.035	0.016	2.1 (1.1, 3.8)
Prevalence analysis					
Boundary (p)	0.0005	0.0005	0.0013	0.0067	
Neuropathy at 5 y	0.0009	0.00045	<0.0001	<0.0001	2.3 (1.3, 5.4)

Results nominally significant with a p-value (0.05 are shown; NS = not nominally significant). Group sequential boundary critical p-values at the 0.05 significance level (two-sided) are also shown.

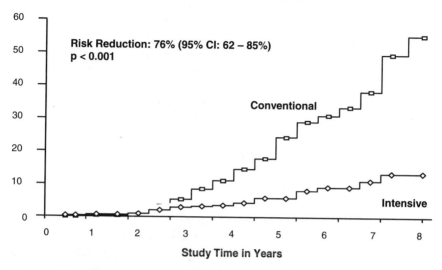

Figure 1 Cumulative incidence of sustained progression of 3 or more steps on the ETDRS scale of retinopathy severity separately within the DCCT primary prevention and secondary intervention cohorts, with the associated risk (hazard) reduction for intensive versus conventional therapy. Reproduced from DCCT (1993) with permission of the *N. Engl J Med*.

ingfully lower levels of blood glucose (HbA$_{1c}$) and a constant three-fold greater risk of hypoglycemia, as expected; there were no clinically significant increased risks of adverse outcomes with intensive therapy. Accordingly the DSQRG recommended that the trial continue.

In June 1991, at the 12th interim analysis, the lifetable analysis of the incidence of a sustained 3+ step progression within the secondary, but not the primary, trial reached group sequential significance. The analysis of clinically significant neuropathy at five years was nominally statistically significant but did not meet the group sequential criterion for significance. The DSQRG did not find these data to be compelling and recommended that the trial be continued. However, additional analyses were requested, some based on the criteria specified in Table 2.

In December 1991 group sequential significance was observed in the lifetable analysis of a sustained 3+ step progression within both the primary and secondary trials, and in the prevalence of clinically significant neuropathy at five years of follow-up. A nominally statistically significant difference was observed in the lifetable analysis of photocoagulation among all subjects combined.

At this meeting, a variety of additional analyses were presented. The first concerned the patterns of events leading up to the emergence of the significant difference in the lifetable analysis of sustained 3+ step progression. It was determined that the increase in the number of events observed in recent meetings could not be explained by any methodologic factors and was largely due to the increasing accumulation of subject-years of exposure.

Another analysis showed that the observation of a single 3+ step progression at any one visit was associated with an 8.6-fold increase in the risk of developing severe non-proliferative diabetic retinopathy at a future visit (95% confidence limits: 2.7, 14.5) during the study; and a sustained 3+ step progression with a 13-fold increase in this risk (95% CI: 2.5, 23.3). This analysis, therefore, confirmed the predictive importance of 3+ step progression. However, the treatment effect on the risk of severe non-proliferative diabetic retinopathy itself was not statistically significant.

For the first time, the DSQRG entertained a serious discussion of the potential for early termination of the trial. The consensus was that there was a conclusive reduction in risk of the principal outcome, a sustained 3+ step progression in retinopathy, with intensive versus conventional therapy within both the primary and the secondary trials. However, these results alone were not considered clinically compelling because they would not provide a sound basis for treatment recommendations. Therefore, the DSQRG concluded that the study should be continued, but also asked that the Coordinating Center initiate more extensive analyses of retinopathy to address the additional considerations specified in the *Operating Procedures of the DSQRG* (Table 2).

In June 1992 the differences previously observed in 3+ step retinopathy progression and neuropathy persisted, but that in photocoagulation did not. For the first time, the lifetable analyses of severe non-proliferative diabetic retinopathy and of albuminuria were nominally significant in the combined trial. Additional analyses demonstrated that beneficial effects of intensive therapy on retinopathy progression were observed to some degree within specified subgroups of subjects and that there were no major differences among clinics, and that no one or two clinics accounted for the treatment effect.

The general conclusion of the DSQRG was that these analyses satisfied all the criteria necessary for a clinically meaningful treatment group difference in retinopathy. Nevertheless, the DSQRG did not think that all of the major research questions had been answered and questioned whether the current results would be sufficient to inspire a general change in clinical practice. The DSQRG recommended continuation of the study but requested further analyses of hypoglycemia and other adverse effects to better define the benefit to risk ratio of intensive versus conventional treatment.

In December 1992 the analyses of retinopathy progression and neuropathy were group sequentially significant, and those of other more severe outcomes were nominally significant. Table 3 presents the estimated relative risk for conventional versus intensive treatment. The treatment benefit in risk of retinopathy progression was somewhat greater in the primary than the secondary trials. In the total study, the relative risk was 2.5 with 95% confidence limits (1.9, 3.3). This represents a 60% reduction in risk with intensive treatment (95% limits: 47%, 70%). The lifetable analysis of more severe and clinically significant levels of retinopathy and neuropathy also achieved nominal significance within the secondary trial and for both trials combined. In each case, there were too few events within the primary trial to achieve significance, but the observed relative risk was comparable to that within the secondary trial.

Additional analyses of nephropathy demonstrated that beneficial effects of intensive therapy were observed to some degree within subgroups of subjects and that there were no major differences among clinics. Additional analyses also demonstrated that the three-fold increase in the risk of severe hypoglycemia with intensive versus conventional therapy persisted over the full duration of follow-up, was present more or less in all subgroups of the cohort, was relatively stable over time, and was inversely related to the mean HbA_{1c} in both groups.

Overall, therefore, both trials provided strong evidence of clinically meaningful benefit with intensive treatment, and all of the criteria specified in Table 2 were addressed and satisfied. Accordingly, the DSQRG voted unanimously to recommend that the DCCT initiate close-out procedures. At a subsequent meeting in June 1993, based on a preliminary final data set, the DSQRG and Policy Advisory Group jointly recommended that the trial be terminated. Those preliminary results were presented at the national meeting of the American Diabetes Association within weeks of this decision. The final data set was subsequently closed and the major results published in the three months after the final decision to terminate the trial.[2]

LESSONS LEARNED

Methodological Research

One of the major lessons from the DCCT is that the Coordinating Center should be funded to conduct methodological research to address issues posed by the study. The DCCT started with a feasibility trial with a sample size of 278 determined for the analysis of a feasibility outcome. Lachin and Foulkes[9] describe procedures for sample size evaluation for the Mantel-logrank test that allowed for stratification and losses to follow-up, and that provided the total target sample size of 1,400 necessary for the full-scale DCCT given the initial feasibility study sample size.

The treatment assignments in the DCCT were unmasked, thus admitting the potential for selection and experimental biases. Lachin[16] and Wei and Lachin[17] describe the statistical properties of randomization procedures in general, and Wei's urn randomization procedure, respectively. Based on this and other research, the urn procedure was selected for the DCCT randomization to minimize these biases.

For the longitudinal analysis of the ordinal retinopathy scores in the DCCT, and other measurements, Wei and Lachin[12] developed a family of multivariate rank tests. This approach was further generalized by Thall and Lachin[13] and Lachin.[14] Su and Lachin[15] then described a group-sequential procedure for the Wei-Lachin multivariate rank test that was employed in the interim analyses of the DCCT.

The distribution of rates of hypoglycemia had an excess of zeros and a long tail, relative to a Poisson distribution. Bautista, Lan, and Lachin explored methods for the analysis of such over-dispersed count data. Chapter 8 of Lachin[18] describes the method that was employed for the analyses of hypoglycemia and other event rates in the interim and final analyses of the study data.

The group sequential boundary for the primary outcome had been crossed many times before the study was terminated. However, the group sequential critical values were not used in the publication of the final results.[1] Rather, all results were cited as "nominally significant" at $p \leq 0.05$ (two-sided). Lan, Lachin, and Bautista[19] showed that if the boundary is crossed but the trial continues, then it is conservative simply to employ the fixed sample size critical values in the final analyses, as done in DCCT.[1]

Other Lessons

There were many other lessons from the DCCT of a more practical nature.

When planning the study, diabetic retinopathy was selected as the primary outcome because previous studies had demonstrated that it could be reliably assessed and that it was a highly sensitive measure of retinal abnormalities. While no prior study had used 3+ step progression as an outcome, duplicate gradings had shown that this level of progression was highly reproducible, sensitive, and specific. Further, longitudinal epidemiologic studies had provided a basis for estimation of the expected hazard rate in the conventional group that formed the basis for the sample size evaluation for the study. As it turned out, this estimate was too high. This underscores the importance of sound epidemiologic data for the natural history of the primary outcome in the planned population in designing a clinical trial, and for being conservative in the assessment of sample size when there is uncertainty regarding the available data.

The power of a study of incidence (time-to-event) is a function of the number of events observed; that in turn is a function of sample size and study duration. From preliminary studies it was estimated that the median time to retinopathy progression was 3.5 years. In order to ensure that any difference in cumulative incidence documented by the trial could reasonably apply to the entire cumulative incidence curve, ranging up to at least the 75th percentile, the study was designed to have an average duration of follow-up of at least seven years. This precaution proved fortuitous since no difference in risk was observed over the first five years of follow-up.

Recognizing the uncertainty of the estimated hazard rate in the conventional group, there was some concern that losses to follow-up and non-compliance would erode the power of the study. Thus the study group insisted on a conservative assessment of sample size that provided at least 90% power using a two-sided test at the 0.05 level after adjusting for 10% losses to follow-up and 20% non-compliance using the model in Lachin and Foulkes.[9] However, these are adjustments for the loss of information, not the bias that can be introduced by losses or non-compliance. To limit the erosion of power and the introduction of bias, the study was implemented using an *intent-to-treat design* in which all patients are followed to the planned study end regardless of adherence to the assigned therapy or side effects of therapy. Extensive subject education was conducted during the recruitment phase[20] to promote compliance with the assigned treatment and complete follow-up, and no subject was permanently withdrawn from study follow-up. The success was remarkable. Of the 1,441 subjects randomized, 32 were declared temporarily inactive at some point during the study, but most of these later returned to follow-up and their assigned treatment. Only eight of those surviving did not attend a final close-out visit in 1993. During the study, subjects adhered to the assigned treatment for 97% of scheduled visits.

This was fortunate because the hazard rate for the primary outcome in the conventional group was substantially less than that projected—0.05 and 0.07 per year in the primary and secondary trials, respectively, versus a projection of 0.2 in each. Thus the loss of power due to the lower hazard rate was offset by the gains in power due to higher than projected rates of follow-up and compliance.

While the hazard rates of such progression within the two treatment groups were not proportional over time, it would be cheating to assess the pattern of the hazards first and to then select the test that appears to be optimal for that pattern. In fact the hazard increased exponentially in the conventional group, while it remained nearly constant in the intensive group. While the power of the Mantel-logrank test was degraded due to the non-proportional hazards, it was still more sensitive to such patterns than other possible rank tests, such as the Wilcoxon, and in many respects was robust to departures from this assumption. The combination of the conservative assessment of sample size and a relatively robust statistical test helped to ensure that the trial was not underpowered to detect effects of interest.

One of the most important elements in the successful interim monitoring for the DCCT was the selection of DSQRG and PAG members with expertise in all of the areas relevant to the DCCT. These included adult and pediatric diabetes, endocrinology, ophthalmology, nephrology, neurology, cardiology, neuropsychology, ethics, and biostatistics. While many studies have a single statistician member of a DSMB, in the DCCT it was highly advantageous to have three statistician members with different areas of expertise.

Another important step was the development beforehand of a Manual of Procedures[1] for the operation of the DSQRG that covered all aspects of group responsibilities and functions, with input from the study group. This also included a pre-specification of the statistical monitoring plan. No one can foresee the patterns of data that will be observed in a study. What is important, however, is to try to think through the criteria to be used as the basis for a decision to terminate or modify a trial. To the extent possible supplemental analyses, such as subgroup analyses, should be pre-specified.

Despite all these steps, it took many years for the beneficial effects of intensive therapy to evolve. While some might consider that there was cause to consider termination for futility during the early years, this was not the case. The DSQRG realized that these early looks only represented a minor amount of the planned information to be accrued. While it might have been predicted that the benefits of intensive therapy would become manifest sooner, we now understand that hyperglycemia has long-term pervasive physiologic effects that are neither quickly nor completely erased by the implementation of near-normal glycemia, and likewise that the effects of a period of near-normal glycemia are longlasting.[21,22]

It is interesting to note that early in the DCCT, the DSQRG observed a worsening of retinopathy during the first year or so of treatment among subjects assigned to intensive therapy, principally in the secondary intervention trial, where subjects who entered with micro-aneurysms, the earliest sign of retinopathy, developed somewhat more serious sub-clinical lesions. This so-called "Early Worsening" of early retinopathy in patients where tight glucose control is rapidly implemented had been observed in a previous but much smaller trial. The DSQRG reflected on this observation but recommended continuing the trial. With continued follow-up, this excess risk appeared to dissipate with time; however, there was no evidence of any benefit of intensive therapy for at least the first four years of follow-up, in either the primary prevention or secondary intervention trials. Had a great deal of emphasis been placed on this early worsening, and lack of benefit, the DCCT might have terminated early for harm or futility, missing one of the major advances in the treatment of type 1 diabetes.

While the PAG played an essential role in the DCCT, there is rarely the need for a separate unmasked DSQRG and a PAG that remains masked until a decision is pending. However, while the DCCT was underway there were reports from many smaller studies, some randomized, and it was important to have an independent body charged with continual assessment of the progress (feasibility) of the trial and its relevance in light of other emerging data.

The setting, operational scope, and complexity of the DCCT may have been very atypical. However, every clinical trial is unique in some respects, and these differences may impact the choice of the approach to be adopted for the interim monitoring of the study. While only some of the lessons from the DCCT might apply to another study, we hope that future trials may benefit from our experience.

ACKNOWLEDGEMENTS

John Lachin was Director and Patricia Cleary Co-Director of the Coordinating Center, Oscar Crofford was Chair and Saul Genuth Vice-Chair of the Study, David Nathan was Editor in Chief, Charles Clark was Chair and Frederick Ferris member of the DSQRG, and Carolyn Siebert was NIDDK DCCT Program Director. The members of the research group are presented in DCCT (1993).

The historical account of the DCCT is based on the work of the study group, including the Coordinating Center staff; the Data, Safety, and Quality Review Group; and the Policy Advisory Group. The members of the study group, the DSQRG. and the PAG are presented in the appendix to the DCCT (2) article. Patricia Cleary served as the Co-Director of the Coordinating Center (CoC) for the study duration. Other CoC statisticians (chronologically) included Max Halperin and K.K. Gordon Lan as senior statistical advisors; James Knoke, Desmond Thompson, and Oliver Bautista as research faculty; Peter Gilbert, David Kenny, ShuPing Lan and Jye-yu Backlund as staff statisticians. L.J. Wei and Peter Thall provided statistical consultation. The statistician members of the DSQRG who provided guidance to the committee and the coordinating center on statistical matters were Gary Cutter, David DeMets, and Anastasios Tsiatis.

REFERENCES

1. DCCT Research Group. 1993. The effect of intensive treatment of diabetes on the development and progression of long-term complications in insulin-dependent diabetes mellitus. *N Engl J Med* 329:977–986.
2. Siebert C, Clark CM. 1993. Operational and policy considerations of data monitoring in clinical trials: The Diabetes Control and Complications Trial Experience. *Control Clin Trials* 14:30–44.
3. DCCT Research Group. 1986. The Diabetes Control and Complications Trial (DCCT): Design and methodological considerations for the feasibility phase. *Diabetes* 35:530–545.
4. DCCT Research Group. 1988. The Diabetes Control and Complications Trial (DCCT): Update. *Diabetes Spectrum* 1:187–190.
5. DCCT Research Group. 1990. The Diabetes Control and Complications Trial (DCCT): Update. *Diabetes Care* 13:427–433.
6. DCCT Research Group. 1987. The Diabetes Control and Complications Trial (DCCT): Results of the feasibility study (Phase II). *Diabetes Care* 10:1–19.
7. Early Treatment Diabetic Retinopathy Study Research Group. 1991. Grading diabetic retinopathy from stereoscopic color fundus photographs: an extension of the modified Airlie House Classification: ETDRS report No.10. *Ophthalmology* 98:786–806.
8. Lachin JM. 2000. Statistical Considerations in the Intent-to-treat Principle. *Control Clin Trials* 21:167–189.
9. Lachin JM, Foulkes MA. 1986. Evaluation of sample size and power for analyses of survival with allowance for non-uniform subject entry, losses to follow-up, non-compliance and stratification. *Biometrics* 42:507–519.
10. Lan KKG, DeMets DL. 1983. Discrete sequential boundaries for clinical trials. *Biometrika* 70:659–663.
11. Lan KKG, DeMets DL. 1989. Group sequential procedures: Calendar versus information time. *Stat Med* 8:1191–1198.
12. Wei LJ, Lachin JM. 1984. Two-sample asymptotically distribution-free tests for incomplete multivariate observations. *J Am Stat Assoc* 79:653–661.
13. Thall PF, Lachin JM. 1988. Analysis of recurrent events: Nonparametric methods for random interval count data. *J Am Stat Assoc* 83:339–347.
14. Lachin JM. 1992. Some large sample size distribution-free estimators and tests for multivariate partially incomplete observations from two populations. *Stat Med* 11:1151–1170.
15. Su JQ and Lachin JM. 1992. Group sequential distribution-free methods for the analysis of multivariate observations. *Biometrics* 48:1033–1042.
16. Lachin JM. 1988. Statistical properties of randomization in clinical trials. *Control Clin Trials* 9:289–311.
17. Wei LJ, Lachin JM. 1988 Properties of the Urn randomization in clinical trials. *Control Clin Trials* 9:345–364.
18. Lachin JM. 2000. *Biostatistical Methods: The Assessment of Relative Risks.* John Wiley and Sons, New York.
19. Lan KKG, Lachin JM and Bautista OM. 2003. Over-ruling a group sequential boundary–a stopping rule versus a guideline. *Stat Med* 22:3347–3355.
20. DCCT Research Group. 1989. Implementation of a multi-component process to obtain informed consent in the Diabetes Control and Complications Trial. *Control Clin Trials* 10:83–96.
21. The DCCT/EDIC Research Group. 2000. Retinopathy and nephropathy in patients with type 1 diabetes four years after a trial of intensive therapy. *N Engl J Med* 342:381–389.
22. The DCCT/EDIC Research Group. 2002. The effect of intensive therapy on the microvascular complications of type 1 diabetes mellitus. *JAMA* 287:2563–2569.

Data Monitoring in the AIDS Clinical Trials Group Study #981: Conflicting Interim Results

Dianne M. Finkelstein

ABSTRACT

In 1989, the NIH sponsored AIDS Clinical Trials Group (ACTG) mounted a large prospective randomized trial (known as ACTG 981) to compare fluconazole (200 mg daily) with clotrimazole lozenges (10 mg, five times daily) for prevention of invasive fungal infections in patients with advanced HIV disease. At the fourth DSMB review of the study in November 1992, the patients on fluconazole had a significantly lower risk of invasive, serious and superficial fungal infections, but a higher mortality rate than the patients on clotrimazole. The DSMB recommended keeping the study open in spite of the fact that a boundary had been crossed for the primary endpoint. The final analysis of this study, published in the New England Journal of Medicine, reported that the trial gave evidence of the superiority of fluconazole in preventing the most serious fungal infections, but did not show an advantage in reducing overall mortality, thus vindicating the recommendations of the DSMB to keep the trial open until the planned follow-up had been completed. This paper is a review of the DSMB process for this study, and how the Board dealt with the challenges of interpretation of apparently contradictory evidence on treatment efficacy.

INTRODUCTION AND BACKGROUND

In 1989, the standard therapy for the primary infection in patients with advanced human immunodeficiency virus (HIV) infection was zidovadine (called ZDV or AZT). Optimal prophylaxis against opportunistic infections was a major unresolved issue in clinical care, as patients were susceptible to several life-threatening infections, but available treatments were disease-specific and each had associated treatment-limiting complications. Early large cooperative group trails tested the effectiveness of prophylactic treatment of *Pneumocystis carinii* pneumonia (PCP) to prevent initial episodes as well as relapse, and to prolong survival.[1,2] The effectiveness of preventive therapy for *Mycobacterius avium* infection had also been demonstrated.[3] There was no widely accepted practice for prevention of fungal infections, even though invasive fungal infections, especially with *Cryptococcus neoformans* occurred in 5-10% of patients with acquired immunodeficiency syndrome (AIDS) and were associated with a substantial mortality risk.[4] In addition, mucocutaneous candidiasis was common in these patients with recurrence causing substantial morbidity. Fluconazole is an oral antifungal agent that was shown to be effective in preventing a relapse of cryptococcal meningitis.[5] There was also evidence that it prevented recurrence of oropharyngeal candidiasis (thrush), which was associated with some degree of mortality.[6] However, in 1989, there was no clear evidence on the effectiveness of fluconazole for primary prophylaxis, and there was concern about the long-term toxicity, cost, possibility of drug interactions, and eventual drug resistance that could develop with prolonged use.

PROTOCOL DESIGN

In 1989, the NIH sponsored AIDS Clinical Trials Group (ACTG) mounted a large prospective randomized trial (known as ACTG 981) to compare fluconazole (200 mg daily) with clotrimazole lozenges (10 mg, five times daily) for prevention of invasive fungal infections in patients with advanced HIV disease. Clotrimazole was selected for the control group, rather than placebo, in order to offer patients an effective local therapy for oral thrush, which would enable investigators to study the long-term effects of fluconazole use. This study enrolled subjects, as a nested sub-study, from participants of ACTG 081, which was a phase III comparison of ZDV (500 mg) plus aerosolized pentamidine (300 mg every four weeks), or Bactrim (1 D.S. tab orally BID), or Dapsone (50 mg orally BID) for prevention of *Pneumocystis carinii* pneumonia. Patients were excluded from participating in ACTG 981 if they had a history of systemic fungal infection, had indications for an allergy or intolerance to fluconazole, an active mucosal fungal infection, or were already receiving an anti-fungal agent.

Patients were randomly assigned to treatment in a 1:1 ratio, and continued treatment until an invasive fungal infection developed or the patient withdrew or died. There was no expectation that this trial would detect a survival advantage to either therapy. Thus, in the absence of a survival difference, the primary endpoint of the study was deemed to be the time to development of an invasive fungal infection (such as cryptococcosis and histoplasmosis). Secondary endpoints included time to development of an invasive or serious fungal infection (including esophageal candidiasis), time to development of superficial fungal infection (primarily oral thrush), and global effect on health status (as measured by the *HIV-PARSE* instrument). As it was not always possible to obtain a positive culture or biopsy for diagnosis, the investigators relied on *presumptive* diagnosis, which was determined by a syndrome of symptoms. The study was initially designed to enroll 240 patients, which would ensure 80% power to detect a difference of 7.5% (10% versus 2.5%), with a one-sided alpha of .05 in the 18-month rate of invasive fungal infections. The calculations were made using a one-sided test because there was no expectation that fluconazole would be worse with regard to prevention of systemic infections, and the investigators anticipated a very low fungal infection rate. During this era, AIDS trials had to recruit and close very quickly, as the window of opportunity was limited by a rapidly changing treatment options, and an impatient and mobile patient population. The trial was designed to allow for four interim and a final analysis, utilizing Lan–DeMets boundary stopping criteria (with an O'Brien–Fleming spending function). The nominal (one-tail) p-values were calculated assuming that there would be a total of 25 events. All reported endpoints underwent a blind review by the data manager and study chair. All p-values in this report are two-sided unless otherwise noted.

DATA MONITORING EXPERIENCE

ACTG 981 underwent four reviews by a data safety monitoring board (DSMB). Each review consisted of an Open Session that provided an opportunity for study investigators to participate by answering questions from the DSMB members. This was followed by a Closed Session that included none of the study team except the statisticians. At this review, treatment codes were partially blinded (i.e., A versus B for all tables), but a sealed envelope provided the codes, and the DSMB members were allowed to be unblinded at their own discretion. The DSMB review of the parent study ACTG 081 was completed prior to that of ACTG 981.

The first review was in November 1990. The design of the study was discussed. There was a concern that the rate of the primary outcome of the study was anticipated to be very low, and the number of patients impacted by a positive trial of a prophylaxis treatment was expected to be substantial. Therefore there was a sense that a larger study, with more observed serious fungal infections, would be more compelling. The study was accruing well (enrollment was at 301), and a recommendation was made that the trial should be expanded to include any patient enrolled in ACTG 081 and willing to participate in ACTG 981. This expansion of the trial would ensure sufficient power to detect a 4.5% difference (6% versus 1.5%) in the 18-month rate of a specific invasive fungal infections (such as cryptococcosis). Patients enrolled in ACTG 981 were to be followed until the closure of the parent study, ACTG 081 in 1992. The only concern that was raised in this DSMB meeting was the fact that there was an imbalance of 981 participation by 081 treatment arm, which could impact 081 if there was any effect of 981 treatments on 081 endpoints. Since intent to participate in 981 was a stratification factor for 081, it was believed that decision on 981 participation was being made after 081 treatment assignment was known. The 081/981 investigators were advised to educate patients on the independent benefit of fungal prophylaxis regardless of which PCP prophylaxis was the patient was using. At the time of this DSMB, there were no invasive fungal infections, one reported (unconfirmed) case of esophageal candidiasis and six cases of systemic infection (fungemia). Twenty-seven patients had experienced at least one episode of albicans candidiasis (superficial thrush). The recommendation of the DSMB was to continue the trial as planned.

The second DSMB review was in November 1991. At that time, there were 418 patients enrolled in the study (98% complete accrual). There were eight cases of invasive fungal infections, including four cases of cryptococcus (one in the fluconazole group, and three in clotrimazole). There were also nine cases of esophageal candidiasis (one in fluconazole and eight in clotrimazole), and 42 cases of thrush (8 in fluconazole and 34 in clotrimazole). The endpoint of this and subsequent reviews is summarized in Table 1. The toxicity was not substantially different across treatments, but compliance was better on fluconazole than clotrimazole (94% versus 58% had taken 6/7 of their doses). A treatment difference was emerging at this point, with fluconazole patients experiencing a lower rate of invasive, systemic, and superficial fungal infections. However, while there was no clear survival advantage to either treatment, the trend for a mortality benefit was in the opposite direction, as 14 clotrimazole patients and 20 fluconazole patients had died. Although all analyses reported in the closed review were partially blinded (i.e., A vs. B for all tables) with regard to treatment, most felt that they could decipher this information from the profile of outcomes and toxicities.

The third review was of this study was in early May 1992. At that time, there were 16 invasive fungal infections (2 in fluconazole and 14 in clotrimazole), of which ten cases were cryptococcus (one in fluconazole and nine in clotrimazole). The one-sided p-value for the treatment comparison of all 16 invasive fungal infections was $p = 0.0014$. Patients on fluconazole suffered fewer cases of esophogael candidiasis and superficial thrush infections than those on clontrimazole as well (see Table 1). However, 37 of the patients assigned to fluconazole and 27 to clotrimazole had died (two-sided p = 0.177). The groups were imbalanced with respect to median baseline CD4 count and so a CD4-adjusted p-value for the treatment comparison on survival was

Table 1   Frequency of Fungal Infections by Treatment and DSMB Report Date

	Review Date							
	November 1991		March 1992		November 1992		June 1993	
Outcomes	Flu	Clo	Flu	Clo	Flu	Clo	Flu	Clo
Invasive fungal infections	2	6	2	14	4	18	9	23
Cryptococcosis	1	3	1	9	2	13	1	15
Serious fungal infections	1	3	1	9	2	13	2	15
Esophageal candidiasis	1	8	2	13	4	17	3	17
Superficial infection (Thrush)	8	34	30	82	40	101	33	100
Death	20	14	37	27	56	43	98	89

reported (as p = 0.601). The survival advantage for clotrimazole was greater in the patients assigned to ACTG 081 treatments AP and dapsone than in TS. Although the p-value for the treatment comparison on invasive fungal infections had crossed the boundary (of p = 0.0140), indicating a clear advantage for patients assigned to floconazole, the DSMB was concerned about the fact that the survival advantage had a trend in favor of clotrimazole. They asked for further analyses of survival, and a conference call was convened in late May, 1992. On this call, the DSMB recommended that on the basis of the fact that the patients on the more effective prophylactic treatment were experiencing the higher mortality, the trial should be allowed to continue in spite of the fact that a boundary for the primary outcome had been crossed.

The fourth review of this study was in November 1992. At this final interim review, there were 22 invasive fungal infections (4 in fluconazole and 18 in clotrimazole), of which 15 were cryptococcus (2 in fluconazole and 13 in clotrimazole). The one-sided p-value for the treatment comparison of all 22 invasive fungal infections was p = 0.0011. The rates of esophageal candidiasis and superficial infections continued to be lower in the patients on fluconazole than on clotrimazole. However, the mortality rates were still reversed, as fifty-six of the patients assigned to fluconazole and 43 to clotrimazole had died (p = 0.16). The median CD4 count at entry to ACTG 981 was 90 in fluconazole and 114 in clotrimazole (p = 0.13). To account for this imbalance, a baseline CD4-adjusted p-value for the treatment comparison on survival, was calculated and found to be p = 0.41. The survival advantage for clotrimazole was greater in the patients assigned to ACTG 081 treatments aerosolized pentamidine and Dapsone than in Bactrim. The DSMB recommended that the study should remain open until its scheduled closure in June 1993, as the extended follow-up would provide more information on the long-term effects of these treatments on survival. There was some discussion regarding the fact that it was not clear what the stopping boundary would be at this point, as the prescribed boundary had already crossed at the previous review, but the trial continued.

Final Analysis of the Study

The final analysis of the study was based on 428 patients followed from September 1989 until June 1993, with a median follow-up of 34.7 months. For the comparison of the primary endpoint of time to invasive fungal infection, patients were categorized by their treatment assignment at randomization, regardless of compliance or discontinuation. By the end of follow-up, 32 invasive fungal infections had been diagnosed (9 in fluconazole and 23 in clotrimazole, one-sided p = 0.0063). Seventeen of the infections were cryptococcosis (two in fluconazole and 15 in clotrimazole, one-sided p = 0.00095). The estimated two-year rate of invasive fungal infections was 2.8% in fluconazole and 9.1% in clotrimazole, which was not substantially different than the rates anticipated when the study was first designed. The estimated CD4-adjusted relative risk for invasive fungal infections, for patients randomized to clotrimazole was 3.25 that of those randomized to fluconazole (p = 0.0017, 95% lower bound of 1.68). There had been 20 cases of esophageal candidiasis (three in fluconazole and 17 in clotrimazole, one-sided p = 0.0008), and 133 superficial fungal infections (33 in fluconazole and 100 in clotrimazole, p < 0.0001). Ninety-eight patients randomized to fluconazole and 89 patients randomized to clotrimazole had died (unadjusted relative risk 1.18, p = 0.26; CD4 adjusted relative risk 1.04, p = 0.72). An analysis of a combined endpoint of *either* an invasive fungal infection or death indicated that 102 patients in fluconazole and 96 in clotrimazole had experienced an endpoint. The treatment comparison on time to first critical event (infection or death) was not statistically significant (stratified logrank test, p = 0.57).

Exploratory subgroup analyses were performed to try to understand the basis for the fact the treatment effects on mortality and fungal infections so different. Analyses were pursued with regard to treatment provided on the parent study 081 and with regard to baseline CD4 count. Among patients assigned to aerisolized pentamidine (AP) on 081, there was a marginally higher mortality rate for patients assigned to fluconazole as compared to clotrimazole (p = 0.083), while there were no significant differences in the mortality rates for clotrimazole versus fluconazole for patients assigned to Dapsone (p = 0.92) or Bactrim (p = 0.97).

Because systemic PCP prophylaxis can obscure the toxic effects of antifungal therapy, an analysis of toxicity was made in patients on AP (which is delivered as a spray into the airway). This analysis showed that patients on fluconazole required more transfusions (7.4% vs. 2.8%, p = 0.029), and experienced more severe nausea (14.1% on fluconazole versus 3.9% on clotrimazole, p = 0.027), and abdominal pain (18.0% on fluconazole versus 6.5% on clotrimazole, p = 0.03).

It is of interest to note that the 78% of serious fungal infections patients had reached a CD4 of <50. The treatment differences in efficacy are most pronounced in the patients with lower baseline CD4 counts. Seven of the 32 (22%) patients with invasive fungal infections had died of the infection (two in fluconazole and five in clotrimazole).

Patients on clotrimazole discontinued anti-fungal medication significantly earlier than those on fluconazole (p = 0.023). Also, on average 95.3% of patients on fluconazole and 50.5% of clotrimazole patients were compliant at least 6 days a week (p < 0.0001).

In conclusion, this study was specifically designed to allow a comparison of the treatments with regard to rare invasive fungal infections (including cryptococcosis). The *New England Journal of Medicine* article on the study indicated that "study provided a clear indication of the superiority of fluconazole in preventing the these infections, esophageal candidiasis, and superficial fungal infections particularly in patients with CD4 counts below 50, but the drug did not show evidence of reducing overall mortality".[7] It was further noted that this was probably due to the fact that a relatively low rate of mortality was directly attributable to fungal infections. The authors noted that over 11,000 doses of fluconazole were given to prevent each case of invasive infection in the study population, and thus concluded that it was probably best to focus prophylaxis on the population of patients with greatest risk, namely, those with CD4 counts below 50.

LESSONS LEARNED

The study ACTG 981 was an interesting experience both for statisticians and clinicians involved in conduct of this study. There were several issues the study raised which could provide guidance for future study design and DSMB review. First, it would have been helpful to have a more refined and specific judgment on how survival would be considered at each interim review, even though no survival difference was anticipated. This was especially true considering that the treatment delivery was so different (one treatment was systemic, while the other was a lozenge), and thus efficacy, compliance and toxicity patterns could be anticipated to have unsuspected impact on mortality. This could have been decided before the trial began, and perhaps discussed with and agreed to by the DSMB. Thus, instead of stating "in the absence of survival differences, the primary endpoint will be the rate of invasive (and systemic) fungal infections," it may have been better to indicate how survival and fungal infections should be evaluated under all possible scenarios. Instead, when the results of these two analyses disagreed on the optimal treatment for a life-threatening disease, the DSMB needed to draw from the investigators their belief system during the Open Sessions with the study chair while the study was under way.

Second, the interim monitoring was based on a very rare, only mildly lethal infection, and the study was designed to determine the optimal strategy for potential long-term prophylaxis. The cost/benefit issue of the treatment was a factor in the decision, but this had not been formalized in the study design. Thus, when the monitoring boundary was crossed by the primary outcome analyses, and only 22 infections were confirmed in the more than 1,000 patient years of follow-up, the DSMB members did not feel compelled to close the study. However, once the stopping value for the primary endpoint had been ignored, it became difficult to know what or whether there was an appropriate subsequent stopping boundary for the study. In recognition of the importance of the long-term cost/benefit, compliance, and toxicity information, it may have been more appropriate to design the study so that there would not be early stopping except for mortality differences. However, this trial was conducted during the early AIDS era, and there was considerable pressure to reach early decisions on optimal treatment of this life-threatening disease.

Third, in deliberating on whether to terminate this study early, several factors had to be taken into account, including baseline comparability, compliance, internal and external consistency, risk–benefit ratio, multiple outcomes for safety and efficacy, and repeated analyses of each outcome, etc. This simultaneous analysis presented some challenges. With regard to handling baseline treatment imbalances in key variables (such as CD4 count), the primary analysis was supposed to be based on a logrank test comparison of the two treatments with regard to the serious fungal infections. The adjusted analysis required a Cox regression, and there was resistance to shifting the primary analysis at this point to reflect a model-based hypothesis. With regard to the fact that there were really several (correlated) treatment comparisons playing a role in this decision, there was uncertainty about how to weigh each of these, especially when they were not all indicating that the same treatment was optimal.

Finally, noting that the survival differences diminished by the time of publication of the trial results, it would appear that there was basic wisdom shown in this DSMB committee, which decided to recommend that this trial continue rather than close it early with a report of the advantages of fluconazole for prevention of fungal infections in AIDS patients.

In general, the DSMB played an important role in this study which was beyond the goals of monitoring ongoing results for protection of participating patients. In fact, the DSMB served as a scientific advisory committee, guiding the decisions to expand the study and analyzing and interpreting the results. The Open and Closed Session format of the DSMB was useful, as it allowed the DSMB members to draw from the experience and judgment of the PIs, which improved the quality of the analysis and ensured consensus on the final interpretation. This discussion was especially true for a study like ACTG 981, where several different dimensions of treatment efficacy and impact were considered, and the results were not clearly interpretable.

An epilogue to this history can be written by noting that the current standard care of HIV-infected patients aligns with the results and report of this trial. In fact, the 2002 guidelines for prevention of opportunistic infections based on recommendations by the U.S. Public Health Service indicate that routine prophylaxis for fungal infections is not advised, due to a "the relative infrequency of the infection, lack of survival benefit associated with prophylaxis, potential antifungal drug resistance, and cost".[8] ACTG 981 had a lasting and important impact on the care of HIV-infected patients. The scientifically sound trial design and implementation of ACTG 981 and the thoughtful investigators review and prudent recommendations of the DSMB, ensured that the trial provided a compelling and conclusive scientific result.

REFERENCES

1. Hardy WD, Feinberg J, Finkelstein DM, Power ME, He W, Kaczka C, et al. 1992. A controlled trial of trimethoprim-sulfamethoxazole or aerosolized pentamidine for secondary prophylaxis of Pneumocystis carinii pneumonia in patients with AIDS: AIDS clinical trial group protocol 021. *N Engl J Med* 327:1842-1848.
2. Bozzette SA, Finkelstein DM, Spector SA, Frame P, Powderly WG, He W, et al. 1995. A randomized trial of three anti-pneumocystis agents in patients with advanced HIV infection. *N Engl J Med* 332:693-699.
3. Nightingale SD, Cameron DW, Gordin FM, Sullam PM, Cohn DL, Chaisson RE. et al. 1993. Two controlled trials of rifabutin prophylaxis against Mycobacterium avium complex infection in AIDS. *N Engl J Med* 329:828-833.
4. Chuck SL, Sande MA. 1989. Infections with Cryptococcus neoformans in the acquired immunodeficiency syndrome. *N Engl J Med* 321:794-799.
5. Bozzette SA, Larsen RA, Chiu J, Leal MA, Jacobsen J, Rothman P, et al. 1991. A placebo-controlled trial of maintenance therapy with fluconazole after treatment of cryptococcal meningitis in the acquired immunodeficiency syndrome. *N Engl J Med* 324:580-584.
6. Just-Nubling G. Gentschew G. Meissner K. Odewald J. Staszewski S. Helm EB. Stille W. 1991. Fluconazole prophylaxis of recurrent oral candidiasis in HIV-positive patients. *Eur J Clin Microbiol Infect Dis* 10:917-217.
7. Powderly WG, Finkelstein DM, Feinberg J, Frame P, He W, van der Horst C, et al. 1995. A randomized trial comparing fluconazole with clotrimazole troches for the prevention of fungal infections in patients with advanced HIV infection. *N Engl J Med* 332:700-705.
8. Masur H, Kaplan JE, Holmes KK. U.S. Public Health Service. Infectious Diseases Society of America. 2002. Guidelines for preventing opportunistic infections among HIV-infected persons-2002. Recommendations of the U.S. Public Health Service and the Infectious Diseases Society of America. *Ann Intern Med* 137(5 Pt 2):435-478.

Challenges in Monitoring the Breast Cancer Prevention Trial

Carol K. Redmond
Joseph P. Costantino
Theodore Colton

ABSTRACT

The Breast Cancer Prevention Trial (BCPT) was a double-masked, placebo-control, randomized clinical trial designed and conducted by the National Surgical Breast and Bowel Project (NSABP), a National Cancer Institute (NCI)-funded cancer cooperative group. The primary hypothesis tested was whether tamoxifen, a drug that is beneficial for treatment of breast cancer, was effective in preventing the occurrence of cancer in women at increased risk. The Endpoint Review, Safety Monitoring, and Advisory Committee (ERSMAC), the independent data monitoring committee for the BCPT, implemented an innovative monitoring strategy that combined traditional monitoring rules for individual diseases with a global monitoring index in order to weigh the beneficial effects of treatment with known and potential detrimental effects. In addition to developing a monitoring plan tailored for a prevention trial with multiple endpoints of interest, other concerns that were addressed included a reassessment of study sample size and power subsequent to a lengthy suspension of accrual during the trial and handling the occurrence of an unexpected ocular toxicity in association with tamoxifen. Although there were numerous issues that arose during its course, the trial progressed to completion of accrual and successful early termination following the fourth interim analysis, when there was reliable evidence that, not only did tamoxifen prevent breast cancer, but that the beneficial effect outweighed adverse effects of taking tamoxifen.

INTRODUCTION AND BACKGROUND

The BCPT was the first major multicenter randomized clinical trial designed to assess a therapeutic agent for the primary prevention of breast cancer.[1,2] The therapeutic agent was tamoxifen citrate, a drug marketed under the name Nolvadex®, that had been extensively tested and found

118

effective as a treatment in reducing the risk of recurrence and death among women with primary breast cancer. NCI funded the study and the pharmaceutical company, AstraZeneca, provided the medications (tamoxifen and placebo) used in the trial. To be eligible for participation, a woman had to be at least 35 years of age, have no history of an invasive breast cancer or ductal carcinoma in situ, and be at high risk for developing invasive breast cancer. A woman was considered at high risk for developing invasive breast cancer if she met at least one of the three following criteria: (1) was sixty years of age or older; (2) had a prior diagnosis of a lobular carcinoma in situ; or (3) had a five-year predicted risk of developing breast cancer of at least 1.66% as determined by the modified Gail model.[3] Randomization was stratified by age, race, history of lobular carcinoma in situ, and level of predicted breast cancer risk. Women were treated for a planned duration of five years with either 20 mg bid tamoxifen or placebo.

Screening of women for eligibility to the BCPT began in April 1992 and the first participants were randomized in June. Accrual of the 13,388 women randomized to the BCPT occurred between June 1, 1992, and September 30, 1997, although the majority of participants were accrued during the first two years of recruitment. In March 1998, at the time of the fourth interim efficacy analysis, the independent Endpoint Review, Safety Monitoring and Advisory Committee (ERSMAC) for the BCPT recommended that the trial be stopped early due to evidence that tamoxifen was highly beneficial in reducing the incidence of invasive breast cancer. Within a matter of a few days, the trial results were announced by the NCI via the internet and subsequently all participants were unblinded. The formal publication of results in the Journal of the National Cancer Institute occurred a few weeks thereafter.[4]

Throughout the course of the trial, from its initial inception until its early termination with a 45% observed reduction in invasive breast cancer among participants receiving tamoxifen, the BCPT provided many challenges to the study leadership, sponsors, and ERSMAC. The ERSMAC dealt effectively with numerous safety and ethical concerns, often in conjunction with intense public, media, and governmental scrutiny that surrounded the trial. The ERSMAC played a central role in preserving the integrity of the trial that ultimately resulted in determining the effectiveness of tamoxifen for primary prevention of breast cancer. In the discussion that follows, we focus on how the ERSMAC addressed several issues that exemplify the complexity and difficulties in monitoring a large prevention study. These are (1) how to handle an unanticipated ocular toxicity that was identified during the course of recruitment; (2) innovative development of a "global" monitoring strategy to assist in weighing multiple benefits and risks of tamoxifen; and (3) the application of this global monitoring strategy that led to the decision to stop the trial early because of a beneficial effect of tamoxifen therapy.

PROTOCOL DESIGN

Statistical considerations presented in the original protocol established a framework for monitoring data in the BCPT. This section summarizes the salient features of the statistical design, and the major modifications made as the trial progressed, which are important for gaining an understanding of the interim monitoring strategy that evolved during the conduct of the trial.

The design considerations for the BCPT focused on the incidence of invasive breast cancer as the primary endpoint. The original accrual target was to randomize 16,000 women in equal numbers to placebo and tamoxifen within a two- to three-year accrual period with an additional seven years of follow-up to have definitive findings for identifying a 31% reduction in invasive breast cancer incidence (Table 1). During the first year of BCPT accrual, the recruitment rate was consistent with that used in the sample-size calculations, but during the second year of recruitment, in reaction to controversies associated with an NSABP investigator in Canada, randomization to all NSABP trials was suspended for almost a year. When randomization was resumed, the accrual rate was much attenuated from that achieved previously.

The possibility of modifying the sample size in midcourse, depending on the projected baseline breast cancer risk and accrual rate, had been built into the protocol. Because accrual was abruptly halted in1994, the sample size was not formally re-evaluated until 1996, when more than 11,000 women had already been randomized. The participants who entered the BCPT during the first two years had a predicted risk of invasive breast cancer, based on the Gail model, that was approximately double the risk used in the original

Table 1   BCPT Sample-Size Considerations

Parameter Considered	Original	Revised (9/30/96)
Maximal chemoprevention effect	0.40	0.40
Observed chemoprevention effect	0.31	0.31
Significance level (one sided)	0.01	0.01
Power	0.80	0.80
Baseline breast cancer rate (Placebo)	0.033/year*	0.067/year**
Non-adherence to intervention	0.10/year through 5 years*	0.16, 0.14, 0.10, 0.10, 0.10 for years 1 through 5, respectively**
Lost-to-follow-up	1% per year*	1% per year**
Additional years of follow-up	7	5
Sample size (N)	16,000	13,000[†]

* Predicted.
** Observed through 9/30/96.
[†] With 12,029 participants accrued through 9/30/96.

sample-size calculations. Fortunately for the BCPT, which had experienced an increased noncompliance rate and difficulty in recruiting participants after the hiatus in the trial, the Gail model was remarkably accurate in predicting the overall breast cancer incidence rate in the BCPT trial placebo group.[5,6] Recomputing sample sizes using the observed placebo breast cancer incidence and the observed noncompliance rate indicated that a total sample size of 12,820 participants followed for five years after completing accrual would provide 80% power for an observed reduction of 30% in the invasive breast cancer incidence. It would take about 12 months to recruit the requisite additional 2,000 participants at the accrual rate observed when randomization recommenced in 1995. The NCI and FDA approved a formal protocol amendment to modify the sample size to 13,000 in mid-1996. The trial remained a ten-year study with five years of accrual and five years of follow-up rather than the three years of accrual and seven years of follow-up originally planned. Table 1 compares the revised sample-size assumptions with those used in the original design.

Although the primary concern at the design stage of the trial was the reduction in breast cancer incidence, there was interest in evaluating whether tamoxifen might also reduce the incidence of two other important clinical outcomes, coronary heart disease and osteoporosis. In addition, while tamoxifen has antiestrogenic properties in treating breast cancer, it has estrogenic effects on the uterus and vascular system, leading to the need for the trial to monitor for adverse effects such as thromboembolic diseases, including deep vein thrombosis, pulmonary embolus, and endometrial cancer.

The initial BCPT protocol specified stopping guidelines for monitoring of two endpoints, one for interim monitoring of invasive breast cancer and a second guideline for monitoring of coronary heart disease. The preplanned monitoring rule for invasive breast cancer, the primary endpoint, specified that, following the occurrence of a total of 50 breast cancers, the breast cancer incidence would be assessed at yearly time intervals corresponding with preparation of reports for ERSMAC meetings. An O'Brien–Fleming stopping boundary was proposed, employing an exact binomial test assuming an expected difference between treatment groups of the total number of observed breast cancer cases that was based on the distribution of the observed person years at risk.[7] O'Brien–Fleming boundaries were chosen for a one-sided hypothesis with an $\alpha = 0.01$ to be consistent with the sample-size calculations.[8] To protect against the possibility of a finding that tamoxifen treated participants might have a greater breast cancer rate than the placebo, a constant standardized difference of -1.4 was utilized for the lower monitoring boundary for breast cancer. Should the lower boundary be crossed at any interim analysis, the coordinating biostatistician would present to the ERSMAC the findings of an analysis based on stochastic curtailment methods. If the parameters used in the sample size calculations for breast cancer incidence were accurate, then final analysis was to be performed after seven years of follow-up were available on all participants. Otherwise, should accrual goals not be met or the sample size modified, final analysis was planned when sufficient information on breast cancer was obtained to have a power of 0.80 of detecting a maximal chemopreventive effect for tamoxifen of 40%.

The monitoring procedures proposed for coronary heart disease were analogous to those for breast cancer. If at any interim analysis the coronary heart disease incidence crossed the boundaries, the ERSMAC would review the findings and make a recommendation whether the study should continue.

DATA MONITORING EXPERIENCE

The study organization for BCPT included the establishment of an independent monitoring committee that would meet at least twice annually. The membership, as originally constituted, included nine individuals whose areas of expertise encompassed biostatistics, epidemiology, medical oncology, cardiovascular disease, and osteoporosis. Members initially included representatives from two funding agencies, the National Cancer Institute (NCI) and National Heart, Lung, and Blood Institute (NHLBI). The NHLBI withdrew participation in 1994 when it became apparent that the age distribution of the randomized participants was younger than anticipated and, consequently, it was unlikely that sufficient events would be observed for a definitive finding related to coronary heart disease. During the third year after accrual began, the ERSMAC's composition was expanded to 11 members in order to incorporate specialists in gynecology and research ethics. From the beginning statisticians from the NSABP Biostatistical Center participated in the discussions at the meetings but did not vote on action items or recommendations.

The first meeting of the ERSMAC was held on August 7, 1992. During the initial meeting, the committee was charged with monitoring of accrual, study endpoints, safety, and adherence to the protocol and advising the Steering Committee on protocol changes related to participant safety, ethical considerations, or data quality. The committee discussed at that time various organizational procedures related to the open and closed sessions of the meeting, attendance at open and closed sessions, and access to unblinded data. The plan was for the ERSMAC to meet at six-month intervals unless issues related to trial monitoring arose between scheduled meetings, with the next meeting to be arranged for February or March 1993. The ERSMAC also decided that the trial Principal Investigator and NCI Project Officer would not participate in the ERSMAC closed sessions to avoid potential or perceived conflicts of interest influencing committee recommendations.

Combining Stopping Rules with a Global Monitoring Strategy

The stopping guidelines, as originally proposed for BCPT, were similar to the conventional statistical monitoring procedures followed in most treatment trials. Treatment trials generally have statistical stopping rules for the primary efficacy endpoint(s) and perhaps also for a few serious adverse effects known to be associated with the treatment being assessed, but otherwise rely on subjective evaluations by the monitoring committee to interpret informally on whether reported adverse events are likely a consequence of the treatment and should lead to a change or termination of the trial. The ERSMAC members were cognizant that interim monitoring of a prevention trial inherently involved additional considerations that are not a major focus in the conduct of treatment trials. While the protocol stopping rules were helpful in monitoring the primary efficacy endpoints, the need to evaluate the net benefit of a therapy with multiple effects, some positive and some negative, was not an easy task. Participants in BCPT were healthy volunteers, rather than patients with some defined disease, and most clinical outcomes observed were not related to the primary disease of interest. There was a great emphasis in monitoring safety, not only for known or suspect adverse effects, but also for the possibility of unexpected toxicities.

During their meeting in September 1995 members of ERSMAC made plans to hold a special meeting to consider stopping rules and global monitoring procedures for the BCPT prior to their next regularly scheduled interim data review in February 1996. The statistical stopping guidelines for breast cancer and cardiovascular disease encompassed only two among several diseases and conditions to be monitored during the course of the BCPT trial. Since more reliable data had become available at that time on the estimated risk of endometrial cancer, the ERSMAC members believed that it was both desirable and appropriate to have a statistical stopping rule for that outcome to assist in their deliberations. Accordingly, a Bayesian stopping rule was proposed and adopted by ERSMAC, based on the hypothesis that the risk of endometrial cancer among tamoxifen-treated women was not greater than threefold that observed in placebo-treated women.

The NCI statistician on the ERSMAC (Dr. Laurence Freedman) was also involved with the Women's Health Initiative (WHI). The WHI monitoring committee was dealing with similar complex issues in developing the interim monitoring plan for that trial, which had not only multiple endpoints, but also multiple interventions. Recognizing an opportunity to enhance the statistical procedures used in monitoring prevention trials, Freedman devised

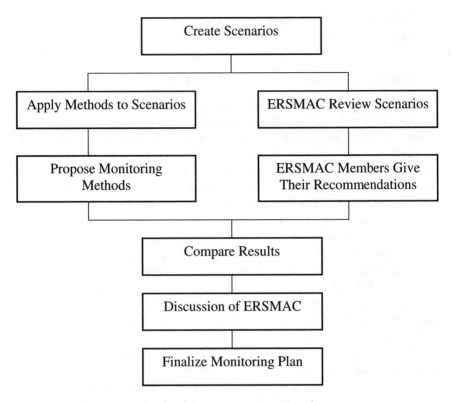

Figure 1 BCPT strategy for developing monitoring procedures.

an innovative approach for developing interim monitoring strategies for both the WHI and BCPT. Additional details on the rationale and procedures proposed for the Women's Health Initiative are given in Freedman et al.[10] Figure 1 summarizes the steps followed by ERSMAC in developing a global monitoring strategy for the BCPT.

Prior to the special session, 12 hypothetical scenarios for interim findings were circulated among members of the ERSMAC to record their decision for each scenario whether they would continue or stop the trial. The scenarios represented potential BCPT findings for five major outcomes constructed at a time when approximately half the follow-up information would be available. The five outcomes included were those used in the protocol to assess risk/benefit ratios for tamoxifen therapy. Figure 2 is an illustration of one scenario in which all endpoints are close to what would be anticipated if all the assumptions employed in designing the trial were correct. Figure 3 is a second scenario where there is a beneficial breast cancer effect, but in which no benefit is evident for coronary heart disease. In both

All Endpoints As Expected			
Type of Event	Placebo (n = 8,000)	Tamoxifen (n = 8,000)	Test Statistic (Z)
Breast Cancer	167	117	3.00
Coronary Heart Disease	52	41	1.07
Endometrial Cancer	13	38	-3.58
Pulmonary Emboli Death	1	2	-0.60
Liver Cancer	1	2	-0.78

Recommendation (Please check one box only)

CONTINUE the trial	
STOP the trial	
Cannot Decide	

Comments

Figure 2 Breast Cancer Prevention Trial: Possible Scenario #1.

All Endpoints As Expected No Benefit for Cardiovascular Disease			
Type of Event	Placebo (n = 8,000)	Tamoxifen (n = 8,000)	Test Statistic (Z)
Breast Cancer	167	117	3.00
Coronary Heart Disease	52	52	0
Endometrial Cancer	13	38	−3.58
Pulmonary Emboli Death	1	2	−0.60
Liver Cancer	1	2	−0.78

Recommendation (Please check one box only)

CONTINUE the trial	
STOP the trial	
Cannot Decide	

Comments

Figure 3 Breast Cancer Prevention Trial: Possible Scenario #2.

scenarios, the test statistic for the reduction in invasive breast cancer exceeds the O'Brien–Fleming boundary. The relative risk for endometrial cancer was about three, which was compatible with the expected level of increased risk. Of the nine ERSMAC members who evaluated the scenarios, six voted to continue the trial and three voted to stop for the two scenarios illustrated, even though the stopping boundary for invasive breast cancer had been reached. During the discussion those who voted to continue the trial expressed the need to have longer follow-up for potential adverse effects before stopping the trial. There was considerable heterogeneity in the votes of the ERSMAC members on the other scenarios as well. There was no scenario for which the ERSMAC members were unanimous that the trial should continue or stop, even if the upper boundary for breast cancer had been exceeded. In the discussion that ensued, it was apparent that many members of the ERSMAC would wish to have more information on long-term adverse events before they would stop the trial, even in the presence of a strong positive effect for breast cancer prevention.

A major distinction between prevention and treatment trials influenced the ERSMAC deliberations. In a treatment trial, continued follow-up after the trial terminates can yield additional insight into long-term deleterious outcomes. In prevention trials, since the participants receiving placebo would likely cross over to tamoxifen therapy if the trial stopped, the opportunity for further follow-up of endpoints would be lost once the trial is stopped. Many of the committee members wanted greater reassurance about long-term net benefit of tamoxifen before they would agree to stop the trial. ERSMAC carried out a second round of reviewing scenarios that had 11 clinical outcomes. The additional outcomes added were hip fractures, colorectal cancer, stroke, transient ischemic attacks, and deep vein thrombosis. The second set of scenarios also included deaths from all other causes as a category. The votes on the second round reflected heterogeneity among ERSMAC members' judgments similar to that observed during the initial round.

In parallel with the evaluation of the scenarios, ERSMAC members discussed the adoption of global monitoring guidelines that would assist in weighing the benefits against the risks of tamoxifen therapy. In developing a global index for the BCPT, members of the ERSMAC had to confront two important issues. The global index (GI) employed was a simple weighted average of the difference in the proportion of events (d_i) between the two groups for each of the 11 individual disease risks (beneficial or adverse) included in the second set of scenarios, i.e., GI $= \Sigma\ w_i d_i$ where GI refers to the global index, w_i is a predetermined weight for d_i. A major consideration was to decide which diseases and conditions to build into the index. Should the index include only those more life-threatening circumstances that had been used in the protocol to project the potential net benefit of tamoxifen therapy or should the index be expanded to include other possible risks and/or non–life-threatening conditions associated with tamoxifen therapy, even if some of them are not well-established? The ERSMAC's decision was to expand the number of diseases in the global index to include the 11 diseases used for the second set of scenarios.

An interrelated consideration was the weights to be used in computing the index, since the availability of data informative for weighting, such as five- or ten-year expected survival, varies considerably depending on the specified disease. Among the options for weighting a global index, if all outcomes were fatal or life-threatening, is to give each outcome equal weight. Alternatively, one might select weights based on the expected survival until some specified time, such as five or ten years (five- or ten-year case fatality). A problem encountered with weighting by expected survival time is that the availability of reliable information on five- or ten-year expected survival varies considerably by the outcome being considered. Furthermore, with this type of weighting, non-life-threatening outcomes could not be included in the determination of a global index. Another suggested approach is to assign weights based upon the stated utilities of the individuals who are participating in the trial.

In the BCPT interim analyses two measures of the GI were routinely calculated for the ERSMAC meetings. The first global index (GI_U) did not employ a weighting by severity of outcome. The second global index (GI_W) employed weights based on the ten-year case-fatality for each outcome. Thus, the weighted GI is similar to a "total mortality" measure.

As shown in Figure 4, the BCPT overall monitoring strategy was a combined approach involving both a conservative stopping rule for the primary outcome, invasive breast cancer, along with a supportive global statistic test.

Level 1 Flagging
ERSMAC Alerted if:
A. Adverse effects are significantly greater in the tamoxifen group for liver cancer, fatal pulmonary embolism fatal or disabling stroke, colorectal cancer or other causes of death.
- OR -
B. Number of endometrial cancers in the tamoxifen group exceeds $3n_p + 1$, where n_p is the number of endometrial cancers in the placebo group.

Level 2 Flagging
A. Benefits
• Flag if both of the following conditions hold:
1. Breast cancer benefit due to tamoxifen is significant according to the O'Brien-Fleming rule;
- AND -
2. The global statistic is supportive (e.g. exceeds some positive value such as 1.96)
B. Harm
• Flag raised if both of the following conditions hold:
1. Adverse effect is observed in any of the disease outcomes according to the O'Brien-Fleming rule;
- AND -
2. The global statistic indicates overall harm (e.g. is less then some negative values such as −1.00).

Figure 4 BCPT guidelines for alerting ERSMAC.

Having these objective guidelines assisted the ERSMAC in carrying out its complex interim monitoring charge in a manner consistent with scientific, ethical, and clinical considerations. An appealing feature of the guidelines was that they provided for two levels of alert. The Level 1 flags covered situations where the ERSMAC's judgment was that, if it reached a decision to continue the trial, it would be necessary to notify and reconsent participants concerning the risks associated with tamoxifen. In particular, using the Bayesian stopping rule established for monitoring endometrial cancer, a Level 1 flag would be raised if there was convincing evidence that the risk of endometrial cancer in the tamoxifen-treated participants exceeded by threefold the risk in placebo participants. The flags at Level 2 were situations where the ERSMAC would consider stopping the trial either because of a convincingly strong beneficial or detrimental effect. ERSMAC members expressed generally positive opinions of the guidelines, but emphasized that they would utilize the global statistic to assist their deliberations rather than as a firm *a priori* stopping rule.

Interim Monitoring of Ocular Effects

The information available from the NSABP treatment trials evaluating tamoxifen, especially the comparison of placebo to tamoxifen in NSABP B-14 study,[10] provided data on the nature and rate of the serious short- and long-term side effects, such as thromboembolic conditions and endometrial cancer, as well as the gynecologic symptoms that could be anticipated in the BCPT. One exception, however, was that data in treatment trials had not been previously collected on the occurrence of ocular effects associated with tamoxifen treatment.

The original consent form for the BCPT stated that an increased incidence of cataracts had been noted in rats, but that there had been no increased incidence reported in humans to that time, although there were scattered reports of other eye problems, such as corneal scarring or retinal changes among a few patients. At the time the BCPT began, routine eye examinations at baseline and follow-up were not part of the usual medical care recommended for women who would receive tamoxifen treatment for breast cancer.

Previous case reports in the literature suggested that long-term low doses of tamoxifen might cause a variety of changes in visual acuity, refractile crystalline deposits in the retina, macular edema, corneal opacities, lens changes, or optic neuritis, but there had been no well-designed studies to evaluate ocular side effects. Since tamoxifen has structural similarities to drugs known to have ocular side effects such as chloroquine, chlorpromazine, thorazine, and amiodarone, there was some rationale to consider monitoring participants for visual problems. Therefore, an opthalmologist researcher was invited to become part of the headquarters team during the planning phase for the BCPT. Concern about vision problems was heightened in early 1992 when an article appeared that stated that there was "clear evidence" of ocular toxicity in association with long term tamoxifen treatment.[11] However, the reported study had serious methodologic flaws and limitations that made it difficult to evaluate the merits of the reported findings. At that time, the NSABP undertook an ancillary study to explore whether there were any vision problems among the patients treated with tamoxifen in the NSABP B-14 treatment trial. In addition, several items were added to the BCPT baseline and follow-up questionnaires to elicit information relating to vision problems, including the findings from routine eye examinations.

In March 1995 interim findings from the NSABP B-14 ancillary eye study, based on the 265 patients in whom vision examinations had been conducted, were presented to the ERSMAC. There remained about 120 patients for whom examinations were still to be done. Of the 188 patients who had received tamoxifen, the average duration of therapy was about 3.5 years. The preliminary findings indicated no difference in visual acuity or ocular edema for patients treated with tamoxifen as compared to those who received placebo. There was an association of tamoxifen with retinal crystal formation, but since the clinical relevance of this condition was unclear, there was, at that time, no recommendation for changes in the BCPT.

In September 1996 a final report of the findings from the ancillary study of ocular disease in NSABP Protocol B-14 was available.[12] The results showed no cases of vision-threatening ocular toxicity in tamoxifen-treated patients. There were also no differences between placebo and tamoxifen-treated patients in visual acuity measures or other tests of visual function except for color screening. The incidence of intraretinal crystals was higher (odds ratio: 3.58; p-value = 0.18). There was, however, an excess of cataracts among women who had received tamoxifen that did not achieve statistical significance (p = 0.07). The ERSMAC members noted that this was a cross-sectional study of long-term survivors in the B-14 trial for whom no baseline ophthalmologic tests were conducted. The clinical recommendations from the study were that neither the occurrence of the retinal crystals, in the absence of macular edema or visual impairment, nor the development of cataracts should be a reason for termination of therapy. The ERSMAC members felt that the association was not sufficiently established at that time to warrant immediate notification of participants and modification of consent forms. Following closed-session review of the safety and outcome data available at that time, the ERSMAC recommended that the trial continue as planned. However, the ERSMAC requested additional analyses be undertaken among the BCPT participants to evaluate this concern utilizing the data collected during BCPT follow-up that dealt with inpatient and out-patient visits.

At the March 1997 meeting of the ERSMAC, data were provided on self-reported cataract diagnosis and cataract surgeries confirmed by discharge summaries of inpatient and outpatient visits among BCPT participants. The review of data from the BCPT participants showed that 311 of 5,890 (5.3%) of women on placebo had reported developing cataracts since their entry into the trial versus 350 of 5,885 (5.9%) of women randomized to tamoxifen. Among women reporting cataracts, 37 participants in the placebo group and 59 in the tamoxifen group, respectively, had undergone cataract surgery. In response to the ERSMAC's recommendation that the findings be provided to the clinical investigators and to the participants in the trial, the NSABP headquarters staff provided the following information for review and approval of the ERSMAC: (1) a letter to all NSABP clinical investigators describing the findings, changes to the consent forms, and procedures to follow in notifying participants; (2) a revised consent form; (3) a letter to oncologists and eye care professionals that could be used to educate health professionals dealing with women receiving tamoxifen; (4) a copy of the BCPT newsletter describing the findings for cataracts; and (5) a copy of the clinical site acknowledgment forms used to document that the clinical site had received the information on cataracts and would review the information with all participants who remained on study.

Decision To Stop the Trial Early Following Sustained Evidence of a Beneficial Effect

The ERSMAC's first review of interim efficacy data occurred in March of 1995, when more than 50 breast cancers were available for analysis. Of the 106 invasive breast cancers that had occurred, 70 were in the placebo group and 36 in the tamoxifen group (test p-value = 0.028; O'Brien–Fleming boundary; p = 0.00013). The ERSMAC's review found no unanticipated side effects or adverse outcomes, and the breast cancer outcome, although favoring the tamoxifen-treated group, did not exceed the prespecified boundary. Therefore, the recommendation at the closed session was for the trial to continue as planned.

The second review of interim efficacy data occurred in April of 1996. At this time, the BCPT population had been followed for an average of two years. During the closed session, the review revealed no unusual or unexpected concerns related to safety. However, of the total 134 incident invasive breast cancers that had been reported, 89 occurred in those randomized to placebo versus 45 among those randomized to tamoxifen. The p-value associated with the statistical test of the difference was 0.00009, a probability that was less than the O'Brien–Fleming boundary of 0.00014 for this second look. The global indices were slightly, but not highly positive. The ERSMAC recommended that the study continue as planned. During the closed ERSMAC session in March 1997, at the third interim efficacy review, the breast cancer benefit had become greater, with approximately a 50% reduction in invasive breast cancer incidence among women randomized to tamoxifen. At that time the number of incident breast cancers numbered 124 in placebo women and 65 in tamoxifen women, yielding a statistically significant p-value of 0.000011 as compared to the O'Brien–Fleming boundary of 0.00015. The global statistic was also more supportive than that at the previous review one year earlier, with both the unweighted and weighted values being about 1.4. the ERSMAC recommended continuing the trial as planned.

The final meeting of the ERSMAC, and the fourth interim efficacy review, occurred in March of 1998. The ERSMAC first carried out a thorough review of all serious toxicities reported as Grade 4 or 5 in the BCPT. There had been 47 such events reported in the placebo group versus 46 in the tamoxifen group. Depression had been scrutinized carefully throughout the trial, and the ERSMAC concluded that there was no meaningful difference between the two treatment groups with respect to the level of depression. There were, as expected, differences between tamoxifen and placebo participants with respect to gynecologic symptoms, which, while frequent in both treatment arms, were reported as more severe for those participants randomized to tamoxifen. The number of participants who reported cataract development after initiation of therapy was greater among those in the tamoxifen group than among those in the placebo group, as was the reported occurrence of cataract surgery. The ERSMAC then considered the interim results analysis with respect to the individual stopping rules and the events included in the global indices. Table 2 presents the global analysis of findings that the ERSMAC reviewed. With a total of 239 incident breast cancers reported, there were 154 in the placebo group versus 85 in the tamoxifen group. The p-value for the test statistic was now significant at a level of 0.000006, which again was much lower than the O'Brien–Fleming boundary of 0.00017 specified in the stopping rule.

The relative risk of endometrial cancer associated with tamoxifen was 2.6, which did not exceed the boundary for the Bayesian stopping rule. All but one of the endometrial cancers diagnosed had a FIGO Stage I at diagnosis. There was one placebo participant with a Stage IV cancer. The ERSMAC came to the unanimous decision that the trial should stop, the participants should be unblinded and the results of the trial disseminated to the public and scientific community as soon as possible. They based this action on several considerations: (1) more than half the participants had been followed for four or more years; (2) the interim monitoring boundary for breast cancer

Table 2 BCPT Global Analysis (Data cutoff: 1/31/98)

	Participants with Events					
	Placebo		Tamoxifen			Test Statistic
Outcome	N	%	N	%	Difference	(Z)
Breast cancer	154	2.296	85	1.272	1.024	4.27
Heart disease	59	0.880	61	0.913	−0.033	−0.20
Hip fracture	20	0.298	9	0.135	0.164	1.94
Endometrial cancer	14	0.209	33	0.494	−0.285	−2.66
Colorectal Cancer	12	0.179	14	0.210	−0.031	−0.38
Liver cancer	0	0	0	0	0	0
Pulmonary embolism	6	0.090	17	0.254	−0.165	−2.20
Stroke	24	0.358	34	0.509	−0.151	−1.27
Transient ischemic attack	21	0.313	18	0.269	0.044	0.45
Deep vein thrombosis	19	0.283	30	0.449	−0.166	−1.51
Other deaths	54	0.805	40	0.599	0.060	1.35
TOTAL	383	5.710	341	5.104	0.606	1.45*

* unweighted Global Index = 1.45; weighted global index = 1.58.

had been crossed for some appreciable time and the global statistic, although not reaching statistical significance, was supportive of an advantage for participants on tamoxifen; and (3) the large reduction in breast cancer, which had been evident for some time, appeared for all age groups and across all years of follow-up. The ERSMAC's collective view was that it was no longer justifiable to withhold the knowledge that tamoxifen had a strong beneficial effect that had at this point been well established and that showed consistent trends to substantiate the findings.

LESSONS LEARNED

Throughout its course the BCPT afforded many opportunities to appreciate the importance of the role that an independent data monitoring committee may have in the conduct of a controversial public health clinical trial. ERSMAC's major contributions include (1) handling of issues in connection with disruption of the trial prior to its completion, including how the committee dealt with the impact of the lengthy hiatus in accrual on the study design considerations; (2) the approach utilized in addressing an unexpected toxicity, indicating an association of tamoxifen with cataracts, that emerged during the course of the trial; and (3) the innovative global monitoring strategy that took into account not only the multiple endpoints, but also weighed concerns related to favorable and unfavorable effects.

The ERSMAC was able to provide reassuring responses to numerous parties, including NIH, FDA, and congress, about the appropriateness of the design and conduct of the trial without violating the confidentiality and integrity of the interim findings. Their recommendations played a major part in keeping the design intact when questions were raised about participant eligibility. In addition, the ERSMAC was an important sounding board for a number of proposed trial changes, including the reduction in the sample size. When designing clinical trials, it is not unusual that there may be considerable uncertainties about various parameters needed to estimate the requisite sample size. In calculating the original sample size and study power for the BCPT, the statisticians made relatively conservative assumptions about the projected baseline incident breast cancer rate and the potential rate of protocol non-adherence. However, there was no way to anticipate that recruitment of participants would be suspended toward the end of the second year of accrual with a concomitant decrease in protocol compliance. When the trial resumed participant recruitment was greatly attenuated from what it had been earlier, and a reevaluation of sample size considerations was clearly warranted. As it happened, the average breast cancer risk of the trial participants was substantially higher than assumed when making the original sample-size estimate. Thus, even with a rise in non-adherence, it was possible to reduce the sample size and still maintain the integrity of the original study hypothesis. Because a reduction in sample size might seem contradictory in light of all that had happened, the ERSMAC's support, as an impartial informed advisory group, was important in providing credibility for the proposed action.

The unexpected observation that cataracts were more commonly diagnosed in women on tamoxifen during the course of the trial was another instance in which the ERSMAC contributed through their detailed review of the evidence both external and internal to the BCPT. Further, they made helpful suggestions for communication of the risk to the clinical investigators, participants, and public in an accurate and prompt manner.

In general, the global monitoring plan devised by the ERSMAC for the BCPT gave considerable flexibility by providing quantitative measures that could be utilized to guide the decision-making process. At the same time the guidelines helped to stimulate thoughtful deliberations on the most relevant findings, without mandating specific rules for when the trial should stop. The adoption by the ERSMAC of a Bayesian rule for Level 1 flagging of the observed excess cases of endometrial cancer was an important addition to the monitoring of data on adverse effects. While many trials have monitoring rules for the primary efficacy outcomes, often there is reliance on *ad hoc* judgments about adverse risks rather than having formal monitoring rules. Since information about the estimated risk for endometrial cancer among women receiving tamoxifen became more reliable after the trial commenced, it was helpful for the ERSMAC to formulate a monitoring guideline that conditioned stopping or modifying the trial for this serious adverse effect based on the current evidence as to the magnitude of the risk rather than simply evidence of a statistically significant increased risk. The asymmetry in the guidelines for adverse versus beneficial effects appropriately reflected that the ERSMAC should concentrate on issues of safety and human subjects as paramount in their recommendations.

There might be some question that the trial continued for almost two years following the crossing of the boundary for a positive breast cancer effect. The rationale for continuation was not related to doubt within the committee that there was a substantial underlying decrease in incident breast cancer for participants who received tamoxifen that might diminish over time. Rather the ERSMAC members believed that there should be more reliable evidence relating to long-term adverse effects in order to predict the net benefit both for women who had participated in the BCPT and for women who might consider taking tamoxifen as a preventive after the trial ended. The recommendation to continue the trial was not only consistent with the overall monitoring plan, but also placed appropriate importance on safety considerations. In retrospect, it may be obvious that the stopping rules for benefit that would have been sufficient for the early termination of a cancer treatment trial provided necessary, but not sufficient, evidence for the same decision in a prevention trial where most of those treated would never develop the disease even if they were at greatly increased risk.

The strategy employed for developing the global monitoring procedures worked well for the BCPT. The interdisciplinary discussion of the scenarios was a worthwhile exercise for the ERSMAC in anticipating issues that would be important for arriving at recommendations as more reliable patterns of disease risks emerged. The combined monitoring strategy not only provided a more comprehensive approach for monitoring, but also took into account that stopping the trial for benefit is not a symmetric situation to stopping the trial because of adverse effects. While the methodology appears promising based on experience in the BCPT, the issues involved in monitoring large prevention trials such as the BCPT are complex and additional practical examples are needed to evolve the procedures more fully.

ACKNOWLEDGMENTS

The authors wish to thank the other members of the ERSMAC for their many valuable contributions and dedicated efforts throughout the monitoring of the BCPT. Members of the ERSMAC, which was chaired by author Theodore Colton included: Martin Abeloff (Johns Hopkins University); Michele Carter (University of Texas at Galveston); Polly Feigl (Fred Hutchinson Cancer Research Center); Laurence Freedman (National Cancer

Institute); Lawrence Friedman (National Heart, Lung, and Blood Institute); Barbara Hulka (University of North Carolina at Chapel Hill); Howard Judd (University of California at Los Angeles); Elliot Rapaport (University of California at San Francisco), and Barbara Tilley (Medical University of South Carolina). The BCPT was supported by Public Health Service cooperative agreements U10-CA-37377 and U10-CA-69974 from the National Cancer Institute, National Institutes of Health, Department of Health and Human Services.

REFERENCES

1. Fisher B, Costantino JP. 1997. Highlights of the NSABP breast cancer prevention trial. *Cancer Control* 4:78-86.
2. Redmond CK, Costantino JP. Design and current status of the NSABP breast cancer prevention trial (BCPT). 1996. In SennHJ, Gelber RD, Goldhirsch A, Thurlimann B (ed.): *Recent Results in Cancer Research.* Springer, New York, 140:309-317.
3. Gail MH, Brinton LA, Byar DP, Corle DK, Green SB, Schairer C, Mulvihill JJ. 1989. Projecting individualized probabilities of developing breast cancer for white females who are being examined annually. *J Natl Cancer Inst* 81:1879-1886.
4. Fisher B, Costantino JP, Wickerham DL, Redmond CK, Kavanah M, Cronin WM, Vogel V, et al. 1998. Tamoxifen for prevention of breast cancer: Report of the National Surgical Adjuvant Breast and Bowel Project P-1 Study. *J Natl Cancer Inst* 90:1371-1388,
5. Costantino JP, Gail MH, Pee D, Anderson S, Redmond CK, Benichou J, Wieand HS. 1999. Validation studies for models projecting the risk of invasive and total breast cancer incidence, *J Natl Cancer Inst* 91:1541-1548.
6. Gail MH, Costantino JP. Editorial. 2001. Validating and improving models for projecting the absolute risk of breast cancer. *J Natl Cancer Inst* 93:334-335.
7. Rosner B. 1999. *Fundamentals of Biostatistics*, ed 4, Boston, 1995, Duxbury Press.
8. Fleming TR, Harrington DP, O'Brien PC. 1984. Designs for group sequential tests. *Control Clin Trials* 5:348-361.
9. Freedman L, Anderson G, Kipnis V, Prentice R, Wang CY, Rossouw J, Wittes J, DeMets D. 1996. Approaches to monitoring the results of long-term disease prevention trials: Examples from the Women's Health Initiative. *Control Clin Trials* 17:509-525.
10. Fisher B, Redmond C, Dimitrov NV, Bowman D, Legault-Poisson S, Wickerham DL, Wolmark N, Fisher ER, Margolese R, Sutherland C, et al. 1989. A randomized clinical trial evaluating tamoxifen in the treatment of patients with node-negative breast cancer who have estrogen-receptor positive tumors. *N Engl J Med* 320:479-484.
11. Pavlidis N, Petris C, Briassoulis E, Klouvas G, Psilas C, Rempapis J, Petroutsos G. 1992. Clear evidence that long- term, low-dose tamoxifen treatment can induce ocular toxicity. A prospective study of 63 patients. *Cancer* 69:2961-2964.
12. Gorin MB, Day R, Costantino JP, Fisher B, Redmond CK, Wickerham L, et al. 1998. Long-term tamoxifen citrate use and potential ocular toxicity, *Am J Ophthalmol* 125:493-501.

Data Monitoring Experience in the Metoprolol CR/XL Randomized Intervention Trial in Chronic Heart Failure: Potentially High-Risk Treatment in High-Risk Patients

Jan Feyzi
Desmond Julian
John Wikstrand
Hans Wedel

ABSTRACT

The Metoprolol CR/XL Randomized Intervention Trial in Chronic Heart Failure (MERIT-HF) was a double-blind, randomized, placebo-controlled trial in 3,991 patients with New York Heart Class II–IV heart failure and LVEF ≤0.40.[1,2] The two primary objectives were to determine the effect of metoprolol CR/XL on all-cause mortality and on the combined endpoint of all-cause mortality or all-cause hospitalizations (time to first event). There was a two-week placebo run-in period. after which patients were randomized to either metoprolol CR/XL at a dose of 12.5 mg (NYHA III–IV) or 25 mg (NYHA II) once daily or matching placebo. The randomized treatment was titrated up to 200 mg once daily or to the highest tolerated dose over an eight-week titration phase. The trial was designed to follow patients for a total mean follow-up of 2.4 years. The Data and Safety Monitoring Board (DSMB) had two tasks. The first was to review all reported Serious Adverse Events (SAEs) on a monthly basis and produce a short report to the sponsor aimed for regulatory agencies. This was done because the sponsor had received a waiver for expedited reporting of SAEs from regulatory agencies including the U.S. Food and Drug Administration (FDA). The second was to perform three pre-specified interim analyses of total mortality. After the second interim analysis, at the point of observing one-half of the targeted number of deaths, the trial was stopped early by the International Steering Committee on recommendation of the DSMB (mean follow-up time 1 year). Final results showed that all-cause mortality was lower in the metoprolol CR/XL group compared to the placebo group (145 deaths, corresponding to 7.2% per patient-year of follow-up for the metoprolol CR/XL group versus 217 deaths, 11.0% per patient-year of follow-up for the placebo group, p = 0.0062 adjusted for interim analyses, p = 0.00009 nominal).[2] The second primary endpoint of all-cause mortality combined with all-cause hospitalizations was also lower for the metoprolol CR/XL group (641 events) compared to placebo (767 events), p = 0.00012 nominal.[3] The procedures developed by the DSMB to implement the required intense safety follow-up will be described.

INTRODUCTION AND BACKGROUND

Chronic heart failure is a progressive clinical syndrome arising from a variety of pathological processes. The central mechanism is the heart's inability to meet the circulatory and metabolic demands of the body. The most common etiology of chronic symptomatic systolic heart failure is coronary heart disease, often complicated by hypertension and diabetes mellitus.

Heart failure is a major and growing public health problem in industrialized countries worldwide, and has a significant impact on the health care system. Estimates of the prevalence of heart failure in the general population in the Western countries range from 0.4% to 2%.[4-8] A conservative estimation indicates that about four million patients in Europe and two million patients in the U.S. have chronic heart failure, and the numbers are expected to increase substantially in the next few decades. An increased proportion of elderly in the population and improved survival after acute myocardial infarction very likely explain this. It is estimated that 90% of new cases of heart failure occur in patients above the age of 60 years.[5]

The prognosis of heart failure is, in general, poor. Approximately half of those patients diagnosed with chronic heart failure will die within four years, and of those with severe chronic heart failure, half will die within one year.[6,9] Chronic heart failure accounts for a considerable proportion of all cardiovascular related hospitalizations; about 20% of admissions and 30% of hospital days are due to this condition. The total economic burden amounts to 1% to 2% of total health care expenditure, of which hospitalization costs make up two-thirds.[7]

Therapy of chronic heart failure caused by left ventricular systolic dysfunction is mainly based on inhibition of neurohormonal stimulation secondary to pump failure. Angiotensin-converting enzyme (ACE) inhibitor treatment in combination with diuretics was initially found to improve survival and symptoms;[10] however, mortality (especially due to sudden death) remained high.[11] Thus, there was a need for continued improvements in reducing mortality and morbidity in this patient population.

Beta-Blockers in Chronic Systolic Heart Failure

For more than two decades after the first positive report was published,[12] use of beta-blockers in chronic heart failure was avoided because of concerns about adverse effects. Three survival studies were then run in parallel investigating the effect of beta-blockers in systolic heart failure: CIBIS II, MERIT-HF, and COPERNICUS. CIBIS II[13] studied bisoprolol an immediate release beta$_1$-selective beta-blocker, MERIT-HF[1] utilized controlled-release/extended-release metoprolol succinate (metoprolol CR/XL, beta$_1$-selective), and COPERNICUS[14] utilized carvedilol, a non-selective beta-blocker with a weak α_1-blocking property. The data and safety monitoring by the DSMB in MERIT-HF was conducted in this context.

PROTOCOL DESIGN

The MERIT-HF trial was designed to evaluate the effect of metoprolol CR/XL in patients with mild to moderate chronic systolic heart failure. The trial had two primary endpoints, total mortality and total mortality plus all-cause hospitalization (time to first event).[1] In MERIT-HF, a total of 3,991 patients were randomized from February 1997 through April 1998 at 313 sites in the US and 13 European countries. Eligibility criteria included patients with NYHA class II–IV heart failure, left ventricular ejection fraction of 0.40 or lower, age between 40 and 80 years, and heart rate of at least 68 beats per minute at enrollment. Patients with acute myocardial infarction or unstable angina within 28 days before randomization were excluded. In addition, patients with a supine systolic blood pressure below 100 mm Hg at enrollment were excluded. The intention of the protocol was that no more than 40% NYHA class II patients were to be randomized.

The randomization was performed according to an optimal allocation procedure which balanced the metoprolol CR/XL and placebo groups for pre-specified baseline factors. The study medication was up-titrated during eight weeks, starting with 12.5 mg (NYHA functional class III–IV) or 25 mg once daily (NYHA II). The target dose was 200 mg once daily or highest tolerated dose. Follow-up visits then occurred every three months. Data on mortality, hospitalizations, and adverse events were collected during these visits. All predefined endpoints were classified by an independent endpoint committee using available medical records.

The trial was initially designed to randomize 3,200 patients over a 14-month period. When recruitment had been ongoing for ten months, the number of randomized patients was higher than expected. The Steering Committee then decided to continue recruitment for the planned 14-month recruiting period, thereby increasing the sample size of the trial. This was done partly in order to increase the power of the trial.

The first-draft Study Protocol defined one primary endpoint, which was total mortality analyzed on an intention-to-treat principle with an alpha-value of 0.05 and a power of more than 80%. After discussions with the U.S. FDA in September 1996, it was decided when planning the trial, to define two primary endpoints: total mortality, and a combined endpoint of total mortality or all-cause hospitalizations (time to first event).[1] The reason for this was that if the trial had failed to show a statistically significant effect on total mortality, there would be a second option for a combined endpoint when filing for registration. An alpha-value of 0.04 was set aside for all-cause mortality and 0.01 for the second primary endpoint.[1] However, the two primary endpoints are related, which means a total alpha-spending of less than 0.05 altogether. The cumulative alpha-value (0.0015) spent on interim analyses at the final analysis of total mortality should be covered by the saving of alpha caused by the correlation between the first and second primary endpoint.

THE DATA MONITORING EXPERIENCE

The DSMB monitored safety issues during the trial based on safety reports prepared by an independent statistical analysis center. The task was to meet each month (via phone conference) to monitor all reported serious adverse events (transferred electronically each month from the sponsor) and adverse events leading to discontinuation of blind study medication, and also to perform three pre-planned interim analyses of total mortality. The procedures were governed by pre-specified DSMB monitoring guidelines stating that the second primary endpoint, i.e., the combined endpoint of total mortality or all-cause hospitalizations (time to first event) should not be monitored with interim analyses during the course of the trial. The stopping rule for efficacy was based on the total number of expected deaths, analyzed based on the intention-to-treat principle.

The trial used an asymmetric group sequential procedure to monitor total mortality.[15] A Peto-type boundary was used for monitoring a positive trend.[16] This approach favors a large critical Z-value for all interim tests before the end of the trial. The cumulative alpha for benefit was set to be 0.0012, 0.0024, and 0.0036 at the first, second, and third interim analyses to take place when 25%, 50%, and 75%, respectively, of the total number of the expected 581 deaths had occurred. It was felt that these boundaries were too conservative for harm, the cumulative probability of early stopping for harm was therefore set to be 0.005, 0.010, and 0.015 at the first, second, and third interim analyses, respectively. The sequential boundaries for MERIT-HF are shown in Figure 1, including the mortality results for each formal interim DSMB analysis.

Safety reports were prepared by the independent statistical analysis center and consisted of a primarily graphical examination of accrual data, baseline characteristics, and adverse event data (including serious adverse events and all-cause mortality). All data were presented in a blinded manner to the DSMB (i.e. with treatments denoted as "A" and "B"). The DSMB initially remained blinded to the corresponding treatment assignment; however, they elected to unblind themselves during the February 1998 safety teleconference due to a widening difference between the two treatments in number of deaths (37 on arm A and 64 on arm B).

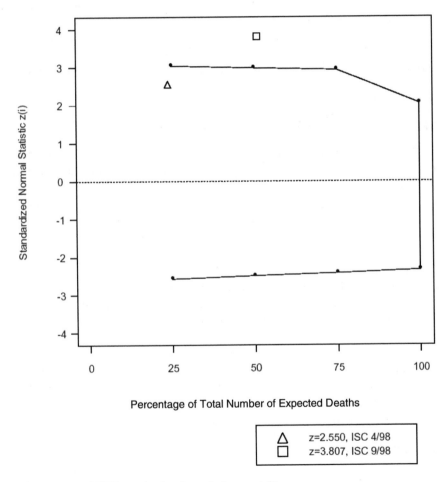

Percentage of Total Number of Expected Deaths

| △ | z=2.550, ISC 4/98 |
| □ | z=3.807, ISC 9/98 |

Figure 1 MERIT-HF monitoring bounds for mortality.

The first formal interim analysis occurred in April 1998, when 24.3% of the expected deaths had been observed. At that time, preliminary results from the CIBIS II trial had been presented (March 1998). This trial was closed prematurely, with positive results showing that bisoprolol reduced mortality. The MERIT-HF DSMB discussed the impact of this trial's early closing and the possible impact on the MERIT-HF trial. The DSMB noted the differences between these trials, especially that the CIBIS II trial studied patients with NYHA Class III–IV heart failure (contrasting to MERIT-HF, with approximately 40% NYHA Class II patients). The logrank Z-value for MERIT-HF at this point was 2.550, below the pre-specified monitoring bound (3.04) for benefit at this point in the trial. Hence, the DSMB recommended to continue the trial; however, it was noted that the Z-value was fairly close to the upper bound and may cross at the time of the next interim analysis if the trend was to continue. Trial randomization was to stop on April 14, 1998. The full CIBIS II results were to be presented in August, 1998, near the time of the next interim analysis.

In scheduling the second formal interim analysis, the DSMB decided to wait until the pre-specified 50% point (September 1998) in order to give the DSMB time to understand and reflect on the CIBIS II results. MERIT-HF safety reviews prior to this scheduled meeting did not show any unexpected safety concerns in the metoprolol CR/XL arm. Updated numbers for deaths and hospitalizations were given and the trend for a lower number of both deaths and hospitalizations for patients on metoprolol CR/XL continued.

The Second Interim Analysis

The second interim analysis meeting of the DSMB was held on September 21, 1998. The chairman of the DSMB had informed the chairman of the Executive Committee that the DSMB wanted to meet with the Executive Committee directly after their second interim analysis. At that time, the CIBIS II results had been already presented and confirmed the initial reports that bispropolol reduced all-cause mortality in patients with NYHA Class III–IV heart failure.[13] The mean follow-up time for patients in the MERIT-HF trial was 10.8 months at this point in the trial. There were 115 deaths on the metoprolol CR/XL arm and 181 deaths on the placebo arm, representing 51% of the expected number of deaths. The logrank Z-value was 3.807, substantially exceeding the upper monitoring bound for benefit of 2.98 pre-specified in the DSMB monitoring guidelines. Although not formally tested, the results for the second primary endpoint of all-cause mortality and all-cause hospitalization were consistent with the mortality results. After discussion of these results and a thorough examination of consistency of results over protocol-specified subgroups, the DSMB unanimously voted to recommend termination of the trial.

The DSMB prepared a brief initial statement and the limited results on mortality were immediately presented to members of the MERIT-HF Executive Committee. The Executive Committee then deliberated as to whether to accept the recommendations of the DSMB, based on these limited data. The Executive Committee voted to accept the DSMB recommendations. The DSMB then fully debriefed the Executive Committee as to the overall results, including baseline data, compliance, mortality, mortality plus hospitalization, adverse events and several pre-specified subgroups.

The DSMB then issued the following statement:

On September 21, 1998, the Independent Safety Committee undertook the secondary interim analysis of the MERIT-HF study. The Committee found that the previously defined criteria for termination of the study for mortality reduction had been met and exceeded (z = 3.807 versus 2.98 as defined in the protocol). These mortality results were consistent across the predefined subgroups. The findings with regard to the second primary endpoint of death and/or hospitalization were consistent with the mortality results. Discontinuation of study medication was similar in the two groups. Serious adverse effects were commoner in the placebo group than in the metoprolol CR/XL treated patients. In view of the highly significant benefit observed, the Independent Safety Committee recommend termination of the study as soon as practicable.

This statement was given to the Executive Committee and kept secret until the Executive Committee met with the Steering Committee of MERIT-HF two weeks later (see below). Furthermore the DSMB recommended that mortality data be published as soon as possible.

Early Stopping

The International Steering Committee of MERIT-HF met October 2, 1998, and decided to close the trial on October 31, 1998, on the recommendation made by the DSMB. However, for regulatory reasons and as previously decided by the Steering Committee, the blind study medication code could not be broken until all data were in, and clean file had been declared, which would take many months after trial closure. The solution was a controlled down-titration of blind study medication in parallel with an optimal up-titration of open label metoprolol CR/XL according to the recommendation made by the Steering Committee of the trial. Since it would take some time to declare clean file at the sponsor it was agreed to base the publication on mortality results on analyses performed by the independent statistical analysis center.[2]

The Executive Committee and sponsor recommended that the DSMB remain functional throughout the close-out period of the trial in order to ensure patient safety. This would also allow the Executive Committee and sponsor to remain blinded for individual patient assignments during the final data collection period. The DSMB continued to monitor patient safety until the database was locked (June 1999). The final published mortality[2] and mortality plus hospitalization results[3] are summarized in Table 1. Kaplan–Meier plots of the time to death and time to death plus hospitalization can be found in Figures 2a,b. Baseline characteristics are summarized in Table 2.

LESSONS LEARNED

The MERIT-HF monitoring experience provided a number of lessons for the monitoring of patient safety in future trials. First, because of the waiver for expedited reporting of SAEs, the DSMB had to meet more often than usual in order to provide reports to regulatory agencies. In order to comply with this request, the independent statistical analysis center provided the DSMB with monthly safety reports with subsequent discussion by the DSMB via teleconference. Scheduling of such meetings could be potentially problematic; however, a time convenient to all DSMB members was established at the onset and remained predictable throughout the trial to encourage consistent participation. Any early trends, both positive or negative, could be addressed with such monitoring.

In addition, because of the lack of data for long-term exposure to betablockers in this patient population, asymmetric monitoring bounds were established with a conservative upper bound for benefit and a less conservative lower bound for harm. This allowed for less stringent statistical criteria to be met in the case of a negative trend. However, the pre-defined DSMB

Table 1   Mortality and Mortality Plus Hospitalization Results

Endpoints (N, %)*	Metoprolol CR/XL (n = 1990)	Placebo (n = 2001)	Relative risk (95% CI); p-value[†]
Total mortality	145 (7.2%)	217 (11.0%)	0.66 (0.53–0.81); p = 0.0062 (adj)
Cardiovascular mortality	128 (6.4%)	203 (10.3%)	0.62 (0.50–0.78); p = 0.000022
Sudden death	79 (3.9%)	132 (6.7%)	0.59 (0.45–0.78); p = 0.0002
Total mortality or all-cause hospitalization	641 (38.8%)	767 (48.0%)	0.81 (0.73–0.90); p = 0.0001
Total mortality or hospitalization for CHF	311 (16.5%)	431 (23.5%)	0.69 (0.60–0.80) p = 0.0000008

* Percentage per patient year of follow-up (2,004 vs. 1,977; 1,651 vs. 1,599; and 1,882 vs. 1,837 patient years for the different endpoints, respectively).
† For total mortality, p-value adjusted for interim analysis is given; otherwise the nominal p-value is given.

(a)

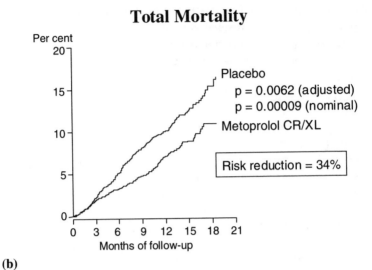

(b)

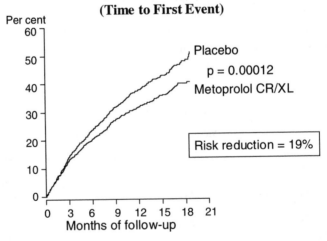

Figure 2 Kaplan–Meier estimates of the first primary endpoint of total mortality (a), and of the second primary endpoint of total mortality or all-cause hospitalization (time to first event; b). From references 2 and 3, with permission.

Table 2   Baseline Characteristics

Baseline characteristics	Metoprolol CR/XL (n = 1,990)	Placebo (n = 2,001)
Age, mean, yr	64	64
Sex, % female	23	22
White, %	94	94
Ischemic etiology of heart failure	65	66
NYHA class, %		
II	41	41
III	56	55
IV	3.4	3.8
Ejection fraction, mean	0.28	0.28
Previous myocardial infarction, %	48	49
Time since last myocardial infarction <1 yr, %	8	7
Hypertension, %	44	44
Diabetes mellitus, %	25	24
Medications, %		
Diuretics	91	90
ACE inhibitor	89	90
A-II-blocker	7	6
ACE inhibitor or A-II-blocker	95	96
Digitalis	63	64
Spironolactone	7	8

Revised from MERIT-HF (2000) with permission from JAMA.

monitoring guidelines stated that in the event that a negative mortality trend would emerge during the course of the MERIT-HF study, the DSMB should proceed until a definitive result had been obtained. Although the negative trend may be sufficient to rule out any possible positive benefit, the DSMB should continue the trial until a harmful effect could be distinguished from neutrality. The rationale for this was that being able to distinguish between a harmful mortality effect and a neutral mortality effect was important in this patient population since metoprolol may be used for other beneficial effects than mortality.

The release of the results from other similar trials can both simplify and complicate the decision-making process. The CIBIS II results provided confidence that the effect of beta-blockers on survival in patients with heart failure is a real phenomenon. However, there was a real concern that the early release of results of CIBIS II to the medical community could have adversely affected completion of the MERIT-HF trial. Luckily, randomization was near complete and would not have been compromised. However, had the patient populations in the two trials been more alike regarding their heart failure profiles, an ethical dilemma as to whether to continue the trial in light of the CIBIS II results could have arisen. The results of the COPERNICUS trial (of carvedilol in patients with severe heart failure) were released shortly after the closure of the MERIT-HF trial and further established the efficacy of beta-blockers in the treatment of patients with heart failure. Thus, external consistency of the effects of beta-blockers on both mortality and mortality plus hospitalization is reassuring.

The method used by the DSMB to reveal the results to the Executive Committee is of interest. This process was discussed in closed-session by the DSMB after the unanimous vote to recommend termination of the trial. It was decided that the first information to be given to the Executive Committee was that the DSMB had recommended that the trial be terminated and to ask whether the Executive Committee would like to be unblinded to the trial results. Members of the Executive Committee who were present met in closed-session to further discuss this issue. They decided that they indeed wanted more information. The DSMB immediately informed them of additional results.

Finally, in order to speed up the publication of the mortality results,[2] the independent statistical analysis center generated all the analyses for the MERIT-HF Steering Committee while the sponsor was still working on the clean file process.

Subsequent to the publication of the MERIT-HF trial, regulatory review raised a question regarding the consistency of results across geographic areas.[17] In particular, for mortality, the hazard ratio for the U.S. patients was near 1.0 in contrast to the non-U.S. (European) results of 0.55. For mortality plus hospitalization, the results were in fact consistent.[3] The FDA asked whether or not the trial could have been terminated early in the non-U.S. sites and allowed the U.S. sites to continue with blinded treatment. While the DSMB did not in fact deliberate on this issue, in retrospect, some members of the DSMB have conjectured that they do not believe that MERIT-HF could have been continued in the U.S. alone, given the striking overall results of MERIT-HF as well as the results of other beta-blocker studies, which did not have this anomaly. It was concluded that the best estimate of the treatment effect on total mortality for any subgroup is the estimate of the hazard ratio for the overall trial.[17]

REFERENCES

1. The International Steering Committee on behalf of the MERIT-HF Study Group. 1997. Rationale, design, and organization of the metoprolol CR/XL randomized trial in heart failure (MERIT-HF). *Am J Cardiol* 80:54–58J.
2. MERIT-HF Study Group. 1999. Effect of metoprolol CR/XL in chronic heart failure: Metoprolol CR/XL Randomised Intervention Trial in Congestive Heart Failure (MERIT-HF). *Lancet* 353:2001–2007.
3. Hjalmarson A, Goldstein S, Fagerberg B, Wedel H, Waagstein F, Kjekshus J, et al. 2000. Effects of controlled-release metoprolol on total mortality, hospitalizations, and well-being in patients with heart failure: The Metoprolol CR/XL Randomized Intervention Trial in Congestive Heart Failure (MERIT-HF). *JAMA* 283:1295–2007.

4. Cohn, JN. *1996*. The management of chronic heart failure. *N Engl J Med* 335: 490-498
5. MattsonJack EpiOnline database accessed on 21.03.02 at http://www.epidb.com/epiOnline/Phase1/fmeLayout.asp
6. Senni M, Tribouilloy CM, Rodeheffer RJ, et al. 1999. Congestive heart failure in the community. Trends in incidence and survival in a 10-year period. *Arch Intern Med* 159:29-34.
7. McMurray J, Hart W, Rhodes G. 1993. An evaluation of the economic cost of heart failure to the National Health Service in the United Kingdom. *Br J Med Econ* 6:99-110
8. Task Force on Heart Failure of the European Society of Cardiology. 1995. Guidelines for the diagnosis of heart failure. *Eur Heart J* 16:741-751.
9. The CONSENSUS Trial Study Group. 1987. Effects of enalapril on mortality in severe congestive heart failure. Results of the Cooperative North Scandinavian Enalapril Survival Study (CONSENSUS). *N Engl J Med* 316:1429-1435.
10. Garg R, Yusuf S. Collaborative group on ACE Inhibitor Trials. 1995. Overview of randomized trials of angiotensin-converting enzyme inhibitors on mortality and morbidity in patients with heart failure. *JAMA* 273:1450-1456
11. Goldstein, S. 1997. Clinical studies on beta-blockers and heart failure preceding the MERIT-HF trial. *Am J Cardiol* 80(9B):50J-53J.
12. Waagstein F, Hjalmarson Å, Varnauskas, Wallentin I. 1975. Effect of chronic beta-adrenergic receptor blockade in congestive cardiomyopathy. *BMJ* 37:1022-1036.
13. CIBIS-II Investigators and Committees. 1999. The cardiac insufficiency bisoprolol study II (CIBIS II), *Lancet* 353:9-13.
14. Packer M, Coats AJS, Fowler MB, et al. 2001. Effect of carvedilol on survival in severe chronic heart failure. *N Engl J Med* 344:1651-1658.
15. Lan KKG, DeMets DL. 1983. Discrete sequential boundaries for clinical trials. *Biometrika* 70:649-653.
16. Peto R, Pike MC, Armitage P, et al. 1976. Design and analysis of randomized clinical trials requiring prolonged observations of each patient. I. Introduction and design. *Br J Cancer* 34:585-612.
17. Wedel H, DeMets D, Deedwania P, Fagerberg B, Goldstein S, Gottlieb S, Hjalmarson Å, Kjekshus J, Waagstein F, Wikstrand J on behalf of the MERIT-HF Study Group: 2001 Challenges of subgroup analyses in multinational clinical trials: Experiences from the MERIT-HF trial. *Am Heart J* 143:502-511.

Stopping the Randomized Aldactone Evaluation Study Early for Efficacy

Janet Wittes
Jean-Pierre Boissel
Curt D. Furberg
Desmond Julian
Henri Kulbertus
Stuart Pocock

ABSTRACT

The Randomized Aldactone Evaluation Study (RALES) was a randomized double-blind placebo-controlled trial designed to test the hypothesis that addition of daily spironolactone to standard therapy would reduce the risk of all-cause mortality in patients with severe heart failure as a result of systolic left ventricular dysfunction. The Data Safety Monitoring Board (DSMB) for RALES reviewed data on safety and efficacy throughout the trial using pre-specified statistical stopping boundaries for efficacy. To ensure that the data were complete, the DSMB requested successive "mortality sweeps." At the time of these sweeps, all RALES investigators determined the vital status of participants at their clinics. Therefore, the data that the DSMB saw included a much higher percentage of the deaths than would have been observed without these sweeps. At the DSMB's fifth meeting, the data showed 351 deaths in the placebo group and 269 in the spironolactone group for an estimated hazard ratio of 0.78 (p = 0.00018). The board recommended early termination of the trial because the observed Z-value of 3.75 exceeded the pre-specified critical value of 2.79 and the data on mortality showed consistency among subgroups and across time. The sweeps had identified 31 deaths that likely would not have been reported by the time of the meeting. Subsequent data collection identified an additional 46 deaths that had occurred by the time the study ended. Even when the endpoint of a randomized clinical trial is mortality, routine methods of data collection and reporting are unlikely to identify all events in a timely manner. The experience from RALES provides an example of the importance of active follow-up of patients to ensure that a DSMB is observing a high proportion of the events that have actually occurred.

INTRODUCTION AND BACKGROUND

In "heart failure," the heart is incapable of maintaining cardiac output adequate to accommodate metabolic requirements and venous return. The heart fails either because it is subjected to an overwhelming pressure or volume overload, because myocardial contractility is depressed (e.g., in myocardiopathy or intoxication), or because a significant loss of contractile tissue has occurred (e.g, after a myocardial infarction).[1] The condition can lead to a rise of pressure in the return veins, both on the systemic and the pulmonary sides. The resulting engorgement of pulmonary veins and capillaries can cause dyspnea, a difficulty with breathing, which is the most common symptom of heart failure. Heart failure also involves a fall of cardiac output, which can cause fatigue and activate the sympathetic nervous system with, consequently, an increase in heart rate and vasoconstriction of arteries and veins.

The fall in cardiac output and the increase in sympathetic drive lead to reduced effective renal blood flow. Through the renin–angiotensin system, this reduced flow induces a rise in the levels of angiotensin II, a vasoconstrictor, which stimulates aldosterone secretion by the cortex of the adrenal gland. Aldosterone is a hormone that, by its action on the distal renal tubule, promotes retention of sodium and accompanying water, while increasing potassium excretion. Consequently, blood volume increases, leading to the potential development of peripheral edema and pulmonary congestion. In addition to its renal action, aldosterone exerts a large number of potentially deleterious effects on the cardiovascular system. The New York Heart Association categorizes patients with heart failure into four classes depending on the severity of their symptoms, principally, dyspnea:[2]

Class I   patients withstand normal physical activity without symptoms;
Class II patients develop symptoms on moderate or severe exertion only;
Class III symptoms are present even on mild exertion;
Class IV symptoms are present at rest.

A relationship between functional capacity and survival in heart failure is well established. In the early 1990s, studies showed the annual mortality rate of Class IV patients to be above 50% while the annual mortality rate in Class III patients varied between 10% and 45%.[3]

Until the mid-1980s, treatment was not evidence-based. Because fluid retention is the hallmark of heart failure, diuretics were the principal agents used for its treatment. Digitalis, a positive inotrope that boosts cardiac contraction, was also commonly prescribed. Vasodilators, in particular, nitrates, prazosin, and ACE inhibitors, were recently introduced with a view to unload the heart, thereby improving cardiac function. In 1986 and 1987, the first trials to demonstrate a benefit of vasodilator therapy on mortality were published.[4,5]

On the basis of the then understood physiopathology of heart failure, a logical approach to treatment would have been to add a drug that blocks aldosterone receptors. At that time, however, physicians were reluctant to prescribe aldactone, an aldosterone inhibitor, to patients with heart failure because of the potential for serious elevations in potassium levels (hyperkalemia) among those receiving an ACE inhibitor, a class of agents that had quickly become one of the mainstays of treatment. Addressing this potential problem, a study published in 1996 showed that treatment with a low dose of spironolactone, an aldosterone-receptor blocker, in conjunction with standard dose of an ACE inhibitor, a loop diuretic, and digoxin was well tolerated and did not lead to serious hyperkalemia.[6]

PROTOCOL DESIGN

The establishment of the safety of low-dose spironolactone in patients with heart failure led to the design of the double-blind Randomized Aldactone Evaluation Study (RALES), a trial that aimed "to test the hypothesis that daily treatment with 25 mg of spironolactone would significantly reduce the risk of death from all causes among patients who had severe heart failure as a result of systolic left ventricular dysfunction and who were receiving [the then] standard therapy, including an ACE inhibitor, if tolerated."[7]

RALES took place in 195 centers from 15 countries. Sponsored by Searle, the manufacturer of spironolactone, the study had an academic executive committee chaired by Bertram Pitt, M.D., and an independent Data Safety Monitoring Board (DSMB) chaired by Desmond Julian, M.D. Collectively, the DSMB had expertise in cardiology, epidemiology, biostatistics, and clinical trials. Spironolactone had been in use since 1960, so its adverse event profile was well known. The most common adverse events are gynecomastia and other feminizing symptoms in males. As described above, the most serious expected adverse event associated with spironolactone is hyperkalemia. The role of the DSMB was to monitor safety, especially with respect to the potential for hyperkalemia, and to assess whether to recommend stopping the study early for efficacy.

The DSMB was originally blind to treatment code. Several of the members argued for unblinding the groups immediately, but given that the opinion was not unanimous the reports to the DSMB were designed with the treatment groups for most variables labeled as A and B. Because increased rates of gynecomastia and hyperkalemia would unmask the A and B assignments, these two adverse events were labeled X and Y. The DSMB reserved the right to unblind itself should it feel the need.

DATA MONITORING EXPERIENCE

During the trial, Searle provided data to Statistics Collaborative, which prepared reports to the DSMB. The board had a predefined statistical guideline for stopping for efficacy. The guideline specified that early in the trial, stopping for efficacy would require very strong evidence favoring spironolactone. As the trial progressed, the standard for efficacy would become less stringent. Overall, the probability of declaring benefit if spironolactone and placebo had identical effects on mortality was 0.025. Technically, the guidelines were based on an O'Brien–Fleming boundary[8] for efficacy at a two-sided α-level of 0.05. Because the standard O'Brien–Fleming boundary requires looking at the data at equal increments of numbers of deaths and there was no practical way to schedule the meetings to ensure equal numbers of deaths at each meeting, the Lan–DeMets use function[9] was employed. This function allows flexibility in planning meetings without sacrifice of the stringency of the type I error rate. Figure 1 shows the boundaries used.

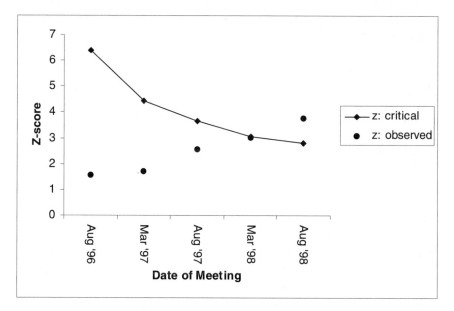

Figure 1 Monitoring boundaries and observed Z-values at the five interim analyses.

The board did not specify a boundary for safety; instead it relied on its collective judgment to recommend early termination if spironolactone showed a net adverse effect.

The original protocol specified an event-driven trial. Investigators would randomize patients 1 : 1 to spironolactone or placebo and stop recruitment at a pre-specified number of events. A trial with this design is called an "information time" trial because the design specifies the number of deaths, defined as the "total information." At each look, the DSMB would calculate the "information time" as the fraction of deaths that had occurred thus far relative to the total planned deaths.

The first patient was randomized on March 24, 1995. A protocol amendment, approved in early 1996, changed the planned end of the trial to December 31, 1999. Thus, the trial was now based on calendar time instead of total events. Consequently, the calculations for the interim analysis had to be based on an unknown total number of deaths.

Each DSMB meeting began with an open session for the investigators and the sponsor to report about the status of the trial. At the closed session, attended only by the DSMB and the statisticians reporting to it, the DSMB reviewed the data.

The Emerging Data

On August 24, 1996, at the DSMB's first meeting with an interim analysis, a difference in mortality between the two groups emerged, with 70 deaths in one group and 52 in the other (see Table 1). The Z-value was far from statistically significant ($z = 1.58$; critical $z = 6.38$, nominal p-value = 0.11 Note: the "critical Z" is the predetermined boundary that must be exceeded for the drug to be deemed effective.); nonetheless, the board expressed the view that such a large difference in the direction of increased mortality in the spironolactone group would lead to concern about safety. Consequently, the DSMB unblinded itself and learned that the lower event rate was occurring in the treated group. The board recommended continuing the trial with no change in protocol.

Recruitment ended as planned on December 31, 1996. At that time, a total of 1,663 patients had been randomized, 841 to receive placebo and 822 to receive spironolactone.

At the second meeting, which took place on March 17, 1997, the reported deaths were now 136 and 109 in the placebo and spironolactone groups, respectively, for a hazard ratio of 0.83 ($Z = 1.69$; critical $Z = 4.43$; nominal p-value = 0.092). Again, the board noted the reduction in mortality; however, in light of the non-statistically significant finding, it again recommended continuing the trial with no change in protocol.

Table 1   Observed and Projected Number of Deaths and Summary Statistics at Each Interim Analysis

Look number	Meeting date	Observed Deaths		Hazard ratio	Estimated information time	Z-value		Observed two sided p-value
		Placebo	Spironolactone			Critical	Observed	
Interim analyses with the sweeps as they occurred								
1	24-Aug-96	70	52	0.76	0.12	6.38	1.58	0.11
2	17-Mar-97	136	109	0.83	0.24	4.43	1.69	0.092
3	25-Aug-97	224	175	0.80	0.34	3.67	2.55	0.011
4	30-Mar-98	304	241	0.81	0.48	3.04	3.02	0.0026
5	24-Aug-98	351	269	0.78	0.57	2.79	3.75	0.00018
Estimated interim analyses that would have occurred without the sweeps								
4a	30-Mar-98	281	222	0.81	0.45	3.16	2.93	0.0034
5a	24-Aug-98	333	256	0.79	0.55	2.81	3.59	0.00034
Interim analysis cutoffs that would have occurred had the true numbers and times of deaths been known								
1b	24-Aug-96	81	59	0.75	0.14	5.88	1.80	0.072
2b	17-Mar-97	189	140	0.76	0.26	4.24	2.75	0.0060
3b	25-Aug-97	257	201	0.80	0.38	3.46	2.82	0.0048
4b	30-Mar-98	330	254	0.79	0.51	2.95	3.56	0.00038
5b*	24-Aug-98	383	283	0.76	0.60	2.72	4.46	0.000008

* These are the data in the paper describing the final results.[8]

At the time of the third meeting on August 25, 1997, data were still strongly favoring spironolactone, with 224 deaths in the placebo group and 175 in the spironolactone group for a hazard ratio of 0.80. Although the p-value was now nominally statistically significant ($p = 0.011$), the observed Z-statistic of 2.55 was quite far from the critical value of 3.67 defined by the O'Brien–Fleming boundary. At that meeting the board prepared itself for a crossing of the boundary. Given the strong trends observed thus far and the consistent patterns emerging over subgroups of interest, the board predicted that the data would cross the pre-specified stopping boundaries before the planned end of the study. It was, however, somewhat uncertain about the reliability of the data. According to the protocol, investigators were to report deaths within 24 hours of occurrence; because the interval between protocol-specified visits was every three months through one year of study follow-up and every six months thereafter, the DSMB suspected that information about deaths might be delayed. The board believed it highly likely that the number of deaths was being undercounted. If the probability of late reporting of deaths were equal in the placebo and spironolactone groups, this delay would reduce the power of the statistical tests at the interim analyses. More seriously, if deaths in the placebo group were reported with more, or less, alacrity than deaths in the spironolactone groups, the apparent effect size might be either over- or underestimated. While the double-blind nature of the study should afford considerable protection against differential reporting; nonetheless, if adverse events or better functioning were leading one group to have more frequent contact with the study staff than the other group, a bias in the reporting of events, including deaths, could occur.

The board was concerned lest it make a decision at one of the next meetings to recommend stopping the trial only to learn later, when all the deaths were reported, that the observed effect size was incorrect. To prevent crossing the statistical boundary with uncertainty remaining about the number of unreported deaths, the board requested that each investigator provide a census, or a "sweep," of vital status as of December 31, 1997. To avoid alerting the sponsor and the investigators of the reason for its request, the board worded its request in terms of the need for a "standard two-year" accounting of data. Anticipating a crossing of the boundary for efficacy, it also requested that at each meeting of the DSMB, the sponsor and the Principal Investigator routinely remain available for another open session at the end of the closed session.

The request for a sweep required considerable effort on the part of the sponsor and the investigators. Each investigator had to contact every participant, a task that was somewhat daunting, partly because it was unexpected.

After the March 1998 meeting, where the boundary was almost crossed (observed $Z = 3.02$; critical $Z = 3.04$), the board requested another "sweep" just prior to its subsequent meeting. It also discussed the data it wanted to see at the next meeting with the view toward assuring that, should it recommend stopping, it would have considered all reasonable likely criticisms of an early stop. It discussed writing a press release, methods of informing the investigators of the early stop, and approaches to early publication of the results.

Finally, at the fifth meeting in August 1998, the observed Z-value was 3.75 while the critical Z-value required to cross the boundary was 2.79. The board's planning at its previous meeting allowed it to proceed deliberately at this last meeting. Although the data had crossed the boundary, the DSMB carefully considered the totality of the evidence available to it in deciding whether to recommend stopping the trial for efficacy. In particular, it reviewed effects in subgroups of interest; it considered the strength and internal consistency of the secondary endpoints; and it assessed the likelihood that the data would be reversed when the complete information became available. Given the consistency of the results and the strong effect on mortality, the board recommended early termination. Because it had requested that the sponsor and the Principal Investigator be present after the closed session, the board was able to report the data to them immediately. The board, the sponsor, and the Principal Investigator drafted a letter to the Steering Committee and a press release describing the data.

Ending the Study

The study ended smoothly because, having anticipated that the study would stop early, the DSMB set in motion actions to facilitate the process. The sweeps had identified a sizable increase in the number of deaths reported at the fourth and fifth interim analysis. While no can one know how many deaths would have been reported had the sweeps not occurred, the statistical group performed computer simulations to assess the likely effect of the sweeps. The simulations showed about an 8% increase in the number of reported deaths at each of the fourth and fifth meetings.[10] When several months later all the data were complete, another 46 deaths were identified. These deaths strengthened the inference so that the Z-statistic changed from 3.75 (for a p-value of 0.00018) at the DSMB meeting to 4.46 (p = 0.000008) when all the data had been collected. The estimated hazard ratio was 0.78 when the DSMB recommended stopping the study; the final estimate was 0.76.

LESSONS LEARNED

Several lessons emerged from the RALES trial. First, blinding in a study of this type is difficult. Even if one believes that a DSMB should be blind to treatment (which most of the authors of this chapter do not), the actual process of blinding is cumbersome. The nature of the adverse events are often so clear that blinding requires complicated efforts on the part of the statistical center. Moreover, this process clouds the ability of the DSMB to weigh the risks and benefits of therapy.

Another lesson related to ascertainment of the endpoint during a study. In trials of mortality, one might assume that because ascertainment of the primary endpoint–death–is simple, the accruing data should be complete. RALES provides an example where this assumption does not hold. Ideally, studies should devise methods to ensure a very short delay between the occurrence of an event and its reliable documentation in the dataset. One such method is performing periodic sweeps assessing the primary endpoint for each person. Such a process, while cumbersome, can be essential to decision-making. RALES showed some evidence of differential reporting in the two groups. In the placebo group, 32 of the total of 383 deaths, or 8.4%, were reported after the last sweep; the comparable numbers for the spirono-lactone group were 14 of 283, or 4.9% (p = 0.09). Differential reporting is likely greater in unblinded studies.

The choice of how to monitor the study–by information time or calendar time–may seem statistically arcane, but in RALES we had to confront the choice explicitly because the study changed from one based on information time (800 deaths) to one based on calendar time. Even though the study was based on calendar time, we chose to monitor it on the basis of information time because in a long-term follow-up study, monitoring by information time is more statistically efficient. We, of course, did not know the number of deaths that would have occurred if the study were to continue until its planned end. Therefore, at each meeting of the DSMB, the statistical group calculated the expected total number of deaths projected from the observed survival patterns thus far. To ensure that the decision to stop early was insensitive to the estimated total, the statisticians provided a range of information fractions consistent with the data thus far and reported the boundaries for this range. Had the DSMB used calendar time instead, the boundary would have been crossed at the meeting of March 1998 (data not shown).

Finally RALES confirmed the importance of careful planning and of frequent communication with the study sponsor and the Principal Investigator. The DSMB's foresight enhanced its ability to recommend stopping the trial early and to make clear conclusions. Data from trials rarely leap over the monitoring boundaries; instead, a DSMB usually has highly suggestive evidence several meetings before the boundary is crossed. Positioning itself to make an orderly decision helps the credibility of a study. Furthermore, the availability of the sponsor and the Principal Investigator at the DSMB's meetings helped foster mutual understanding of the roles of everyone involved.

ACKNOWLEDGMENTS

The authors of this chapter consist of the members of the DSMB for RALES and the statistician (J.W.) who presented the data to the DSMB. Dr. Bertram Pitt was the Principal Investigator; Dr. Alfonso Perez and Dr. Barbara Roniker were the clinical monitors at Searle.

REFERENCES

1. Julian DG, Cowan JC, McLenachan JM. 1998. *Cardiology*, 7th Edition. WB Saunders, London.
2. Criteria Committee of the New York Heart Association: Diseases of the Heart and Blood Vessels (Nomenclature and Criteria for Diagnosis). 1964. Little, Brown, Boston.
3. Gradman AH, Deedwania PC. 1994. Predictors of mortality in patients with heart failure. *Cardiol Clin* 12:25-35.
4. Cohn JN, Archibald DG, Ziesche S, Franciosa JA, Harston WE, Tristani FE, Dunkman WB, Jacobs W, Francis GS, Flohr KH, et al. 1986. Effect of vasodilator therapy on mortality in chronic congestive heart failure. Results of a Veterans Administration Cooperative Study. *N Engl J Med.* 314:1547-1552.
5. The CONSENSUS Trial Study Group. 1987. Effects of enalapril on mortality in severe congestive heart failure. Results of the Cooperative North Scandinavian Enalapril Survival Study (CONSENSUS). *N Engl J Med.* 316:1429-1435.
6. The RALES Investigators. 1996. Effectiveness of spironolactone added to an angiotensin-converting enzyme inhibitor and a loop diuretic for severe chronic congestive heart failure (the Randomized Aldactone Evaluation Study [RALES]). *Am J Cardiol* 78:902-907.
7. Pitt B, Zannad F, Remme WJ, Cody R, Castaigne A, Perez A, Palensky J, Wittes J for The Randomized Aldactone Evaluation Study Investigators. 1999. The effect of spironolactone on morbidity and mortality in patients with severe heart failure. *N Engl J Med.* 341:709-717.
8. O'Brien P, Fleming T. 1979. A multiple testing procedure for clinical trials. *Biometrics* 35:549-556.
9. Lan K, DeMets D. 1983. Discrete sequential boundaries for clinical trials. *Biometrika* 14:1927-1931.
10. Wittes J, Palensky J, Asner D, Julian D, Boissel J, Furberg C, Kulbertus H, Pocock S, Roniker B. 2001. Experience collecting interim data on mortality: an example from the RALES study. *Curr Control Trials Cardiovasc Med* 2:59-62.

Data Monitoring in the Heart Outcomes Prevention Evaluation and the Clopidogrel in Unstable Angina to Prevent Recurrent Ischemic Events Trials: Avoiding Important Information Loss

Janice Pogue
David Sackett
DG Wyse
Salim Yusuf

ABSTRACT

Caution should always be exercised in considering early termination for any randomized clinical trial not only to avoid reacting to a temporary trend in the data, but also to avoid the loss of important treatment information concerning secondary outcomes, key subgroups, and patient safety data. For the Heart Outcomes Prevention Evaluation (HOPE) and Clopidogrel in Unstable Angina to Prevent Recurrent Ischemic Events (CURE) trials, their Data and Safety Monitoring Boards (DSMBs) ensured that this information was complete prior to making their decisions. For the HOPE trial, the DSMB did unblind the principal investigator early, who agreed with their assessment and stopped the trial before its scheduled conclusion. For CURE trial, the DSMB decided not to recommend early termination but allowed the trial to continue to collect important safety data to its planned end. DSMBs play a vital role in ensuring that information that effects clinical practice is ultimately obtained.

INTRODUCTION AND BACKGROUND

While all randomized controlled trials have primary outcomes, the vast majority also hope to address important secondary hypotheses as well. Although it is extremely important to obtain the correct answer to the primary question, given the effort, skill, time, and money required to launch a large-scale randomized controlled trial, it is truly worthwhile that these secondary hypotheses are answered in a reliable manner as well. These questions typically include determining whether the effects of treatment vary in different subgroups and whether any potential adverse effects outweigh the benefits. Although the early termination of a clinical trial draws attention from investigators, trial participants, physicians, and the media, this should be counterbalanced by the potential information lost from stopping a study too early, even when the result on the primary outcome is clear.

We were involved in two trials, the HOPE and CURE trials, where the benefits of treatment were clear and each crossed their pre-specified monitoring boundaries. The actions of each DSMB ensured that important additional questions about the treatments were also reliably addressed.

PROTOCOL DESIGN

The HOPE trial was a double blind two-by-two factorial design studying both ramipril versus placebo and vitamin E versus placebo in patients at high risk for cardiovascular outcomes. HOPE was a large, simple, multi-center, international clinical trial enrolling 9,541 patients from 19 countries at 267 clinical centres. Patients had to be at least 55 year old with either a history of coronary artery disease, stroke, peripheral vascular disease, or have diabetes with one additional risk factor (hypertension, elevated total cholesterol levels, low high-density lipoprotein cholesterol levels, cigarette smoking, or documented microalbuminuria). Patients were due to be followed for an average of five years. The primary outcome was first occurrence of myocardial infarction, stroke, or cardiovascular death. The design and results of the trial are described elsewhere.[1-3] The study deliberately enrolled a broad population and was interested in demonstrating clear answers not only overall but also in a number of subgroups of clinical interest (women as well as men, young as well as old, and those with and without diabetes) and whether the benefits were consistent in various subgroups who were already receiving other effective therapies. Furthermore, the individual components of the composite primary outcome were of sufficient clinical importance by themselves that it was important to obtain clear answers as to the effect of each treatment on each of them. Finally, a number of secondary clinical outcomes (e.g., heart failure, renal progression, etc.) were of great clinical interest, and the investigators wished to demonstrate unambiguous results on these outcomes as well.

The CURE trial was a randomized, double-blind, placebo-controlled trial comparing clopidogrel with placebo given with aspirin in patients who presented with acute coronary syndrome without ST-segment elevation. These patients presented to hospital within 24 hours of symptom onset. A total of 12,562 patients were randomized at 482 centers in 28 countries. Patients were followed for an average of 9 months. The design and results have been reported previously.[4,5] The primary study objective was to evaluate whether clopidogrel is superior to placebo in preventing ischemic complications in patients receiving aspirin therapy. The first of two co-primary outcomes was the first incidence of the composite of cardiovascular death, myocardial infarction, and stroke. The second co-primary outcome was time to the first co-primary outcome or refractory ischemia. The secondary objective was to evaluate the safety of clopidogrel in patients receiving aspirin as observed through rates of hemorrhagic stroke and bleeding.

DATA MONITORING EXPERIENCE

For both HOPE and CURE, the DSMBs had adopted statistical monitoring guidelines at the beginning of each trial. These guidelines were conservative and required convincing evidence of benefit or harm before they would be triggered. The guideline was a modification of the original Haybittle–Peto stopping rule.[6,7] The boundary for reduction in the primary outcome was set at equivalent to a Z-value of 4 during the first half of the trial and a Z-value of 3 in second half. For excess in primary outcome, the boundary was set at equivalent to a Z-value of 3 in the first half of the trial and Z-value of 2 in the second half. The boundary had to be crossed on two consecutive looks. This approach is conservative, avoids making decisions on temporary fluctuations in the data, requires extreme evidence before it is triggered, and uses negligible amounts of type 1 error rate or alpha. Plans were to have interim analyses at four time points in HOPE and twice in CURE, equally spaced with respect to the accumulating follow-up and events.

Each committee met at regular intervals and observed a monitoring boundary crossing at the last planned interim analysis. For the HOPE trial, a beneficial trend for ramipril was present at each interim analysis, and the data crossed the warning boundary at the fourth look, indicating a robust treatment effect for the primary outcome. (See Figure 1 for the treatment effect at each interim and the final analyses.) This boundary crossing triggered a detailed examination of the totality of evidence. First was the treatment benefit consistent across all components of both the composite primary outcome and key secondary outcomes. The treatment patterns over

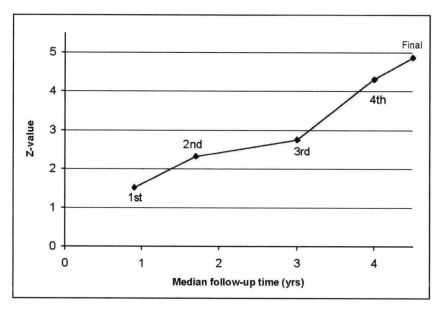

Figure 1 Interim and final results for HOPE for the primary outcome of cardio-vascular death, myocardial infarction, and stroke.

time for each of these are presented in Figure 2. Notice that only by the fourth interim analysis did the treatment effect become clear for each of these components. Second, given this consistency across outcomes, the DSMB then examined the treatment pattern in pre-specified subgroups and found no indication of important differences in the treatment effect. (See Figure 3 for the interim pattern of results by these subgroups.) Third, the DSMB requested that these analyses be repeated after accumulating four more months of follow-up, to be certain that these extreme results were not simply temporary fluctuations. At this follow-up meeting (but still 8 months before the expected trial end date) the DSMB decided to unblind the Principal Investigator (PI). The PI studied the unblinded data, shared it with the other members of the HOPE Steering Committee, and a decision was made to terminate the ramipril arm of the trial early, due to efficacy.

For CURE, there was also a trend toward benefit due to clopidogrel at the first interim analysis point, but the boundary was crossed at the second interim look for the first co-primary outcome (see Figure 4). It was also clear very early that there was an increased risk of bleeding, and the DSMB was faced with making a judgment about whether bleeding events were clini-cally important enough to offset the trajectory of benefit seen in the co-primary outcome. Clearly minor bleeding was of concern but the DSMB

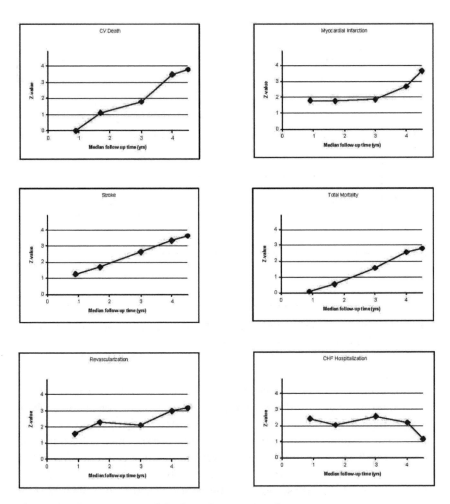

Figure 2 HOPE interim and final results over time by outcome.

decided to focus on major hemorrhage and in particular intracerebral hemorrhage as events more comparable to death or myocardial infarction. The DSMB then had another meeting three months after this time point to ensure that this trend was not a temporary one and to reassess bleeding events. Even though the benefit remained robust and the monitoring boundary had been crossed, they decided that given that there were only three months left before trial completion, that the adjudication of outcomes was incomplete, and there was a desire to have more information about safety events, particularly intracerebral hemorrhage, they did not unblind the study PI but instead let the trial close as originally planned. The treatment pattern for safety outcomes did change importantly from this interim look to study end.

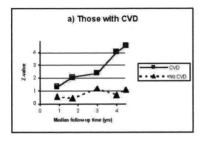
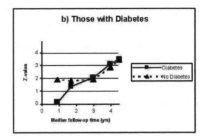

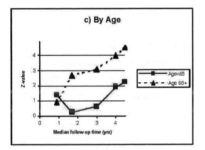
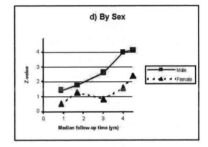

Figure 3 HOPE interim and final results for the primary outcome over time by subgroups.

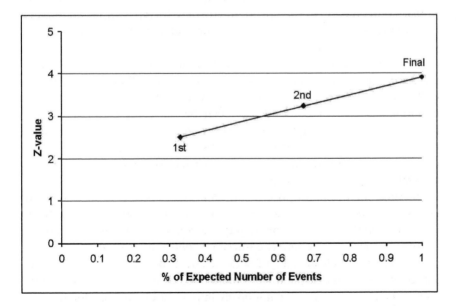

Figure 4 Interim and final results for CURE of first co-primary outcome of cardio-vascular death, myocardial infarction, and stroke.

Of concern to the DSMB was that there were seven and one intracerebral hemorrhages in the clopidogrel and placebo arms, respectively, at the last interim analysis, which fortunately changed to seven and five at the study close.

LESSONS LEARNED

The DSMBs for both trials displayed caution when observing a treatment effect that crossed the pre-specified statistical monitoring boundary for the first time. In doing so, they ensured that important questions in each trial did get answered, and thus each committee was vital in helping these trials provide comprehensive results that would assist physicians in making decisions concerning the treatment of their patients. The clear results of both trials resulted in a rapid acceptance of study results worldwide.

Physicians often wish to see evidence of consistency of treatment effect across a variety of clinically important subgroups and a range of important outcomes. Therefore, a decision to continue a trial can be justified as worthwhile, at least for certain outcomes in certain subgroups, until sufficient evidence is present. In both trials, we think it was the consistency of the results across subgroups and secondary outcomes, in addition to the overall results, that lead to uptake of this therapy in populations at risk. We acknowledge that some consider it to be unethical to the patients within the trial to continue blinded study medications once a treatment effect is observed for the primary outcome. However, uptake of any new therapy within the medical community is the one factor that will truly influence patient care for trial participants and all future patients.

Also, the time to obtain reliable answers for primary outcomes, on the one hand, and for important safety outcomes, on the other, may differ, especially when the latter are rare. Therefore, when a therapy carries the risk of important adverse outcomes, a case can be made for continuing a trial beyond the point of demonstrating primary efficacy to obtain a more accurate estimate of risks as well as benefits. The CURE trial was continued despite clear demonstration of benefits to learn whether there was a favorable safety profile for clopidogrel in this setting.

Because the prime purpose of any clinical trial is to provide convincing evidence about the efficacy and safety of a treatment, its value to patients, clinicians and the scientific community is lost if it stops before the evidence becomes clear and coherent. The interim evidence must be statistically convincing and medically meaningful, and the effect size must be estimated with sufficient precision that the lower bound of its confidence interval (and not merely its mean) exceeds the minimally important difference. Moreover, the treatment effect also should be assessed for all important secondary outcomes and among all important subgroups of patients. Finally, any treatment effect observed must not be the result of a temporary fluctuation but must be consistent over time. The decision to stop a trial must never be taken lightly, and the HOPE and CURE DSMBs provide examples of how they can contribute to these decisions in such fashion that trial results are compelling and lead to important changes in clinical practice.

REFERENCES

1. The HOPE Study Investigators. 1996. The HOPE (Heart Outcomes Prevention Evaluation) Study: The design of a large, simple randomized trial of an angiotensin converting enzyme inhibitor (ramipril) and vitamin E in patients at risk of cardiovascular events. *Can J Cardiol* 12:127–137.
2. The Heart Outcomes Prevention Evaluation Study Investigators. 2000. Effects of an angiotensin-converting-enzyme inhibitor, ramipril, on cardiovascular events in high-risk patients. *N Engl J Med* 342:145–153.
3. The Heart Outcomes Prevention Evaluation Study Investigators. 2000. Vitamin E supplementation and cardiovascular events in high-risk patients. *N Engl J Med* 342:154–160.
4. CURE Study Investigators. 2000. The Clopidogrel in Unstable angina to prevent Recurrent Events (CURE) trial programme: Rationale, design and baseline characteristics including a meta-analysis of the effects of thienopyridines in vascular disease. *Eur Heart J* 21:2033–2041.
5. The Clopidogrel in Unstable Angina to Prevent Recurrent Events (CURE) Trial Investigators. 2001. Effects of clopidogrel in addition to aspirin in patients with acute coronary syndromes without ST-segment elevation. *N Engl J Med* 345:494–502.
6. Haybittle, JL. 1971. Repeated assessment of results in clinical trials of cancer treatment. *B J Radiol* 44:793–797.
7. Peto R, Pike MC, Armitage P, Breslow NE, Cox DR, Howard SV, et al. 1976. Design and analysis of randomized clinical trials requiring prolonged observations of each patient. I. Introduction and design. *Br J Cancer* 34:585–612.

The Data Monitoring Experience in the Candesartan in Heart Failure Assessment of Reduction in Mortality and Morbidity Program*

Stuart Pocock
Duolao Wang
Lars Wilhelmsen
Charles H. Hennekens

ABSTRACT

The Candesartan in Heart Failure Assessment of Reduction in Mortality and morbidity (CHARM) program was designed as three separate randomized trials comparing candesartan with placebo in patients with chronic heart failure (CHF) who (1) were intolerant to angiotensin converting enzyme (ACE)-inhibitor and had left ventricular ejection fraction (LVEF) ≤ 40%, (2)) were on ACE-inhibitor and had LVEF ≤ 40% or (3)) had LVEF > 40%. CHARM provides an interesting example of the challenges faced by a Data and Safety Monitoring Committee (DSMC).

While the primary efficacy endpoint for each component trial was cardiovascular (CV) death or hospitalization for CHF, the primary outcome for the overall program was all-cause mortality. The DSMC received monthly safety reports and also met every six months (seven times in all) to review interim reports. Statistical stopping guidelines were predefined for all-cause mortality in the overall program. The overarching principle of the DSMC was proof beyond a reasonable doubt that would be likely to influence clinical practice.

There were significant treatment differences in all-cause mortality at several interim analyses, and the statistical stopping guideline was reached on one occasion. The DSMC consistently recommended that the program

* This paper first published in the *Am Heart J* 2005; 149:939–943.

continue as planned. The final published results for all-cause death over a median 3.1 years were a 9% reduction in hazard (95% CI 0% to 17%, p = 0.055), whereas for CV death or hospitalization for CHF there was a 16% reduction in hazard (95% CI 9% to 23%, p < 0.0001). Subsequent exploratory analyses suggest that the hazard reduction in CV death was more marked in the first year after randomization, and that, if real, this apparent treatment-time interaction offers a plausible explanation for why the interim mortality data showed statistically more extreme findings than the overall final results.

The DSMC experience in the CHARM program illustrates the importance of continuing a trial to its scheduled completion unless there is proof beyond reasonable doubt that would influence clinical practice rather than strict reliance on a statistical stopping guideline.

INTRODUCTION AND BACKGROUND

Angiotensin-receptor blockers such as candesartan offer the potential to improve clinical outcomes in heart failure patients as alternatives or adjuncts to those seen with angiotensin-converting enzyme (ACE) inhibitors. Accordingly the CHARM program[1-4] was designed as three independent randomized double blind trials comparing candesartan with placebo in three populations of patients with symptomatic heart failure:

1. *CHARM—Alternative* patients (N = 2,028) had a left ventricular ejection fraction (LVEF) ≤ 40% and were not on ACE inhibitor because of previous intolerance.[2]
2. *CHARM—Added* patients (N = 2,548) also had LVEF ≤40% and were being treated with an ACE inhibitor.[3]
3. *CHARM—Preserved* patients (N = 3,023) had LVEF >40%.[4]

The primary endpoint for each trial was CV death or hospitalization for worsening CHF and each required sample size was based on power calculations for this endpoint. The overall program was designed to evaluate all-cause mortality in the broad spectrum of symptomatic heart failure patients, with the overall sample size (N = 6,500) equal to the sum of all three trials.[1] With an estimated overall annual mortality in the placebo group of 8% the program had over 85% power to detect a 14% reduction in mortality at two-sided 5% significance based on a logrank test.

All three trials were done at the same 618 sites in 26 countries. The CHARM program exceeded its recruitment goal of 6,500 by enrolling 7,599 patients between March 1999 to March 2001, who were followed for a minimum of two years. Hence, all follow-up was concluded on March 31, 2003, resulting in a median duration of 3.14 years. The final results were published in the *Lancet* on September 6, 2003.[1-4] For the overall CHARM program , CV death or hospitalization for worsening CHF had a 16% reduction on candesartan versus placebo, 95% CI 9% to 23%, p < 0.0001. For all-cause mortality there was a 9% reduction, 95% CI 0% to 17%, p = 0.055.

DATA MONITORING EXPERIENCE

The Data Safety and Monitoring Committee (DSMC) had three members, two physicians, Charles Hennekens (chair) and Lars Wilhelmsen, and a statistician, Stuart Pocock. In collaboration with the CHARM Executive Committee, a charter was drawn up, defining the terms of reference, operating procedures as well as guidelines for early termination, which included statistical stopping boundaries. The overarching principle for early termination was proof beyond a reasonable doubt that would be likely to influence clinical practice.

It was agreed that the DSMC would receive a monthly safety report primarily containing data on all serious adverse events and deaths to date. In addition, the DSMC would meet twice a year to evaluate a fuller interim report containing more extensive follow-up data, especially as regards deaths, primary and secondary clinical outcomes, and serious adverse events. Such safety reports and interim reports would present results for the overall program, and also separately for each component trial. The Endpoint Committee verdicts on causes of death and non-fatal major clinical events were used when available, but for events pending Endpoint Committee validation the investigator's classification was used. All six-monthly interim reports and monthly safety reports were produced by a data analyst, Duolao Wang, who was independent of the trial sponsor, Astra Zeneca. Results were presented in a blinded manner, i.e., with coded treatment groups A and B, with the option of unblinding at any stage, i.e., identifying whether candesartan was A or B, if the DSMC thought this was appropriate.[5] Such unblinding in fact occurred at the second interim analysis.

Following each monthly safety report any DSMC member could identify any safety concerns or call for a teleconference or meeting if warranted. No such concerns arose, so each time the DSMC statistician faxed and mailed confirmation to the Executive and Sponsor that the study should continue as planned.

For each six-monthly DSMC meeting there was a closed session attended only by the DSMC members and the independent data analyst. These were the only individuals to see and to discuss any interim results by coded treatment group. At least two DSMC members were always present face-to-face for such meetings, but on two occasions a third member joined by teleconference.

For all but the first DSMC meeting, there was an open session also attended by members of the CHARM Executive Committee and sponsor representatives. Such open sessions were primarily to share information on the study progress and organization. From the fourth interim report onward, a blinded interim report was produced for the Executive Committee containing only the data for both treatment groups combined. The existence of this open session was also helpful should the DSMC have needed to make any recommendations regarding cessation or modification of either the overall program or any specific component trial(s). In fact, no such recommendations needed to be made.

Guidelines for Early Termination

The principle adopted by the DSMC for early termination required a totality of evidence that provided proof beyond a reasonable doubt that would be likely to influence clinical practice. The emerging data would also have to fulfill predefined statistical stopping guidelines.

In the DSMC charter, which was jointly agreed by the DSMC, Executive Committee and sponsor there were no statistical stopping guidelines for the primary efficacy outcome of each trial, i.e., CV death or CHF hospitalization. It was agreed that pre-defined intentions for stopping the program early should focus on all cause mortality.

The Haybittle–Peto rule[6] was employed at each interim analysis, requiring two-sided $p < 0.001$ for the overall program treatment difference in mortality in favor of candesartan using a logrank test stratified by trial. However, two modifications were pre-defined:

1. For each interim analysis occurring within 18 months of the date of first patient's being randomized in the CHARM program, the rule was made more stringent requiring two-sided $p < 0.0001$.

2. Stopping a specific trial required the same trial-specific p-value criteria as above, and also statistical evidence of heterogeneity among trials as regards estimated hazard ratios for mortality of sufficient strength to merit termination of one trial only. In fact, no such statistical heterogeneity arose.

In order to stop for safety (i.e., mortality greater on candesartan) the same general principle applied, except one required $p < 0.001$ for any analysis within 18 months and $p < 0.01$ for any subsequent analysis.

Interim Mortality Results

About three weeks before each six-monthly meeting of the DSMC, a data file was transferred from the sponsor's data management department to the independent data analyst. He then merged the data with the treatment code to produce the interim report that was then couriered to the DSMC members a few days before the meeting.

Table 1 lists for each interim analysis the numbers of deaths by treatment group, both overall and for each constituent trial, and the overall logrank test P-value. Figure 1 plots the consequent hazard ratio and 95% CI at each analysis. The corresponding results for the final published data are also given.

By the *second interim analysis* in March 2000 there was a substantial difference in mortality overall: 76 deaths on candesartan versus 123 on placebo, with hazard ratio 0.63, 95% CI 0.49 to 0.80, p = 0.0007. The DSMB unblinded themselves as to which treatment was which at this point. The formal stopping boundary p < 0.0001 had not been crossed. A total of 5,800 patients had been randomized since patient entry began one year earlier. There were more deaths in CHARM-Added since patient recruitment was more rapid than in CHARM-Alternative, N = 2,548 and 1,212 respectively. CHARM-Preserved had many fewer deaths because recruitment was somewhat slower than in CHARM-Added (N = 2,040) and its population had lower mortality rates.

The situation was broadly similar at the *third interim analysis* in July 2000, though with 67% more deaths. The magnitude of treatment effect was slightly reduced: hazard ratio 0.66, 95% CI 0.53 to 0.82. But with a larger number of deaths, statistical significance was slightly enhanced at p = 0.0002, still just short of the stopping boundary of p < 0.0001.

At the *fourth interim analysis* in March 2001, there were almost twice as many deaths compared to six months earlier. The overall treatment effect

Table 1   CHARM Mortality Results At Each Interim Analysis and At Study Close-Out*

Analysis Date	CHARM-Alternative		CHARM-Added		CHARM-Preserved		Overall Program		p-value
	C	P	C	P	C	P	C	P	
							8	4	0.3
9 Aug 1999	3	0	5	4	0	0	76	123	0.0007
27 March 2000	20	38	45	69	11	16	133	198	0.0002
27 July 2000	39	60	76	113	18	25	260	339	0.0006
1 March 2001	66	100	140	168	54	71	387	474	0.0010
9 Aug 2001	117	148	186	219	84	107	556	631	0.009
22 Feb 2002	166	198	258	285	132	148	682	756	0.015
1 Aug 2002	210	236	298	336	174	184			
Final Report**							886	945	0.055

* Each line gives the number of deaths by treatment group for each constituent trial and overall, plus the overall logrank p-value, stratified by trial (C = candesartan, P = placebo).
** Final report on September 6, 2003, based on follow-up to March 31, 2003.

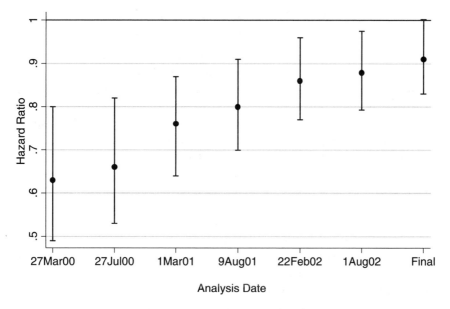

Figure 1 Hazard ratio and 95% for all-cause mortality (candesartan vs. placebo) at each interim analysis and at study close-out.

was further attenuated, hazard ratio 0.76 95% CI 0.64 to 0.87, but being based on more deaths statistical significance was maintained at p = 0.0006. This was well past 18 months from the start of recruitment and hence the stopping boundary p < 0.001 had been crossed. The more rapid recruitment in CHARM-Added (final N = 2,548 completed over a year earlier) meant that it had almost twice as many deaths as in CHARM-Alternative (N = 1,989 with one month of recruitment still to go) while CHARM Preserved had fewer deaths in its lower risk population (final N = 3,023 completed six months earlier). As was the case at all other analyses, there was no statistical heterogeneity in hazard ratios between trials, interaction test p = 0.45. However, it was noted that the treatment difference in mortality only achieved even a conventional level of significance in CHARM-Alternative (66 vs. 100 deaths, p = 0.006) compared with CHARM-Added (140 vs. 168 deaths, p = 0.07) and CHARM-Preserved (54 vs. 71 deaths, P = 0.14).

The DSMC recommended that the program continue without alteration. Thus, as on previous occasions the DSMC requested that the Executive Committee and sponsor ensure that data be as complete as possible for future interim analyses, particular assurance being sought that the Endpoint Committee adjudicate all causes of deaths and major morbid events that had arisen and were available to them.

The DSMC unanimously agreed at this fourth interim analysis that the CHARM program should continue for the following reasons:

1. While the overall mortality result in favor of candesartan reached the statistical stopping guideline, the mortality differences in two of the three component trials did not achieve even a conventional level (p < 0.05) level of statistical significance.

2. Data on the primary efficacy endpoint, CV death and CHF hospitalization, were incomplete at this point with many reported endpoints awaiting adjudication by the Endpoint Committee.

3. The average length of patient follow-up was relatively short and one major goal was to evaluate candersartan's effect over two or more years' treatment.

4. There was no previous trial evidence regarding a survival benefit of candesartan, or indeed other angiotensin-receptor blockers, in patients with CHF. In fact, one earlier small pilot trial RESOLVD[2] had shown possible but inconclusive higher mortality on candesartan (with or without enalapril), compared with enalapril alone.

5. The DSMC was mindful of the likelihood that trials that stop early for efficacy are liable to exaggerate the true treatment effect with the danger that people may infer that the observed result is "too good to be true."[8] Aware that from such a potentially "random high" there may well be some "regression to the truth" of a more modest estimated mortality reduction, the DSMC voted unanimously to continue for at least a further six months.

There did not appear to be proof beyond a reasonable doubt of treatment efficacy that would be likely to influence clinical practice.

At the *fifth interim analysis* there was a further attenuation of the mortality hazard ratio now 0.80, 95% CI 0.70 to 0.91 with stratified logrank p = 0.00103, so the DSMC felt once again that early stopping was not warranted. There were in fact two more interim analyses, each with less statistically convincing evidence of a mortality difference p = 0.009 and p = 0.014, respectively, so that it became increasingly straightforward for the DSMC to recommend continuation of CHARM.

Final Results of CHARM

Patient follow-up continued for a further seven months after the last planned interim analysis. Published results were available 5 months later as follows: the numbers of deaths were 886 on candesartan versus 945 on placebo, hazard ratio 0.91, 95% CI 0.83 to 1.00, p = 0.055. The predefined secondary analysis adjusting for 33 baseline covariates had hazard ratio 0.90 p = 0.032.

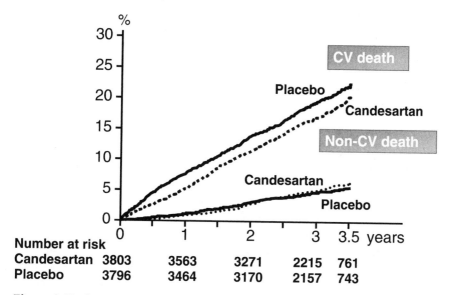

Figure 2 Kaplan–Meier curves for cardiovascular and non-cardiovascular deaths.

This treatment difference could be entirely attributed to cardiovascular deaths 691 versus 769, hazard ratio 0.88, 95% CI 0.79 to 0.97, p = 0.012 as shown in Figure 2. Subgroup analyses revealed no relevant interactions between treatment and baseline features, and there was no evidence of heterogeneity among trials.

Trial continuation to its intended conclusion enabled clear results for the primary efficacy endpoint, CV death or CHF hospitalization. Over a mean 3.14 years follow-up there were 1,150 (30.2%) vs. 1,310 (34.5%) cases, hazard ratio 0.84 95% CI 0.77 to 0.91, p < 0.0001. There was no statistical heterogeneity among trials, interaction p = 0.33, though this efficacy appeared somewhat less pronounced in patients with preserved LV systolic function.

The investigators concluded that "candesartan was generally well tolerated and significantly reduced cardiovascular deaths and hospitalizations for heart failure. The clinical evidence we report . . . offers the opportunity to further reduce cardiovascular mortality and morbidity in this expanding segment of our aging population."[1]

LESSONS LEARNED

The DSMC experience in the CHARM program illustrates the crucial importance of continuing a trial to its scheduled termination unless there emerges evidence of proof beyond a reasonable doubt that would influence clinical practice. Indeed, early termination of CHARM based solely on a statistical guideline would have been misleading. During March 2000 to August 2002 there were six interim analyses, followed by the final analysis in 2003. For these seven successive analyses the difference in the numbers of deaths (candesartan vs. placebo) were 47, 65, 79, 87, 73, 74, and 59 respectively. Thus, the early mortality difference persisted but was not increased by further follow-up.

The final data indicate that mortality benefit was confined to CV deaths, as one would expect. Closer inspection of Figure 2 reveals that the treatment difference in CV deaths was substantial by one year of follow-up, 199 versus 285 deaths on candesartan and placebo, respectively, an absolute difference of 2.29% mortality. Beyond one year the numbers of subsequent deaths in candesartan and placebo groups are very similar: 492 and 484, respectively, and the estimated absolute treatment difference in CV deaths at 3 years is 2.31%. This indicates that the early benefit in CV mortality reduction attributed to candesartan was maintained but not enhanced by further follow-up. It is worth noting that a similar pattern emerged in the SOLVD trial[9] comparing enalapril and placebo in patients with chronic heart failure: the mortality reduction due to enalapril occurred within 18 months of randomization, with no additional benefit over a further mean two years of follow-up.

This post hoc exploratory finding, if real, offers a plausible explanation as to why the early interim results, based exclusively on short-term follow-up gave the greatest reduction in hazard.

1. The experience of the DSMC in the CHARM program emphasizes the importance of judging early mortality differences in the context of the totality of evidence and not relying exclusively on a statistical stopping guideline when a trial is designed to determine the overall longer-term benefits (if they exist) of a treatment for a chronic condition that is intended to be given for several years.

2. The CHARM experience illustrates the complexity of simultaneously monitoring these inter-related trials in one overall program. In particular, it is difficult to pre-specify a statistical stopping guideline that will correct all contingencies that may arise.

ACKNOWLEDGEMENTS

We are grateful to members of the CHARM Executive Committee for their helpful comments.

REFERENCES

1. Pfeffer MA, Swedberg K, Granger CB, Held P, McMurray JJV, Michelson EL, et al. 2003. Effects of candesartan on mortality and morbidity in patients with chronic heart failure: the CHARM-Overall Programme. *Lancet* 362:759–766.

2. McMurray JJV, Östergren J, Swedberg K, Granger C B, Held P, Michelson EL, et al. 2003. Effects of candesartan in patients with chronic heart failure and reduced left-ventricular systolic function taking angiotensin-converting-enzyme inhibitors: The CHARM-Added Trial. *Lancet* 362:767-771.

3. Granger CB, McMurray JJV, Yusuf S, Held P, Michelson EL, Olofsson B, et al. 2003. Effects of candesartan in patients with chronic heart failure and reduced left-ventricular systolic function intolerant to angiotensin-converting-enzyme inhibitors: The CHARM-Alternative Trial. *Lancet* 362:772-776.

4. Yusuf S, Pfeffer MA, Swedberg K, Granger CB, Held P, McMurray JJV, et al. 2003. Effects of candesartan in patients with chronic heart failure and preserved left-ventricular ejection fraction: the CHARM-Preserved Trial. *Lancet* 362:777-781.

5. Pocock S, Furberg CD. 2001. Procedures of Data and Safety Monitoring Committees. *Am Heart J* 141:289-294.

6. Peto R, Pike MC, Armitage P, et al. 1976. Design and analysis of randomised clinical trials requiring prolonged observation of each patient: I. Introduction and design. *Br J Cancer* 34:585-612.

7. McKelvie RS, Rouleau JL, White M, Afzal R, Young JB, Maggioni AP, et al. 2003. Comparative impact of enalapril, candesartan or metoprolol alone or in combination on ventricular remodelling in patients with congestive heart failure. *Eur Heart J* 24:1727-1734.

8. Pocock SJ, White I. 1999. Trials stopped early: Too good to be true. *Lancet* 353:943-944.

9. SOLVD Investigators. 1991. Effect of enalapril on survival in patients with reduced left ventricular ejection fractions and congestive heart failure. *N Engl J Med* 325:293-302.

General Harm

Introduction to Case Studies Showing Harmful Effects of the Intervention

David L. DeMets
Curt D. Furberg
Lawrence M. Friedman

Based on the Declaration of Helsinki and established principles of ethics in research, one major objective of data monitoring is the protection of trial participants from being harmed by the study intervention. This section presents nine cases of clinical trials showing evidence of harm attributed to a trial intervention, eight of which were terminated earlier than planned. Three of the trials tested more than one active intervention (the Coronary Drug Project (CDP—Case 12), the Cardiac Arrhythmia Suppression Trial (CAST—Case 13). and the Antihypertensive and Lipid-Lowering Treatment to Prevent Heart Attack Trial (ALLHAT—Case 18). In this section, we focus on the treatment arms associated with harmful effects. The complexities behind the decision to recommend trial termination are illustrated.

Eight of the nine trials were placebo-controlled, a design feature that facilitates determination of harm. The ninth trial, ALLHAT (Case 18), was an active-control trial designed to determine whether any of three newer and costlier antihypertensive drugs was superior to a generic diuretic. Due to the lack of a placebo group, this trial evaluated the treatment effect along the axis of superiority-indifference-inferiority rather than the axis efficacy-indifference-harm, which applies to placebo-controlled trials. In active-control trials, inferiority does not automatically mean harm, since an inferior intervention could be less beneficial or neutral. The magnitude of the inferiority may indirectly shed some light on the question of harm. The two-fold higher risk of congestive heart failure (CHF) in the doxazosin group of ALLHAT compared to the chlorthalidone group, in spite of only a small difference in systolic blood pressure reduction, suggests a harmful effect of doxazosin on CHF risk. All-cause mortality was the pre-specified primary outcome in four trials (CDP, the Prospective Randomized Milrinone Survival Evaluation Trial [PROMISE—Case 14], the Diaspirin Cross-Linked Hemoglobin for Emergency Treatment of Post-Traumatic Study [Baxter DMC—Case 16] and the Moxonidine

Congestive Heart Failure Trial [MOXCON—Case 19]) and a pre-specified secondary outcome in the other five trials (CAST, the Carotene and Retinol Efficacy Trial [CARET—Case 15], the Heart and Estrogen/progestin Replacement Study [HERS—Case 17], ALLHAT, and the Placebo-Controlled Trial of Daclizumab in Acute Graft-versus-Host Disease [ECOG—Case 20]). Five trials had a disease-specific primary outcome (CAST, CARET, HERS, ALLHAT, and ECOG).

The CDP (Case 12) may have been the first clinical trial with external monitoring, although the Data Monitoring Committee was not appointed until a couple of years after the trial was launched. Many of the methods for data monitoring that we use today were developed during the course of CDP. The other eight trials all had pre-specified monitoring guidelines or "stopping rules."

Two trials were designed with a one-sided hypothesis. The daclizumab trial (Case 20) tested whether active treatment was superior to placebo at a statistical significance level of 0.05. Interestingly, when the trial was terminated due to excess mortality in the actively treated group, there was no difference between the daclizumab and placebo groups for the primary outcome. CAST (Case 13) was also initially designed to determine benefit at the statistical significance level of 0.05. However, the monitoring committee changed the alpha level for benefit to $p = 0.025$ and added the same significance level for the testing of harm. The lesson from these two trials is that an adverse effect of the intervention, however promising, can never be ruled out.

Most trials employed symmetric boundaries during the monitoring process. In other words, they required similar strength of evidence for claim of benefit and harm. One exception was MOXCON (Case 19), which had an asymmetric boundary with stricter criteria for benefit. The monitoring of the moricizine–placebo comparison in CAST (Case 13) also relied on an asymmetric lower boundary.

Five of the trials (CDP [two treatment arms], CAST, PROMISE, CARET, and MOXCON) were terminated due to group differences in the pre-specified primary outcome. In two trials, the recommendations for early termination were based on observed group differences in secondary or other outcomes (CDP [one treatment arm] and ALLHAT). In HERS (Case 17), one of the components of the primary outcome (non-fatal MI plus CHD death) appeared early destined to cross the stopping boundary. An excess of early CHD deaths (a nominal $p = 0.02$) was observed in the hormone therapy group. For a variety of good reasons, the board voted to continue the trial. Later this trend reversed itself and the relative hazard at trial termination was 0.99. In the middle years, the risk of one of the pre-specified secondary outcomes, venous thromboembolic events (VTE), crossed the stopping boundary. Rather than recommending trial termination, the board advised the Steering Committee to inform all participants of this risk, to modify the study protocol to reduce the future risk of thromboembolic complications and to publish the VTE data (*JAMA* 1997;278:477).

Futility was, in addition to harm, a consideration in the recommendation to terminate four trials (CDP [one treatment arm], CARET, ALLHAT, and MOXCON). In two trials (CARET and MOXCON) external scientific evidence was considered in the decision making.

Deciding to terminate a trial is difficult and it is very common that the monitoring committee votes will be split. This leaves the sponsor in a difficult position. One solution to this dilemma is consultation with a second advisory group. In fact, in three of the trials (CDP [one treatment arm], CARET, and ALLHAT), a second committee was formally consulted before a final decision to terminate was made.

Breaking New Ground: Data Monitoring in the Coronary Drug Project

Paul L. Canner

ABSTRACT

Arriving at a decision for early termination of a treatment group or of an entire clinical trial, due to either beneficial or adverse results, is a complex process. It may involve, among other things, the need to (1) determine whether the observed treatment differences are likely to represent real effects and are not due to chance; (2) weigh the importance of different response variables, some possibly trending in favor of the treatment and some against it; (3) adjust for differences in distributions of baseline characteristics among the treatment groups; (4) discern possible biases (due to the study not being double-blind) in the medical management of patients or in the diagnosis of events; and (5) evaluate treatment effects in subgroups of the study participants. Experiences from the Coronary Drug Project in making decisions for early termination and for non-termination of treatment groups are described.

INTRODUCTION AND BACKGROUND

By 1960 evidence had accrued linking elevated blood lipid levels with increased incidence of coronary heart disease (CHD). At the same time the pharmaceutical industry was developing drugs that were effective in reducing blood cholesterol in persons with hyperlipidemia. The time had come to assess whether reduction of lipid levels would be effective in the treatment and possible prevention of CHD. In November 1960 the National Advisory Heart Council asked Dr. Robert Wilkins, a Council member, along with National Heart Institute (now National Heart, Lung, and Blood Institute (NHLBI)) staff to explore the desirability, feasibility, and methodology of a controlled clinical trial of cholesterol-lowering drugs. The ultimate develop-

183

ment and funding in 1966 of the Coronary Drug Project (CDP) from this initiative makes a fascinating story in itself,[1] but is beyond the scope of this book.

PROTOCOL DESIGN

The CDP was a randomized, double-blind, placebo-controlled clinical trial of the efficacy and safety of five lipid-modifying agents in men with previous myocardial infarction (MI).[2] The drugs were mixed conjugated equine estrogens at two dosage levels (2.5 and 5.0 mg/day), clofibrate (1.8 g/day), dextrothyroxine (6.0 mg/day), and nicotinic acid (3.0 g/day). All these and a lactose placebo (3.8 g/day) were dispensed in identical-appearing capsules (9 per day at full dosage). The primary outcome variable was all-cause mortality, with secondary outcomes of cardiovascular death, CHD death, recurrent non-fatal MI, coronary incidence (i.e., CHD death or definite non-fatal MI), stroke, and others.

From March 1966 to October 1969, a total of 8,341 patients were recruited at 53 Clinical Centers—about 1,100 in each of the five drug groups and 2,789 in the placebo group. (The 2.5 : 1 ratio of patients in the placebo group relative to each drug group was designed to minimize the total sample size while achieving a specified power relative to each of the five drug-placebo comparisons.[3,4] To qualify for the CDP, a prospective participant had to be a male aged 30 to 64 years with electrocardiogram-documented evidence of an MI's occurring not less than three months previously. Patients were followed with clinic visits and examinations every four months for a minimum of 5 and a maximum of 8.5 years per patient. The scheduled conclusion of patient follow-up took place during the summer of 1974.

DATA MONITORING EXPERIENCE

The CDP may have been the first clinical trial to have an external monitoring committee. However, even the CDP did not have such a committee from the outset. During the first two years of the study, reports on data, including mortality, morbidity, and side effects by treatment group, were presented to the entire CDP investigator group at its semiannual meetings.[5]

For the two investigator group meetings in 1967, the results were presented with the treatment groups identified by the letters A through F. We may snicker at the naivety and lack of wisdom of the CDP leadership with regard to sharing treatment group data with the study investigators, but in those days there was no precedent for any other approach. The philosophy changed when Dr. Thomas Chalmers wrote a letter dated October 31, 1967, to Dr. Robert Wilkins, chairman of the CDP Policy Board, expressing concern that knowledge by the investigators of early trends (not statistically significant) in mortality, morbidity, or incidence of side effects might result in some investigators—desirous of treating their patients in the best possible manner, i.e., with the drug that is ahead—pulling out of the study and unblinding the treatment groups prematurely. Furthermore, it was feared that if the investigators were continually being shown treatment trends with respect to cardiovascular events, side effects, and physical examination findings, there might be a tendency on the part of the investigators toward over-diagnosis and reporting of these findings at future CDP patient-visits. As a result of this, in 1968, presentation of the treatment-specific data to the CDP investigator group was discontinued and a Data Monitoring Committee was established with the charge of meeting to review an extensive report of the accruing treatment group data at six-month intervals as well as receiving interim reports of the major outcome variables at two or three month intervals.[5] In 1970 or 1971 the name of this CDP committee was changed to Data *and Safety* Monitoring Committee (DSMC).

The CDP DSMC was a large committee composed of persons knowledgeable in the fields of cardiology, clinical medicine, biostatistics, epidemiology, and biochemistry (between 13 and 16 members altogether). Unlike such committees today, the CDP DSMC included persons who were intimately involved in the day-to-day activities of the CDP, including the chairman of the CDP Steering Committee and members of the CDP Coordinating Center, ECG Reading Center, Central Laboratory, and NHLBI Medical Liaison Officers. Since the DSMC did not include CDP Clinical Center physicians, the data reports were no longer coded as to treatment group—a very wise practice in this author's opinion.

In addition to the DSMC, a CDP Policy Board was established from the very outset of the study to act in a senior advisory capacity on policy matters throughout the duration of the study. The board was composed of five voting members who were all well known in their respective disciplines—one clinical pharmacologist, one biostatistician, and three clinician/cardiologists— and all totally independent of the CDP. The DSMC had primary responsibility for in-depth review of the CDP treatment group data and for making recommendations of changes in the treatment protocol based on the accruing data. The CDP Policy Board received copies of all of the DSMC reports prepared by the Coordinating Center, but it never formally reviewed the data unless the DSMC had first made a recommendation for a treatment change; even then, the review tended not to be as detailed as that given by the DSMC. The following lines of authority were followed for making decisions: The DSMC made recommendations to the Policy Board which either affirmed or overturned such recommendations; the Policy Board decision was transmitted to the sponsoring agency (the NHLBI) and then to the CDP Steering Committee and investigator group.[5]

Upon recommendation of the DSMC and ratification by the Policy Board, three of the CDP treatment groups were terminated early, i.e., before the scheduled end of the study; these were both estrogen groups and the dextrothyroxine group.[6-8] The two remaining drug groups—clofibrate and nicotinic acid—and the placebo group were followed until the scheduled conclusion of the trial.[9] There is a unique data monitoring story to be told for each of the five CDP treatment groups.

High-Dose Estrogen

In May 1970 a decision was reached to discontinue the 5.0-mg/day estrogen (ESG2) group because of an increased incidence of cardiovascular events. One of the major considerations in the deliberations over the ESG2 findings had to do with possible bias in diagnosing definite non-fatal MI and non-fatal thromboembolic events as a result of unblinding of the treatment in a large percentage of the patients due to feminizing side effects of the medication. Several special analyses were carried out to assess the possibility and extent of such bias:[6]

1. Incidence and duration of hospitalization for cardiac problems were reviewed. It was considered that any bias in the direction of over-diagnosis of events for the ESG2 group, relative to the placebo group, would be associated with more frequent but shorter-duration hospitalizations for these patients, since they would tend to be admitted more frequently for suspect events, only to be discharged relatively early because of lack of documentation of such events.

2. Incidence of subsequent cardiovascular death in patients with definite non-fatal MI since entry was obtained. Over-diagnosis of MI in the ESG2 group would be expected to result in a lower incidence of subsequent cardiovascular death in such patients than for similar placebo group patients.

3. Incidence of several non-fatal cardiovascular events ranked in order of severity was obtained, counting only the single most serious event for a given patient. This was done to assess whether definite MI was being over-diagnosed in the ESG2 group at the expense of lesser events such as suspect MI, definite or suspect acute coronary insufficiency, or definite or suspect angina pectoris.

4. The findings on the electrocardiograms taken in connection with new MI events and read centrally without knowledge of treatment group were compared for the ESG2 and placebo groups. Again, one would have expected that over-diagnosis of definite MI in the ESG2 group would lead to a lower

Table 1 Mortality and Morbidity in the High-Dose Estrogen (ESG2) and Placebo Groups, Coronary Drug Project

Event	Risk group*	ESG2		Placebo		Z-value
		n	%	n	%	
Total mortality	All	1,118	8.1	2,789	6.9	1.33
	1	738	5.1	1,831	6.1	−0.95
	2	80	13.9	958	8.5	3.02
Definite non-fatal MI	All	1,022	6.2	2,581	3.2	4.11
	1	684	6.7	1,689	2.9	4.30
	2	338	5.0	892	3.7	1.05

* Risk 1 = men with one MI without complications prior to entry into the study; Risk 2 = men with more than one previous MI or one MI with complications prior to entry.
Source: Coronary Drug Project Research Group.[10]

incidence of significant ECG findings than were observed in the placebo group.

These analyses did not yield any evidence in support of the hypothesis of over-diagnosis of non-fatal MI in the ESG2 group.[6,10]

The final decision to discontinue the ESG2 group was by no means clear-cut. At its meeting on May 13, 1970, the DSMC reviewed the subgroup analyses shown in Table 1. For this analysis, Risk 1 comprised men with one previous MI without complications prior to entry into the study and Risk 2 included men with either more than one previous MI or one MI with complications prior to entry. For the total group the Z-value for the ESG2-placebo difference in total mortality was 1.33 and the corresponding Z-value for definite non-fatal MI was 4.11. [A Z-value value is defined here as a drug–placebo difference in proportions of a given event, divided by the standard error of the difference; Z-values of ±1.96 correspond to a conventional p-value of 0.05. However, given the multiple treatment groups, multiple endpoints (here, total mortality and definite non-fatal MI), and multiple reviews of the data during the course of the study, it was judged necessary to require much larger Z-values than these to establish statistical significance.[11,12]] It was largely on the basis of the large Z-value (i.e., 3.02) for total mortality in patients in Risk 2 that the DSMC approved a motion at this meeting to discontinue the ESG2 treatment in Risk 2 patients. The vote was 10 to 1 with 2 abstentions. A further motion was made to discontinue this treatment in Risk 1 patients as well. After a lengthy discussion, this second motion was defeated by a vote of 7 to 5 with 1 abstention. On the following day the Policy Board accepted the decision by the DSMC concerning the Risk 2 patients but overturned the Risk 1 decision. Thus the entire ESG2 treatment group was discontinued. The excessive incidence of definite non-fatal MI (Z = 4.30), thromboembolic events, and other non-fatal cardiovascular events in

Risk 1 patients in the ESG2 group, in spite of the slightly lower mortality in this group compared to the placebo group (Z = −0.95), was an important factor in the Policy Board's decision to reject the DSMC decision concerning Risk 1 patients.

Dextrothyroxine

In October 1971 a decision was reached to discontinue the dextrothyroxine (DT4) treatment group in the CDP. This was based primarily on a higher mortality in the DT4 group compared to placebo, although the Z-value (1.88) for the difference did not achieve conventional statistical significance. The deliberations that led to this decision focused largely on the question of whether the excess mortality was present consistently throughout the total group of DT4-treated patients or whether it was concentrated in certain subgroups.[7]

Table 2 gives the observed DT4 and placebo group findings for total mortality in subgroups defined by baseline risk categorization, history of angina pectoris, and ECG heart rate. Within each of the higher risk subgroups (i.e., Risk 2, history prior to entry of suspect or definite angina pectoris, and baseline heart rate ≥70 beats per minute) there was a substantially higher mortality in the DT4 group than in the placebo group. Conversely, DT4 showed a somewhat lower mortality than placebo in the three lower-risk subgroups. These subgroups showing adverse effects of DT4 were identified following a survey of 48 baseline variables. Some DSMC members insisted that these high-risk subgroups were the very ones in which one might have expected DT4 to perform poorly. However, it was finally agreed that since no *a priori* hypotheses concerning DT4 effects in defined subgroups had been specified, the observed effects would have to be treated as *a posteriori* findings in the evaluation of their statistical significance. It should be noted here that when the DSMC dealt with the ESG2 decision the previous year, the members were not concerned about *a priori* subgroup hypotheses when dealing with data by baseline risk group. The reason for this was that risk group had been the one and only stratification or blocking factor (along with Clinical Center) used in making randomized treatment allocations in the CDP. The DSMC made the tacit assumption at that time that stratification on a particular baseline characteristic was equivalent to having an *a priori* subgroup hypothesis. This issue was considered more carefully in conjunction with the DT4 decision and the DSMC came to the conclusion that stratification for treatment allocation had to be distinguished from *a priori* hypotheses of treatment effects in specific patient subgroups.

The statistical analysis of these subgroup findings lay primarily in two directions.[7] First, since the observed subgroup findings emerged from an

Table 2 Percentage of Deaths in Selected Subgroups, Dextrothyroxine (DT4) and Placebo Groups, Coronary Drug Project

Baseline characteristic	DT4		Placebo		
	n	%	n	%	Z value
Risk Group,* 8/1/71					
Risk 1	719	10.8	1,790	11.0	−0.11
Risk 2	364	22.5	925	15.4	3.06
History of angina pectoris 8/1/71					
Negative	440	7.7	1,142	9.9	−1.33
Suspect/definite	643	19.6	1,573	14.4	3.06
ECG heart rate, 8/1/71					
<70/min	576	9.5	1,482	10.7	−0.74
≥70/min	494	21.3	1,194	14.7	3.32
Combination,** 8/1/71					
Subgroup A	460	6.5	1,210	9.9	−2.17
Subgroup B	623	20.9	1,505	14.6	3.58
Combination, 10/1/70					
Subgroup A	460	4.1	1,210	7.7	−2.60
Subgroup B	623	16.4	1,505	11.2	3.29
Combination in interval 10/1/70–8/1/71					
Subgroup A	441	2.5	1,117	2.4	0.09
Subgroup B	521	5.4	1,337	3.8	1.50

* Risk 1 = men with one MI without complications prior to entry into the study; Risk 2 = men with more than one previous MI or one MI with complications prior to entry.
** Subgroup A = men with baseline ECG heart rate <70/min and either Risk 1 or with no history of angina pectoris prior to entry; Subgroup B = men with either baseline ECG heart rate ≥70/min or Risk 2 plus history of suspect or definite angina pectoris prior to entry.
Source: Coronary Drug Project Research Group.[7]

analysis involving 48 different baseline variables, it was desirable to determine whether the observed differences were any greater than might be expected by chance alone from evaluation of 48 variables. The interaction between each baseline variable and treatment group with respect to total mortality was ascertained and evaluated statistically using a linear regression model. For dichotomous characteristics, this was essentially equivalent to testing whether the drug–placebo difference in mortality at one level of the baseline variable was different from that difference at the other level. If these 48 tests were assumed to be nearly independent (which they were not because of correlations among the baseline variables), the Bonferroni inequality[13] would suggest testing each interaction at a significance level of 0.05/48 or 0.00104 (corresponding to normal deviates of ±3.28). These critical values were refined, taking into account the observed correlation structure among the 48 baseline variables, by use of a computer simulation procedure. In each replication of this procedure, vital status was assigned randomly to each patient in the DT4 and placebo groups and the magnitude of the maximum interaction effect among the 48 baseline variables was determined. By this means it was found that the observed interactions with treatment for baseline heart rate and for history of angina pectoris both fell in the 5% tail of the simulated distribution of maximum interaction effects. It was concluded from this analysis that there very likely was a real difference in the effects of DT4 on mortality between the two subgroups defined by each of these two variables.

The second approach to the statistical evaluation of subgroup findings focused on two rather complicated subgroups based on entry heart rate, history of angina pectoris, and risk categorization. In the data report prepared for a previous DSMC meeting, these two subgroups were defined as a result of a trial and error process of maximizing the treatment-subgroup interaction with respect to total mortality. Patients in Subgroup A had a baseline heart rate less than 70 beats per minute and either were classified as Risk 1 or had no history of angina pectoris prior to entry into the study. Patients in the complementary subgroup, Subgroup B, either had a baseline heart rate of 70 or more beats per minute or had a history of suspect or definite angina pectoris prior to entry and also were classified as Risk 2 at baseline. For Subgroup A the Z-value for the DT4-placebo difference was −2.60 and for Subgroup B it was +3.29 (Table 2). The z value for interaction was 3.96 for these subgroups.

It was considered that if a subgroup decision were to be made for the DT4 treatment, Subgroup B would likely be the best one in which to discontinue DT4. But since this subgroup was constructed solely as a result of analyzing the data many different ways, there was inadequate statistical evidence that this would indeed be the best subgroup to stop. Hence the patients were followed for another few months to see if DT4 continued to do poorly in Subgroup B and well in Subgroup A. During this additional follow-up period, in Subgroup B DT4 continued to show a greater than 40% higher mortality than the placebo group (5.4% vs. 3.8%), thus justifying the choice of this subgroup as one in which DT4 treatment should be discontinued. However, in Subgroup A, there was no longer a mortality benefit with DT4 (2.5% vs. 2.4%; Table 2).[7]

As a result of these and other data analyses, the DSMC, at its meeting on October 21, 1971, unanimously approved a motion to discontinue DT4 medication in Subgroup B. Following this a motion was made to discontinue DT4 medication in Subgroup A as well. This motion was passed by a narrow 7–6 margin. The main reason for not continuing DT4 in Subgroup A or in any other subgroup was the failure to identify any subgroup in which DT4 showed any consistent evidence of benefit. These decisions were affirmed by the CDP Policy Board.[10]

In this case, the decision process might have been somewhat less complicated if hypotheses had been stated in advance—at the beginning of the study—concerning treatment effects in specific subgroups. It is recommended that consideration be given to specification of subgroup hypotheses prior to the start of clinical trials.

Low-Dose-Estrogen

In March 1973 a decision was reached to discontinue the 2.5-mg/day estrogen (ESG1) group.[8] This decision was based on an excess incidence of venous thromboembolism, an excess mortality (not quite statistically significant) from all cancers, and a small, statistically insignificant excess of total mortality in the ESG1 group compared to the placebo group. The last of these reasons will provide the focus of discussion in this section.

The CDP was carried out for the purpose of assessing whether any beneficial effects of study drugs significantly outweighed any adverse effects. For obvious ethical reasons, it did not seek to prove beyond a shadow of a doubt that any drug was positively harmful. As of February 1, 1973, 19.9% of the patients in the ESG1 group had died, compared to 18.8% in the placebo group (Table 3).[8] This difference was not statistically significant, and there was no clear evidence that the drug was doing definite harm. The question was then posed: What is the possibility that this trend could reverse itself with ESG1 showing a statistically significant beneficial effect at the end of the study in summer 1974? It was projected that there would be 670 deaths in the placebo group by the end of the study (Table 3, line C). In order for the ESG1 group mortality to be significantly lower (i.e., 1.96 standard errors lower or a conventional p-value of 0.05) than the placebo mortality, there would have to be no more than 232 deaths in the ESG1 group. (Had multi-

Table 3   Projection of Future Mortality Experience, Low Dose Estrogen (ESG1) and Placebo Groups, Coronary Drug Project

	ESG1	Placebo
A. Current % deaths	19.9	18.8
	(219/1,101)	(525/2,789)
B. Current survivors	882	2,264
C. % deaths at end of study,	21.1	24.0
1.96 SE difference	(232/1,101)	(670/2,789)
D. Future % deaths given	1.5	6.4
1.96 SE difference at end of study	(12/882)	(145/2,264)

Source: Coronary Drug Project Research Group.[10]

ple data reviews, endpoints, and treatment groups been taken into account in this analysis, a larger number of standard errors would have had to be specified.) Given that as of the date of analysis, February 1, 1973, there were 219 and 525 deaths in the ESG1 and placebo groups respectively, this meant that the future mortality in the two groups would have to be 1.5% for ESG1 and 6.4% for placebo (Table 3, line D). Since this was considered to be an extremely unlikely outcome given the experience to date, this analysis plus the other considerations noted earlier led to the early discontinuation of the ESG1 group in 1973.[10]

A statistical refinement of the preceding method has been developed by Halperin and Ware using observed follow-up time and time to death for each study patient, rather than simply life-death status at a given time point.[14] By means of this method it was demonstrated, using the February 1, 1973 data, that it would be not only unlikely but virtually impossible for the ESG1 group to end up with a significantly lower mortality than the placebo group.

Clofibrate

At the conclusion of the CDP, the mortality of the clofibrate group was almost identical to that of the placebo group (25.5% versus 25.4%).[9] However, it was not always this way. Figure 1 shows the Z-values for the clofibrate–placebo differences in proportion of deaths computed at two-

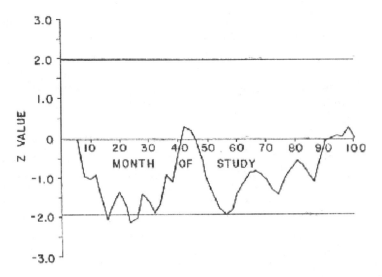

Figure 1 Z-values for clofibrate-placebo differences in proportion of deaths by calendar month since beginning of study (Month 0 = March 1966, Month 100 = July 1974). Reproduced from CDP (1981) with permission of the *Control Clin Trials.* Source: Coronary Drug Project Research Group.[10]

month intervals throughout the course of the study.[10] In this figure, Month 0 corresponds to March 1966, the month in which the first patients were enrolled in the CDP. Month 100 corresponds to July 1974, when patient follow-up was concluded. On three occasions during the first 30 months of the study the Z-value exceeded the −1.96 boundary (signifying a conventional p-value less than 0.05). If the DSMC had decided to stop the study and declare clofibrate therapeutically efficacious on the basis of these early "statistically significant" results, it is evident that in retrospect it would very likely have been the wrong decision. Fortunately, the DSMC was careful not to react quickly and drastically to results that reached "statistical significance" at the conventional 5% level. The reason for this was the committee's realization that the chances of finding significant differences in the absence of true differences became much higher than 5%—perhaps as high as 30 or 35%—when the data were examined repeatedly over time for such differences[15] and when five different drug groups were being compared to placebo at each of these time points.

Several statistical methods were used in the CDP to take account of the repeated analysis of treatment effects in the decision-making process. These included a modification of sequential statistical testing procedures applicable to clinical trials with long response time,[11,12] an approach developed by Cornfield using the likelihood principle,[16-18] and the Halperin–Ware procedure based on a Wilcoxon two-sample test for accumulating survival data.[14] The use of each of these methods required a much more extreme Z-value than −1.96 early in the study to conclude that a statistically significant difference had been found.

Although clofibrate ultimately showed no benefit overall, the question was raised as to whether the patients who adhered well to the clofibrate treatment regimen and those who experienced a lowering of serum cholesterol showed any benefit with respect to mortality and cardiovascular morbidity.[19] However, the DSMC leadership wisely resisted looking at the data in these ways on the grounds that there was no valid way of interpreting these data as there were no similar subgroups among the placebo patients to be used for comparison. It was postulated that the reasons for good adherence and cholesterol lowering would be quite different between the clofibrate and placebo groups. The wise restraint shown by the DSMC members on this issue was justified later when analyses were carried out for the purpose of demonstrating the problems with interpreting such analyses by post-baseline subgroups. Clofibrate and placebo group patients were classified according to their cumulative adherence—the estimated number of capsules actually taken as a percentage of the number that should have been taken according to protocol during the first five years of follow-up or until death, if earlier. For those with ≥80% adherence, five-year mortality was nearly identical in the clofibrate and placebo groups (15.0% vs. 15.1%). For those with

<80% adherence, five-year mortality was somewhat lower for clofibrate (24.6%) than for placebo (28.2%). But the most astounding finding came from focusing on the two figures for the placebo group: 15.1% mortality for good adherers versus 28.2% for poor adherers. The z value for this difference was -8.12 (p = 4.7×10^{-16}). Adjustment for 40 baseline characteristics reduced the mortality difference between good and poor adherers only to 16.4% versus 25.8% (Z = -5.78). In conclusion, it is doubtful that any valid conclusions can be drawn from analyses like these because there is no way of ascertaining precisely how or why the patients in the treated and control groups have selected themselves or have become selected into the subgroups of good and poor adherers.[20]

Niacin

The results in the niacin group were unremarkable. While there were substantial reductions in the niacin group in definite non-fatal MI (Z = -3.09) and the combination of CHD death or definite non-fatal MI (Z = -2.77) at the end of the trial, neither of these were the primary outcome, which was all-cause mortality. Thus, the following conclusion was reported by the CDP Research Group: "The Coronary Drug Project data yield no evidence that niacin influences mortality of survivors of myocardial infarction; this medication may be slightly beneficial in protecting persons to some degree against recurrent non-fatal myocardial infarction. However, because of the excess incidence of arrhythmias, gastrointestinal problems, and abnormal chemistry findings in the niacin group, great care and caution must be exercised if this drug is to be used for treatment of persons with coronary heart disease."[9]

However, "the game's not over till it's over," as the saying goes. Nine years later, the NHLBI provided funding to the CDP Coordinating Center to conduct a mortality follow-up of CDP patients. The main interest was to ascertain whether there continued to be an excess of cancer deaths in the two estrogen groups. The answer to that question turned out to be no. However, most surprisingly, a highly significant reduction in all-cause mortality was seen in the niacin group compared to placebo (52.0% vs. 58.2%; Z = -3.52) as well as to all other CDP treatment groups.[21] Because of this there is renewed interest among cardiologists in prescribing niacin for modification of serum lipid levels in persons at risk for CHD.

LESSONS LEARNED

Some of the lessons learned from the data and safety monitoring experiences in the CDP include the following:

1. First and most fundamentally of all, do not share accruing treatment group data with the Clinical Center investigators.

2. Double-blinding (or masking) is good and wise; triple-blinding (where the members of the DSMC and Policy Board are blinded as to identification of the study treatments in the data monitoring reports) is not so good and wise. This is a lesson that more and more present-day DSMBs are failing, or refusing, to accept. Assimilating hundreds of pages of tables and graphs on a great variety of safety and efficacy outcomes in a short period of time is difficult enough for members of a DSMB without their being blinded to treatment group identification as well. With treatment group blinding, significant patterns in the data with respect to treatment efficacy or safety might easily be missed. Furthermore, decisions concerning treatment efficacy are not symmetrical with those concerning treatment safety, with more evidence required for early stopping for efficacy than for safety.

3. Baseline characteristics used for stratification or blocking of randomized treatment allocations should not automatically be assumed to imply *a priori* subgroup hypotheses.

4. Prior to initiating patient accrual for a clinical trial, hypotheses about treatment effects in specific subgroups of patients should be stated in the study protocol. More precisely, it is preferable to state such hypotheses in terms of baseline characteristics having statistical *interactions* with treatment differences rather than making statements about treatment efficacy in specific subgroups.

5. If, toward the end of the follow-up period, the probability of ending up with a beneficial treatment effect is virtually nil, and there is not even hope of finding sufficient benefit in any subgroup of patients to warrant the design of a new clinical trial, then serious consideration should be given to stopping the study—or treatment arm—early. In the CDP, the patients in the three treatment arms that were stopped prematurely for adverse effects or lack of efficacy were put to good use. A short-term randomized trial of aspirin and placebo was carried out in these patients.[22] The results were promising enough to warrant additional clinical trials of aspirin in patients with CHD, and the rest is history.

6. If a DSMB is reviewing accruing outcome data several times during the course of the trial, then statistical tests need to be adjusted for multiple looks at the data. Adjustment for multiple treatment arms and multiple primary outcome variables may also be necessary.[23]

7. Given the existence of the National Death Index, it would seem generally to be a cost-effective exercise to carry out a mortality surveillance perhaps five years after the conclusion of a clinical trial, especially when the participants are old enough to have a sizable five-year mortality. Even if the

original clinical trial is negative, there is always the potential for long-term surprises, as found in the group treated with niacin in the CDP.

8. Decision-making in clinical trials is complicated and often protracted. Although a number of rather sophisticated statistical tools are available to assist in the decision-making process, these are at best red flags that warn of possible treatment problems and can never be used by themselves as hard and fast decision rules. No single statistical decision rule or procedure can take the place of the well-reasoned consideration of all aspects of the data by a group of concerned, competent, and experienced persons with a wide range of scientific backgrounds and points of view.[10]

REFERENCES

1. Zukel WJ. 1983. Evolution and funding of the Coronary Drug Project. *Control Clin Trials* 4:281-312.
2. Coronary Drug Project Research Group. 1973. The Coronary Drug Project. Design, methods, and baseline results. *Circulation* 47 (suppl. 1):I1-I79.
3. Canner PL, Klimt CR. 1983. Experimental design features of the Coronary Drug Project. *Control Clin Trials* 4:313-332.
4. Dunnett CW. 1955. Multiple comparison procedures for comparing several treatments with a control. *J Am Statist Assoc* 50:1096-1121.
5. Canner PL. 1983. Monitoring of the data for evidence of adverse or beneficial treatment effects in the Coronary Drug Project. *Control Clin Trials* 4:467-483.
6. Coronary Drug Project Research Group. 1970 The Coronary Drug Project. Initial findings leading to modifications of its research protocol. *JAMA* 214:1303-1313.
7. Coronary Drug Project Research Group. 1972. The Coronary Drug Project. Findings leading to further modifications of its protocol with respect to dextrothyroxine. *JAMA* 220:996-1008.
8. Coronary Drug Project Research Group. 1973. The Coronary Drug Project. Findings leading to discontinuation of the 2.5 mg/day estrogen group. *JAMA* 226:652-657.
9. Coronary Drug Project Research Group. 1975. Clofibrate and niacin in coronary heart disease. *JAMA* 231:360-381.
10. Coronary Drug Project Research Group. 1981. Practical aspects of decision making in clinical trials: The Coronary Drug Project as a case study. *Control Clin Trials* 1:363-376.
11. Armitage P, McPherson CK, Rowe BC. 1969. Repeated significance tests on accumulating data. *J R Statist Soc A* 132:235-244.
12. Canner PL. 1977. Monitoring treatment differences in long-term clinical trials. *Biometrics* 33:603-615.
13. Miller RG. 1966. *Simultaneous Statistical Inference*. McGraw-Hill, New York.
14. Halperin M, Ware J. 1974. Early decision in a censored Wilcoxon two-sample test for accumulating survival data. *J Am Statist Assoc* 69:414-422.
15. Armitage P. 1975. *Sequential Medical Trials*, 2nd ed. Wiley, New York .
16. Cornfield J. 1966. Sequential trials, sequential analysis and the likelihood principle. *Am Statistician* 20:18-23.
17. Cornfield J. 1966. A Bayesian test of some classical hypotheses—with applications to sequential clinical trials. *J Am Statist Assoc* 61:577-594.
18. Cornfield J. 1969. The Bayesian outlook and its application. *Biometrics* 25:617-657.
19. Feinstein AR. 1977. Clinical biostatistics. XLI. Hard science, soft data, and the challenges of choosing clinical variables in research. *Clin Pharmacol Ther* 22:485-498.

20. Coronary Drug Project Research Group. 1980. Influence of adherence to treatment and response of cholesterol on mortality in the Coronary Drug Project. *N Engl J Med* 303:1038-1041.
21. Canner PL, Berge KG, Wenger NK, Stamler J, Friedman L, Prineas RJ, Friedewald W. 1986. Fifteen year mortality in Coronary Drug Project patients: Long-term benefit with niacin. *J Am Coll Cardiol* 8:1245-1255.
22. Coronary Drug Project Research Group. 1976. Aspirin in coronary heart disease. *J Chron Dis* 29:625-642.
23. Canner PL. 1984. Monitoring long-term clinical trials for beneficial and adverse treatment effects. *Commun Statist Theor Meth* 13:2369-2394.

The Data Monitoring Experience in the Cardiac Arrhythmia Suppression Trial: The Need to Be Prepared Early

David L. DeMets
Lawrence M. Friedman

ABSTRACT

The Cardiac Arrhythmia Suppression Trial (CAST) was designed to evaluate the hypothesis that suppression of cardiac ventricular arrhythmias in patients with a recent myocardial infarction would reduce the incidence of sudden death and total mortality, using three drugs known to suppress cardiac arrhythmias. Patients were randomized to receive either active drug or a matching placebo. The trial was terminated after only 15% of the planned-for events had been observed with an unexpected but dramatic increase in sudden death and total mortality in those patients receiving two of the active therapies. Later, the third drug was also discontinued.

INTRODUCTION AND BACKGROUND

Premature contractions/depolarizations of the left ventricle of the heart in a patient population surviving a myocardial infarction are a risk factor for sudden death and cardiac mortality. Increases in these premature contractions/depolarizations are associated with a fourfold higher mortality rate.[1,2] Drugs such an encainide, flecainide, and moricizine were established as being very effective in suppressing these premature ventricular contractions; the first two drugs were approved by regulatory agencies for treatment of serious arrhythmias, but moricizine was not yet approved in the United States. Physicians began to treat patients with ventricular arrhythmias during the 1980s, using encainide and flecainide, as they were more effective and better tolerated than other antiarrhythmic drugs.[3] There was widespread belief that these drugs should reduce mortality because of their antiarrhythmic effect, despite the fact that previous trials had not shown that use of these drugs reduced the risk of sudden or cardiac death.[4] Thus, despite increasing use of these drugs, the question remained as to whether anti-arrhythmiac treatment was of clinical benefit to the patient surviving a myocardial infarction but experiencing ventricular arrhythmias.

PROTOCOL DESIGN

Following a pilot trial, the Cardiac Arrhythmia Pilot Study (CAPS),[5] which established the arrhythmia-suppressing effect of encainide, flecainide, and moricizine in a population of post-infarct patients, the Cardiac Arrhythmia Suppression Trial (CAST) was designed.[6] The CAPS pilot study had not indicated any major toxicity. CAST, sponsored by the National Heart, Lung, and Blood Institute (NHLBI), was designed as a randomized, placebo-controlled trial to evaluate the effect of these three drugs in reducing the incidence of sudden cardiac death (primary) or death from any cause (secondary).[6] The patient population consisted of men and women with a myocardial infarction who had asymptomatic or minimally symptomatic ventricular arrhythmias with some reduced ventricular function.

The trial started with an open label titration or run-in period, with patients given, in random order, one or more of the three drugs, to identify those who would respond to treatment by having at least an 80% arrhythmia suppression. Patients with this level of arrhythmia suppression were then eligible to be randomized into the main study to either the effective drug or its matching placebo. Patients who had increased arrhythmias or could not tolerate the drugs were not entered.

The primary endpoint in CAST was death due to arrhythmia. Secondary endpoints included total mortality and cardiac death for any cause. Anticipated potential adverse events included an increase in arrhythmias, electrocardiographic changes, and worsening heart failure. The trial was initially designed to randomize 4,400 patients with 90% power to detect a 30% reduction in sudden death, using a one-tailed 0.05 significance level. This design assumed an 11% cumulative rate of sudden death over the three years of planned follow-up. The primary test statistic to compare time to sudden death between active therapy and placebo was the logrank test. CAST had an independent Data and Safety Monitoring Board (DSMB) which was scheduled to meet twice yearly. The rationale for the one-tailed 0.05 test was that it was not the main objective of CAST to demonstrate a harmful effect and that DSMBs were unlikely to allow trials to continue to that level of evidence.[7]

Patient enrollment began in June 1987 and was scheduled to be completed in June 1990. In April 1989, the DSMB recommended that two of the

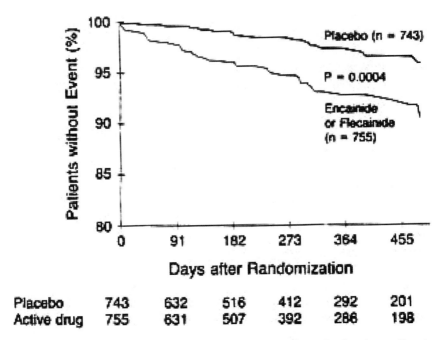

Figure 1 Actuarial Probabilities of Freedom from Death or Cardiac Arrest *Due to Arrhythmia* in 1498 Patients Receiving Encainide or Flecainide or Corresponding Placebo. The number of patients at risk of an event is shown along the bottom of the figure. Reproduced from CAST (1991) with permission of the *N Engl J Med.*

three drugs in CAST, encainide and flecainide, be stopped because of a likely harmful effect from these drugs.[6,8] The final results from these two drugs are shown in Figures 1 and 2, with cause specific mortality shown in Table 1. Later, the DSMB recommended termination of moricizine as well.[9] For the rest of this presentation, we will refer to the first portion of CAST as CAST-I and the subsequent moricizine-alone portion as CAST-II.[9]

DATA MONITORING EXPERIENCE

In March of 1987, the DSMB met for the first time to review the protocol.[10] While the investigators had designed CAST to be a one-tailed 0.05 design, the DSMB voted to recommend a one-tailed 0.025 alpha level to test for treatment benefit, which reduced the power from 90% to approximately 85%. Their rationale was that a trial should require the same level/strength of evidence for benefit, regardless of whether the design was one-tailed or two-tailed. A one-tailed 0.025 requires the same critical value (i.e., 1.96) for

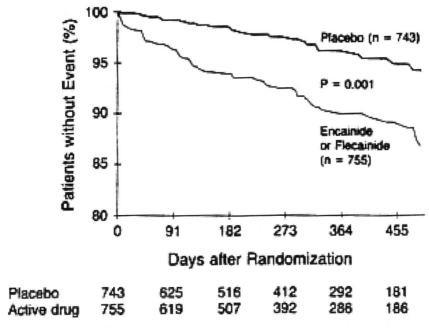

Figure 2 Actuarial Probabilities of Freedom from Death or Cardiac Arrest *Due to Any Cause* in 1498 Patients Receiving Encainide or Flecainide or Corresponding Placebo. The number at risk is shown along the bottom of the figure. Reproduced from CAST (1991) with permission of the *New England Journal of Medicine.*

Table 1 Cause of Death and Cardiac Arrest (with Resuscitation) in the CAST, According to Treatment Group

Cause	Both Groups		Total
	Active Drug	Placebo	
Patients in group	755	743	1498
All deaths and cardiac arrests	63	[†]26	89
Cardiac death or cardiac arrest	60	[‡]21	81
Arrest with resuscitation	7	1	8
Death or arrest due to			
Arrhythmia	43	[§]16	59
Arrest with resuscitation	5	1	6
Death or arrest not due to			
Arrhythmia	17	[¶]5	22
Arrest with resuscitation	2	0	2
Noncardiac death	3	[¥]5	8

[†] $P = 0.0001$ for comparison with patients receiving active drug.
[‡] $P < 0.0001$ for comparison with patients receiving active drug.
[§] $P = 0.0004$ for comparison with patients receiving active drug.
[¶] $P = 0.0107$ for comparison with patients receiving active drug.
[¥] $P = 0.4822$ for comparison with patients receiving active drug.
Modified Table 1. N Engl J Med 324:781–788, 1991.

the test statistic as a two tailed 0.05 level design. A conservative group sequential 0.025 boundary was established to monitor for treatment benefit. At the same time, the DSMB recommended a 0.025 lower symmetric advisory boundary for adverse effects as well. In addition, conditional power methods were to be used for assessing the futility of achieving a beneficial effect with an interim observed negative trend. Both the beneficial and harmful sequential boundaries were implemented using the approach of Lan and DeMets,[11,12] using the expected number of cardiac sudden deaths (initially estimated to be 425 and later revised to 300 due to a lower than expected placebo event rate) to calculate the observed information fraction (observed events/expected total events). The sequential boundaries for the logrank test statistic are shown in Figure 3. These lower boundaries were called advisory because the DSMB did not want to be bound to crossing these thresholds for negative or harmful trends.

At the second meeting in January of 1988, before outcome data were available, the DSMB decided to remain partially blinded in their review of interim data, seeing tables by codes with the intent of maintaining objectivity. However, the DSMB also agreed that it could totally unblind its members should they need to in their deliberations.

In September of 1988, the DSMB met to finalize the monitoring plan and to review very preliminary data on 1,147 patients already randomized, which was approximately one-fourth of the target. Data were provided partially

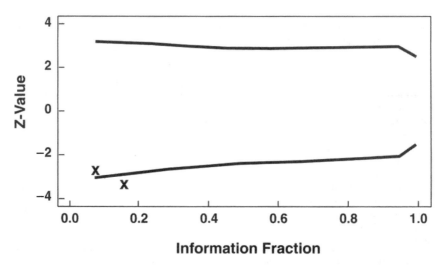

Figure 3 CAST Sequential Boundaries. Reproduced from CAST (1991) with permission of the *N Engl J Med.*

blinded, labeled Drug X and Drug Y. The primary endpoint, sudden death, was 3/576 for Drug X and 19/571 for Drug Y. These 22 events represented approximately 5% of the expected primary events. Since the number of events was very small and the goal of CAST was to evaluate longer/chronic term use of these drugs, the DSMB decided no recommendations were appropriate and remained blinded, with the plan to meet again in six months.

Meanwhile, the CAST Coordinating Center summarized the data monthly for its own internal monitoring and notified the Project Office at the NHLBI in late January of 1989 that the results had become more extreme. On February 13, unblinded updated tables for the primary events were presented to NHLBI. The Chair of the DSMB was notified and a conference call with the board was scheduled for March 2, 1989. The DSMB was informed of the updated analyses and unblinded. The results were substantially trending in a negative or harmful direction. A series of additional analyses were requested including verification of treatment codes and a sweep of the clinical sites for as yet unreported primary events. The DSMB decided to meet at its regularly scheduled meeting on April 16 and 17, 1989, to review all of the available data and the additional analyses.

At the April 1989 DSMB, data presented during the conference call were all confirmed. The advisory boundary for harm, with all three drugs combined, had been crossed. At this time, most of the events were in the encainide and flecainide arms, and their respective placebo controls. Because moricizine was not as effective in suppressing ventricular arrhythmias as were encainide or flecainide, fewer patients were assigned to moricizine or its placebo. Although the initial goal of CAST was to evaluate overall active treatment versus placebo, the DSMB decided to focus on the two treatments that had sufficient numbers of patients and events. In the encainide and flecainide arms, there were 33 sudden cardiac deaths on active treatment and nine on placebo. There were 56 deaths on treatment and 22 on placebo. The DSMB recommended that the encainide and flecainide arms be dropped from the protocol. The DSMB concluded that it was too soon to make judgments about moricizine. Not only were there very few events among those on moricizine or its corresponding placebo, the results were trending slightly in favor of the active drug. That same day, the sponsor of the study— the National Heart, Lung and Blood Institute—was notified. The principal investigators were informed the following day. Because the study was international (clinics in the United States, Canada, and Sweden), the drug regulatory agencies from those countries were also immediately notified. In addition, because of the concerns that many non-study patients were being treated with these drugs, the public was quickly alerted to the findings. A preliminary report was published[6] as rapidly as the data could be assembled.

It should be noted that a subsequent publication[8] reported on the final results, after all outstanding data had been incorporated. At that time, the deaths were 63 in the encainide-flecainide group and 26 in the placebo groups (Table 1).

In retrospect, the observed data (3 vs. 19) on September of 1988 would also have crossed the lower advisory bound for harm. However, if the data sweep had occurred at that time, the updated data (10 versus 22) would not have crossed the lower boundary although still indicating a very negative trend. The interim logrank results are shown on the sequential boundary plot shown in Figure 3.

Following the DSMB recommendation for encainide–flecainide (i.e., CAST-I), the board recommended that CAST be redesigned for the moricizine versus placebo comparison to continue. Moricizine was pharmacologically different from encainide and flecainide, and thus the answer to its effect on sudden death was still unknown. Of the remaining 2,100 patients to be enrolled, half would be randomized to moricizine and the rest to the matching placebo. Patients still on the encainide–flecainide portion could be re-randomized to CAST-II. However, another important design change was made. In CAST-I, the run-in period had patients only on active treatment, so no comparisons with a placebo could be made. The mortality event rate observed during this period appeared to be higher than expected. In the redesign, patients enrolled in the two-week run-in period were randomized to moricizine or placebo. Those who were initially randomized to placebo were subsequently placed on moricizine in order to see if their arrhythmias were suppressed by the drug. If patients had 90% of their arrhythmias suppressed, they were eligible to be randomized to the main study. This redesign allowed the CAST investigators to evaluate the risk of initial exposure to moricizine by having a placebo comparison during the two-week run-in with over 70% power for a two-fold increase in sudden death.[9]

At the April 1991 meeting, the DSMB reviewed interim mortality data, partially blinded as before, for the CAST-II trial. While there were no apparent trends for the moricizine–placebo comparison in the main study, an apparent difference was emerging in the run-in period: 12 versus 3. Given the CAST-I experience, the DSMB decide to unblind and became aware that the 12 sudden deaths were on the moricizine arm, including the last six events.

The advisory lower boundary harm as applied to the run-in period had not been crossed and the confidence intervals around the estimated treatment effect were quite wide. Although at the time that CAST-I ended, moricizine had shown a small, but positive trend, now, with further data, the likelihood of a treatment benefit in the main trial was less than 30%. The DSMB voted to continue CAST-II and meet again in three months.

At the July 1991 meeting, the DSMB recommended that CAST-II be terminated. In the two-week run-in period, there were now 15 sudden deaths on moricizine and still three on placebo, a result that is statistically significant at $p = 0.02$ after adjusting for monitoring. The conditional power for the main study had dropped to less than 10%. Given the total CAST experience, the DSMB felt the results were sufficiently compelling to recommend that moricizine should not be used for these indications. The final data in the run-in period, after all events were accounted for, was 17 to 3.

LESSONS LEARNED

1. The CAST experience has provided both the cardiology and the clinical trial community with many valuable lessons. One fundamental lesson is that conventional wisdom and practice can be wrong. Prior to CAST, the consensus was that suppression of asymptomatic or minimally symptomatic ventricular arrhythmias was beneficial in patients who had survived a myocardial infarction. The fact that the presence of the arrhythmias is correlated with the subsequent risk of sudden or cardiovascular death lead many to view the suppression of arrhythmias as a surrogate for the clinical outcome. CAST proved that suppression of ventricular arrhythmias is not in fact a surrogate for the clinical outcome of sudden or cardiovascular death. Arrhythmia suppression may be important but is clearly not sufficient. This trial is one of many that have demonstrated the challenges and dangers of using invalid surrogate outcomes.[13]

2. A related issue is the one-sided versus the two-sided hypothesis issue that the CAST DSMB raised. Based on conventional wisdom of a treatment's likely effect, it may make sense to consider a one-sided test of the hypothesis of the treatment benefit. However, CAST illustrates that conventional wisdom is not always correct. Many trials may be considered as having two one-sided hypotheses, one for a positive beneficial treatment effect and the other in a negative direction testing for possible harm. The degree of evidence for these two one-sided hypotheses need not be the same. Keeping the level of evidence for treatment benefit to be the same, regardless of whether the hypothesis is posed as one-sided or two-sided hypothesis, seems advisable. For example, the two-sided 0.05 alpha level trial and the one-sided 0.025 alpha level designs both require a test statistic of 1.96 or approximately two standard errors (with no adjustments for interim analysis) to be judged significant and beneficial. The lower boundary for harm could be symmetric as was done for CAST-I or asymmetric as was used in CAST-II. In either case, the lower boundary is more of a guide for the DSMB because clinical judgment is often critical in assessing negative or harmful trends. For example, a DSMB may choose not to wait until a lower sequential boundary

has been crossed depending on other factors observed in the data. For that reason, the CAST DSMB referred to the lower boundary as advisory. Of course, at the time they made those recommendations, they did not anticipate that such boundaries would play a role. It was fortunate that the lower advisory boundary was in place prior to the September 1988 DSMB meeting.

3. Another lesson is that trials must have the DSMB in place prior to the start of the trial. Often DSMBs are convened some months after the trial has started randomizing patients. This may cause two problems. First, the DSMB may have some constructive suggestions regarding the design which are difficult to incorporate once the trial is underway. In CAST, the DSMB made a suggestion as to the significance level that should be required. Furthermore, the negative trends began to emerge at the first DSMB meeting where data were available and got rapidly more negative by the time only 15% of the expected events had been observed. If CAST had waited until 25% or 50% of the expected primary events had been observed, a number of patients would have been unnecessarily harmed. Thus, the DSMB should be appointed and convened prior to the initiation of the trial.

4. In order to support the DSMB, the data management system must be in place and functioning. As CAST demonstrated, having data as early as the first 5% of events and in the months following was critical. While some delay in getting data from the clinics into the database is to be expected, that delay cannot be months. For example, had the CAST DSMB focused on the logrank test statistic at their first analyses, they would have observed that the lower advisory boundary was being approached. Yet, in retrospect, the actual number of events at the point in time would not have been so extreme in the negative direction. The DSMB and CAST would have been in a very awkward situation to have recommended termination due to the extreme test statistic but find that the evidence had weakened with the data cleanup. Fortunately, current informatics technology allows for rapid transmission of key outcome data but unless these are put into place, the DSMB is left vulnerable and consequently current and future patients.

5. Regardless of how detailed the DSMB charter and monitoring plan are, the DSMB will likely have to react to unexpected events and situations. The DSMB has to have contingency plans to react in a timely fashion. For example, the redesign of the run-in period for CAST-II turned out to be extremely important, indicating that simple exposure to these drugs for post infarction patients with ventricular arrhythmias was sufficient to increase the risk of sudden death. The lack of a placebo control in the titration run-in for the pilot and CAST-I made interpretation of initial risk difficult.

6. Finally, the CAST DSMB had to weigh the balance between obtaining convincing and persuasive evidence with ethical responsibility to current and future patients. If the data are not allowed to become convincing, then belief and practice may not change, which would have put even more patients at risk. However, prolonging the trial beyond the point where the data have become persuasive would be placing patients at unnecessary risk. The point at which data become persuasive is largely based on the DSMB's best judgment. Statistical methods such as sequential monitoring boundaries can be very useful for the primary outcome or outcomes but the totality of information must be considered in any DSMB recommendation.[14,15] In CAST, the evidence was accumulating very rapidly so there was not much time for deliberation. This requires that the DSMB and monitoring procedures be put in place at the beginning and that data flow be very current.

REFERENCES

1. Bigger JT Jr, Fleiss JL, Kleiger R, Miller JP, Rolnitzky LM. 1984. The relationships among ventricular arrhythmias, left ventricular dysfunction, and mortality in the 2 years after myocardial infarction. *Circulation* 69:250-258.
2. Ruberman W, Weinblatt E, Goldberg JD, Frank CW, Shapiro S. 1977. Ventricular premature beats and mortality after myocardial infarction. *N Engl J Med* 297:750-757.
3. Morganroth J, Bigger JT, Jr, Anderson JL. 1990. Treatment of ventricular arrhythmia by United States cardiologists: a survey before the Cardiac Arrhythmia Suppression Trials results were available. *Am J Cardiol* 65:40-48.
4. Furberg CD. 1983. Effect of antiarrhythmic drugs on mortality after myocardial infarction. *Am J Cardiol* 52:32C-36C.
5. The Cardiac Arrhythmia Pilot Study (CAPS) Investigators. 1988. Effects of encainide, flecainide, imipramine and moricizine on ventricular arrhythmias during the year after acute myocardial infarction: The CAPS. *Am J Cardiol* 61:501-509.
6. The Cardiac Arrhythmia Suppression Trial (CAST) Investigators. 1989. Preliminary report: effect of encainide and flecainide on mortality in a randomized trial of arrhythmia suppression after myocardial infarction. *N Engl J Med* 321:406-412.
7. Lan KKG, Friedman L. 1986. Monitoring boundaries for adverse effects in long-term clinical trials. *Control Clin Trials* 7:1-7.
8. Echt DS, Liebson PR, Mitchell LB, Peters RW, Obias-Manno D, Barker AH, et al. 1991. Mortality and morbidity in patients receiving encainide, flecainide, or placebo. The Cardiac Arrhythmia Suppression Trial. *N Engl J Med* 324: 781-788.
9. Cardiac Arrhythmia Suppression Trial II Investigators. 1992. Effects of the antiarrhythmic agent moricizine on survival after myocardial infarction. *N Engl J Med* 327:227-233.
10. Friedman LM, Bristow JD, Hallstrom A, Schron E, Proschan M, Verter J, DeMets D, et al. 1993. Data monitoring in the cardiac arrhythmia suppression trial. *Online Journal of Current Clinical Trials* Doc 79, ISSN 1059-2725, July 31.
11. Lan KKG, DeMets DL. 1983 Discrete sequential boundaries for clinical trials. *Biometrika* 70:659-663.
12. Pawitan Y, Hallstrom A. 1990. Statistical interim monitoring of the Cardiac Arrhythmia Suppression Trial. *Stat Med* 9:1081-1090.
13. Fleming TR, DeMets DL. 1993. Monitoring of clinical trials: issues and recommendations. *Control Clin Trials* 14:183-197.

14. Canner PL: 1977. Monitoring treatment differences in long-term clinical trials. *Biometrics* 33:603–615.
15. Ellenberg S, Fleming T and DeMets D. 2002. *Data Monitoring Committees in Clinical Trials: A Practical Perspective*. John Wiley & Sons, Ltd., West Sussex, England.

Data Monitoring in the Prospective Randomized Milrinone Survival Evaluation: Dealing With an Agonizing Trend

Susan Anderson
Robert Cody
Milton Packer
Richard Schwarz

ABSTRACT

The Prospective Randomized Milrinone Survival Evaluation (PROMISE) was conducted to clarify discordant findings in previous experimental and clinical studies with milrinone, a cyclic AMP-enhancing positive inotropic agent. Earlier studies had shown positive effects of milrinone on cardiac function and exercise performance in patients with chronic heart failure. To determine the effect of milrinone on mortality, patients with severe chronic heart failure who remained symptomatic despite conventional therapy were randomized to receive either active drug or a matching placebo. The trial was terminated after 20 months, before its scheduled completion, based on an observed adverse effect of milrinone on survival. This paper describes the experience of the Data Monitoring and Safety Monitoring Board (DSMB) in dealing with an emerging negative trend in survival when there were other known beneficial effects of the drug.

INTRODUCTION AND BACKGROUND

Chronic heart failure is an increasing problem with an aging population. Over 500,000 cases are diagnosed each year, and the mortality risk for these patients remains unacceptably high. In the early 1990s few effective treatments were available and the search for new effective agents was a high priority.

209

Cyclic AMP-enhancing agents are among the drugs developed to enhance the inotropic state of the failing heart. Because the production of cyclic AMP is deficient in patients with advanced heart failure, the use of cyclicAMP-enhancing positive inotropic agents had theoretical appeal.[1-3] Experimental studies of heart failure in rats with milrinone showed an encouraging attenuation in the progression of ventricular enlargement after acute myocardial injury and prolongation of survival.[4,5] Despite the theoretical appeal, clinical studies of positive inotropic agents were largely unfavorable, raising concern that cyclic AMP-enhancing agents may accelerate the progression of disease, ventricular arrhythmias, and possibly shorten survival of patients with chronic heart failure.[5-11]

PROTOCOL DESIGN

Because of three major limitations of the earlier clinical studies[1] (most had been carried out in patients with mild-to-moderate symptoms,[2] most were conducted in patients not taking angiotensin converting-enzyme inhibitors,[3] and all were too small to evaluate influence of therapy on survival), PROMISE was designed to evaluate the effect of milrinone on survival in patients with severe chronic heart failure who remained symptomatic despite conventional therapy, which included digoxin, diuretics, and a converting-enzyme inhibitor.[12] Patients had dyspnea or fatigue at rest or on exertion, left ejection fraction $\leq$35% and symptoms of NYHA functional class III or IV for at least three months (including symptoms at rest within two weeks). Treatment with vasodilator drugs was allowed but not mandated.

Patients who met these and other eligibility requirements in screening assessments were randomized to receive milrinone (10 mg orally four times daily) or matching placebo, in addition to digoxin, diuretics, and a converting-enzyme inhibitor (captopril or enalapril).

The primary endpoint was death due to all causes. Secondary endpoints included cardiovascular mortality, number of hospitalizations, and addition of vasodilators due to worsening heart failure, symptoms, and adverse reactions. In addition, the effect of milrinone on survival was to be assessed in pre-specified subgroups defined by important prognostic baseline variables. The trial was designed to have 90% power to detect a 25% difference in mortality at a 0.05 significance level using a two-tailed logrank test. This design was event-driven and the study was planned to continue until 190 deaths had been observed on the placebo arm.

In order to conduct PROMISE as a model parallel to that conventionally used by the National Institutes of Health (NIH), PROMISE investigators modified the NIH model for application to an industry sponsored trial.[13] PROMISE had an independent statistical analysis center reporting to a Data and Safety

Monitoring Board (DSMB) scheduled to meet every four to six months; a Committee of Investigators, who designed the study; a Steering Committee, and a Clinical Coordinating center responsible for day-today policy decisions, all of whom functioned independently of the sponsor (Sterling Research Group). The organizational structure is shown in Figure 1. PROMISE was one of the first industry-sponsored trials to adopt such a model.[13] The Principal Investigator for the study as well as a few representatives (clinical, regulatory, and statistical) of the sponsor were present throughout the DSMB deliberations but were not voting members of the DSMB.

The trial began recruiting in January of 1989 and was projected (based on total mortality event rates) to be completed in March 1991. In October of 1990, the DSMB recommended to the sponsor that PROMISE be terminated early due to an observed adverse effect of milrinone on survival, particularly among patients with NYHA functional class IV.[12] Selected baseline

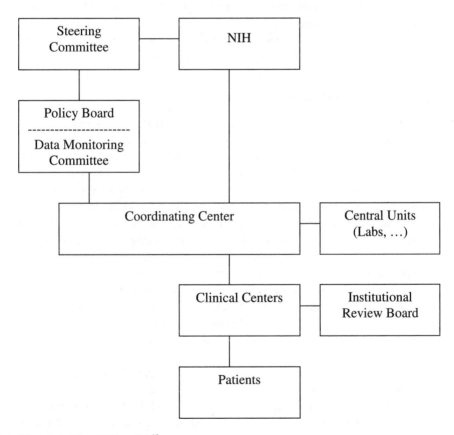

Figure 1 The NIH model.[13]

Table 1 Selected Baseline Characteristics by Treatment Group

Characteristic	Placebo	Milrinone
Number	527	561
Age	64.2	63.1
Gender (%Male)	80%	76%
Principal diagnosis: CHD	54%	54%
Functional class		
III	57%	58%
IV	43%	42%
Angina–previous mycardial infarction	27%	26%
Previous cardiac surgery	41%	39%

characteristics of the 1,088 randomized patients are shown in Table 1. The final results are shown in Figures 2 and 3 and in Table 2, indicating that the milrinone-treated patients had a higher mortality rate than those patients on placebo. The remainder of this discussion will be on the study history and decision process that leading to the recommendation.

DATA MONITORING EXPERIENCE

In November 1988, prior to the start of the study, the DSMB met to review the protocol and establish procedures for monitoring. At the request of the DSMB a written document, or charter, was prepared to specify the general guidelines for interim analysis and evaluation of interim data, including criteria for early stopping. Two-sided symmetric O'Brien–Fleming type boundaries as implemented by Lan and DeMets to allow flexibility in the number and timing of interim analyses while maintaining the total alpha at 0.05 were adopted.[14,15] The O'Brien–Fleming sequential boundaries were truncated at ±3.5 for the very early interim analyses. A number of considerations for the interpretation of the study data as an entirety were explicated and the guidelines stated that recommendation to modify or terminate the trial should not be based totally on statistical grounds. This document also specified procedures to be used to adjust the sample size in order to reach the target of 190 placebo deaths should the initial estimate of placebo mortality rate be incorrect.

In July of 1989, the DSMB met to review study data for the first time. At that time data was available on 233 patients enrolled in the study, and 19 patients had died, 6 on arm A and 13 on arm B. While the DSMB reviewed initially the monitoring report by code (Treatment A and Treatment B), they elected to be informed of treatment identity at this first meeting. Treatment

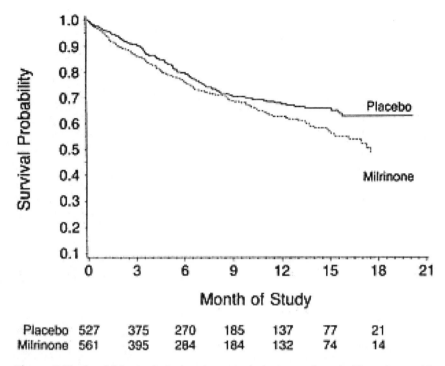

Figure 2 Kaplan-Meier analysis showing cumulative rates of survival in patients with chronic heart failure treated with milrinone or placebo. Mortality was 28% higher in the milrinone group than in the placebo group (p = 0.038). The numbers of patients at risk are shown at the bottom of the figure. Reproduced from Packer, et al. (1991) with permission of the *N Engl J Med.*

arm B was identified as milrinone. Of the 13 deaths in the milrinone arm, most of the adverse effect was in the most severe patients as determined by NYHA class (NYHA III 3 placebo versus 1 milrinone, NYHA IV 3 placebo vs. 12 milrinone). The logrank for the survival comparison at this meeting was −1.14, as shown in Figure 4. The DSMB elected to keep treatments coded in the reports but to maintain the same coding of treatments throughout a given monitoring report and across interim analyses. While the mortality trend was in the wrong or negative direction, the evidence was not judged as being convincing of harm and the DSMB recommended continuation of the trial.

At the second interim analysis in December 1989, a total of 450 patients had been enrolled. The mortality difference (logrank Z = −1.50) remained unfavorable to the treatment arm but was well below the monitoring guideline. The difference in observed deaths remained primarily among the patients who had NYHA class IV symptoms at baseline (NYHA III 11 placebo

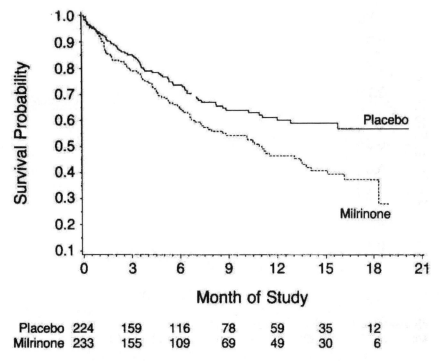

Figure 3 Kaplan–Meier analysis showing cumulative rates of survival in patients with class IV heart failure, According to Treatment Group. Mortality was 53% higher in the milrinone group (p = 0.006). Reproduced from Packer, et al. (1991) with permission of the *N Engl J Med.*

Table 2   Mortality Hazard Ratios by Prognostic Variables

Variable	Hazard ratio	p-value
Ejection fraction		
<0.21	1.26	0.115
>0.21	1.33	0.155
Principal diagnosis		
CHD	1.28	0.101
Other	1.26	0.214
Functional class		
III	1.03	0.859
IV	1.53	0.006
Age/yr		
<65	1.35	0.108
>65	1.34	0.051
Gender		
Male	1.26	0.082
Female	1.33	0.280

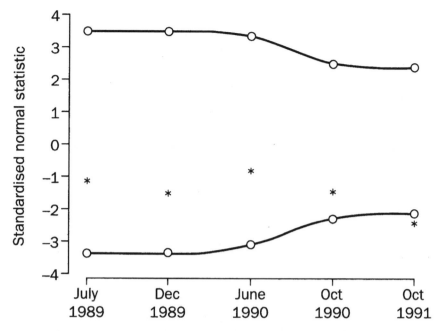

Figure 4 Group sequential boundries for the PROMISE trial. Horizontal axis = information fraction (observed fraction of total expected deaths). Group sequential boundaries set at two-sided 5% significance. Plotted points = logrank test. Crossing upper boundary = benefit, crossing lower boundary = harm. Reproduced from DeMets, et al. (1999) with permission of the *Lancet.*

vs. 11 milrinone, NYHA IV 17 placebo vs. 30 milrinone). Again, the DSMB recommended continuation of the trial.

By the third interim analysis in May 1990, a total of 683 patients of the initial estimated total sample size of 800 patients had been enrolled. The mortality difference was still unfavorable (logrank Z = −0.82) but less significant than at the previous monitoring meeting. Among patients with baseline NYHA class III symptoms, the mortality difference (logrank Z = 0.29) was very slightly in favor of the treatment arm but among patients with class IV symptoms the difference (logrank Z = −1.14) was still unfavorable though not nominally significant. At this analysis the DSMB considered two sets of projections. One set, the conditional power calculations, evaluated the likelihood of reaching a positive or negative conclusion (crossing of either the upper monitoring boundary indicating benefit or the lower boundary indicating harm) by the end of the trial given the current observed mortality and under a range of assumptions about the underlying mortality treatment difference. For example, the projected milrinone effect for the remainder of the trial included the beneficial effect assumed in the design, half of that effect, a null effect, and the observed negative effect.

The second set of projections addressed the necessity for extension of enrollment and/or total study length due to a smaller overall event rate than expected in order to obtain the target 190 placebo arm observed deaths. These calculations indicated that in order to reach the target by the expected completion date of March 1991 enrollment would need to be continued at least through October 1990, the time of the next scheduled DSMB review. The DSMB recommended continuation of enrollment and continuation of the study.

At the fourth interim monitoring meeting in October 1990, data were now available on 1,013 randomized patients. The negative trend in mortality continued, with 114 deaths on placebo and 143 deaths on milrinone. Although the overall mortality comparison (logrank $Z = -1.50$) was still within the monitoring guidelines, the comparison within the NYHA class IV subgroup (65 placebo versus 93 milrinone) was nominally statistically significant (logrank $Z = -2.55$, $p = 0.01$) and in fact was larger than the monitoring bound in place for the overall comparison, as shown in Figure 4. The DSMB recommended that the sponsor terminate the trial and initiate a complete surveillance of all patients for mortality status at the end of the trial. The sponsor and study chair were present at this DSMB meeting, participated in the discussion, but did not vote on the recommendation.

The trial was stopped promptly by the sponsor and Clinical Coordinating Center contacted the investigators to determine survival at the close of the study. In total 1,094 patients were enrolled in PROMISE. The final mortality experience was 127 deaths among 527 patients randomized to placebo and 168 deaths among 567 patients randomized to milrinone. The normalized logrank statistic ($Z = -2.08$) for the comparison of survival was just across the monitoring boundary for the final analysis. The final mortality difference in the NYHA class III subgroup slightly favored placebo (logrank $Z = -0.17$) but was not as striking as the difference in the NYHA class IV subgroup (logrank $Z = -2.77$).

LESSONS LEARNED

In the PROMISE trial the observed estimate of milrinone on survival was negative from the first monitoring meeting onward. As monitoring progressed and information (total deaths) accumulated. It seemed increasingly unlikely that PROMISE would show a mortality benefit for milrinone. However discouraging the mortality evidence, the drug milrinone was believed to improve other clinical measures of heart function, which could improve quality of life for patients with severe heart failure and thus perhaps could be beneficial even without a survival benefit. A neutral mortality result might not be a reason to abandon use of milrinone. However, a truly harmful or negative effect of milrinone on mortality would be an important deterrent. Thus, the DSMB felt the need to purse this agonizing negative trend to distinguish between a neutral mortality effect from a truly harmful effect. This situation in general has been recently been discussed.[16] Throughout the PROMISE trial, the DSMB reviewed quality-of-life measures and changes from baseline in symptoms and measures of heart function. The DSMB recommended closing the trial when a significant negative effect on survival was apparent and outweighed any observed potential symptomatic benefit. In addition, the likelihood of acceptance of conclusion and disease background against which the trial is conducted were other factors seriously considered.

PROMISE was one of the first industry-sponsored trials to implement a fully independent data and safety monitoring board, supported by an independent statistical analysis center. The goal was to obtain the benefits of the clinical trial model pioneered by the NIH, especially with respect to credibility and acceptability by the cardiology community and to provide adequate monitoring for overall patient safety. While the results of milrinone were not expected, in fact the modified NIH clinical trial achieved the goal and performed well with the observed negative harmful treatment effect. This PROMISE model has been modified and adopted by several other trials.[13] Furthermore, this type of independent statistical center has also been suggested by the Food and Drug Administrtion (FDA) guideline on data monitoring committees.[17]

In PROMISE, the study chair and sponsor attended all parts of the DSMB meeting. The current practice of open, closed, and executive sessions was not yet widely practiced. Open sessions typically allow sponsor and investigator participation. In closed sessions, the DSMB and the statistical center independent statistician are in attendance. In the executive session, only the DSMB members attend and form their final recommendations. In PROMISE, study chair and sponsor attendance did not appear to interfere with any of the DSMB deliberations, but it would be hard to claim there was no influence at all. In hindsight, and with further experience using DSMBs for industry-sponsored trials, the open, closed, and executive session format would be the preferred or recommended practice.[13,17,18]

Analysis of subgroups is always a challenge due to the vulnerability of multiple comparisons and false claims. Monitoring overall results as well as selected subgroups is even more challenging. Not only are their typically several subgroups but these are now reviewed repeatedly, which further increases the chances for false claims. Subgroups also have smaller samples sizes; results are subject to the variability of a smaller number of events and possible imbalances in risk factors. Terminating a subgroup alone may also have the effect of essentially terminating the entire trial. For PROMISE, the DSMB followed the high-risk (NYHA IV) heart failure subgroup but chose not to terminate this subgroup alone at earlier meetings. Rather, the DSMB sought to have a convincing overall result.

As described previously,[18-20] termination of a trial for benefit or harm is a complex decision process and depends not only on statistical analysis and monitoring boundaries but many other factors. These include internal consistency across various outcomes and subgroups, external consistency with other trials and preclinical data, and impact of the results on the practicing clinicians. In the case of PROMISE, the trial provided a definitive answer that has been accepted, providing important information on the use of the specific drug in the treatment of moderate to severe chronic heart failure.

REFERENCES

1. Packer M. 1988. Vasodilator and inotropic drugs for chronic heart failure: distinguishing hype from hope. *Am J Cardiol* 12:1299-1317.
2. Feldman MD, Copelas L, Gwanthmey JK, et al. 1987. Deficient production of cyclic AMP: pharmacologic evidence of an important cause of contractile dysfunction in patients with end-stage heart failure. *Circulation* 75:331-339.
3. Wilmshurst PT, Walker Jm, Fry CH, et al. 1984. Inotropic and vasodilator effects of amrinone on isolated human tissue. *Cardiovasc Res* 18:302-309.
4. Jain P, Brown EJ Jr, Langenback EG, et al. 1991. Effects of milrinone on left ventricular remodeling after acute myocardial infarction. *Circulation* 84:796-804.
5. Sweet CS, Ludden CT, Stabilito II, Emmert SE, Heyse JF. 1988. Beneficial effects of milrinone and enalapril on long-term survival of rats with healed myocardial infarction. *Eur J Pharmacol* 147:29-37.
6. Packer M, Leier CV. 1987. Survival in congestive heart failure during treatment with drugs with positive inotropic actions. *Circulation* 75:Suppl IV:IV-55-IV-63.
7. DiBianco R, Shabetai R, Kostuk W, Moran J, Schlant RC, Wright R. 1989. A comparison of oral milrinone, digoxin, and their combination in the treatment of patients wiht chronic heart failure. *N Engl J Med* 320:677-683.
8. Baim DS, McDowell AV, Cherniles J, et al. 1983. Evaluation of a new bipyridine inotropic agent—milrinone—in patients with severe congestive heart failure. *N Engl J Med* 309:748-756.
9. Simonton CA, Chatterjee K, Cody RJ, et al. 1985. Milrinone in congestive heart failure: acute and chronic hemodynamic and clinical evaluation. *J Am Coll Cardiol* 6:453-459.
10. Chesebro JH, Browne KF, Fenster PE, Garland WT, Konstam MA. 1988. The hemodynamic effects of chronic oral milrinone therapy: a multicenter controlled trial. *J Am Coll Cardiol* 11:144A. abstract
11. Packer M. 1989. Effect of phosphodiesterase inhibitors on the survival of patients with chronic congestive heart failure. *Am J Cardiol* 63:41A-45A.
12. Packer M, Carver JR, Rodeheffer RJ, Ivanhoe RJ, DiBianco R, Zeldis SM, et al. 1991. Effect of oral milrinone on mortality in severe chronic heart failure. *N Engl J Med* 325:1468-1475.
13. Fisher MM, Roecker EB, DeMets D. 2001. The role of an independent statistical analysis center in the industry-modified National Institutes of Health model. *Drug Information Journal* 35:115-129.
14. Lan KKG, DeMets DL. 1983. Discrete sequential boundaries for clinical trials. *Biometrika* 70:659-663.

15. O'Brien PC, Fleming TR. 1979. A multiple testing procedure for clinical trials. *Biometrics* 35:549–556.
16. DeMets DL, Pocock S, Julian DG: 1999. The agonising negative trend in monitoring clinical trials. *Lancet* 354:1983–1988.
17. US Food and Drug Administration (2001) Draft Guidance for Clinical Trial sponsors on the establishment and operation of Clinical Trial Data Monitoring Committees. Rockville, MD: FDA. http://www.fda.gov/cber/gdlns/clindatmon.htm
18. Ellenberg S, Fleming T, DeMets D. 2002. *Data Monitoring Committees in Clinical Trials: A Practical Perspective.* John Wiley & Sons, Ltd., West Sussex, England.
19. Canner PL. 1983. Monitoring of the data for evidence of adverse or beneficial treatment effects. *Control Clin Trials* 4:467–483.
20. Friedman LM, Furberg CD, DeMets DL. 1998. Fundamentals of Clinical Trials. Third Edition, Springer-Verlag, New York.

Stopping the Carotene and Retinol Efficacy Trial: The Viewpoint of the Safety and Endpoint Monitoring Committee

Anthony B. Miller[†]
Julie Buring
O. Dale Williams

ABSTRACT

We describe our experience with the events that occurred when it began to be suspected that beta-carotene in non-physiological doses had an unexpected adverse effect on the incidence and mortality from lung cancer. Initially, we delayed a decision to recommend stopping the Carotene and Retinol Efficacy Trial (CARET) for a year, until we were convinced that an adverse trend seen in the first interim analysis of the trial persisted. In hindsight, this seems to have been the correct decision.

INTRODUCTION AND BACKGROUND

The hypothesis that ingestion of beta-carotene was protective for lung cancer arose from a series of observational epidemiology studies, both case-control and cohort (reviewed in IARC).[1] Although there was a possibility that consumption of beta-carotene was an index for a diet high in beta-carotene-containing foods, and that the protective effect was due to other substances in plant foods, it was felt important that the putative protective effect should be assessed by randomized intervention trials in humans. Therefore, in the 1980s, a series of trials were designed to assess the beta-carotene hypothesis.

[†] Dr. Frank Iber was also a member of the SEMC during the events described in this paper, but could not be reached by the first author and therefore had no opportunity to participate in the preparation of this manuscript.

The Carotene and Retinol Efficacy Trial (CARET) was funded in July 1988 to determine the efficacy of a daily combination of 30 mg beta-carotene and 25,000 IU retinal (as retinyl palmitate) in preventing lung cancer in high-risk populations. These populations were heavy smokers and asbestos-exposed workers. The asbestos-exposed workers eligible were men aged 45–69, who were current smokers or quit within 15 years of enrollment, and who had their first exposure to asbestos on the job at least 15 years prior to enrollment. The heavy smokers were men and women aged 50–69 with at least 20 pack-years of cigarette smoking, and who were current smokers or had quit within the previous six years.

CARET was a multi-center trial based on two pilot studies that commenced in Seattle in 1985, one of heavy smokers (N = 1,029), and the other of asbestos-exposed workers (N = 816). These initial entrants were retained in the trial as the Vanguard cohort, who were evaluated more intensively for potential side-effects of the treatment regimen than the participants in the main trial. In the main trial, recruitment continued in Seattle, and centers were opened in Baltimore, New Haven, Portland and San Francisco that recruited asbestos-exposed workers, and the center in Portland recruited heavy smokers, as did another center in Irvine. Each center only entered the trial after their participation had been approved by their relevant Institutional Review Board. Accrual to the trial was completed in September 1994.

DATA MONITORING EXPERIENCE

The Safety and Endpoint Monitoring Committee (SEMC) was established early in the course of the main trial to act as an independent advisor to the investigators and the National Cancer Institute on all aspects of the conduct of the trial. Our mandate was largely ethical; we were initially primarily concerned with the potential toxicity of the regimens, both in the short and long term. For example, given some concerns that the incidence of prostate cancer might be adversely affected by the regimen, we early on instructed the investigators to provide us with regular data on the incidence of prostate cancer, as well as the primary endpoint of the trial, lung cancer. We met on a semi-annual basis, and were provided with coded data (i.e., masked as to regimen). We decided to use the O'Brien-Fleming[2] multiple testing procedure for clinical trials, to facilitate decisions relating to a possible early cessation of the trial, as well as the time when results would be reported. The SEMC initially had five members—two epidemiologists expert in clinical trials, a biostatistician, an expert on the pharmacology of the agents used, and a basic science researcher. After a few years, the last resigned and was not replaced. The SEMC met together with the principal investigator and statistician to the trial, and representatives of the NCI, but none of these had voting rights within the committee, and when judged necessary, the committee met in executive session without them.

In practice, the SEMC encountered few problems, our regular meetings continued over the years, we were provided with all the information we requested, and we received copies of the semi-annual reports provided by the investigators to NCI. Overall, we were very knowledgeable as to the progress of the trial.

Circumstances Surrounding the Stopping of the Trial Regimens

The investigators have already published details of the cessation of the trial from their perspective, especially concentrating on the administrative issues involved.[3] Here, we provide our perspective, a perspective largely influenced by our ethical responsibilities, but also influenced by the wider aspects of science that concerned us at the time.

In April 1994, the Chairman of the SEMC had a call from NCI requesting his participation in a conference call that also include the CARET principal investigator, the director of the supporting NCI Division, and an external expert in epidemiology who was not a member of the SEMC, but who had been extensively involved in the theoretical discussions that eventually led to the trials initiation. We were informed that the initial results of the Finnish Alpha-Tocopherol Beta Carotene (ATBC) trial were about to be published.[4] This showed an unexpected significant increase in the incidence of lung cancer, rather than the protective effect anticipated. Lung cancer mortality was consistent with the lung cancer incidence. We agreed that although the regimens evaluated in CARET and the ATBC trial were not the same, the overlap in both with the use of beta-carotene made it essential that there should be an immediate review of the current status of CARET. An urgent meeting of the SEMC was called, and we requested the investigators and the statistical center to immediately proceed with an analysis of the CARET outcome data, which in effect meant the advance of the first intermediate analysis already planned for the fall of that year. The investigators and statistical center worked extremely hard, so that we were able to meet again in August 1994. We were surprised that there was a significant difference between the regimens, and although the excess incidence of lung cancer did not cross the pre-specified O'Brien–Fleming early-stopping boundary, we unanimously agreed that we should be unblinded as to the nature of the regimens given to the coded groups. We then learned than CARET was the second trial to show an increase in incidence of lung cancer following the use of a regimen including a high (pharmacologic) dose of beta-carotene.

Our decision to recommend to NCI that the trial regimen should be stopped (but that the follow-up continue) was not immediate. Indeed, there was initially a considerable difference of opinion within the SEMC. When we eventually decided to take a vote at that meeting, we were evenly divided, and the chair decided not to use his casting vote, because of the validity of the contrasting views held.

These views may be summarized as follows. In favor of not stopping the trial:

- The statistical significance of the difference had not crossed the O'Brien–Fleming boundary (i.e., this could still be a chance finding).
- The effect was surprisingly rapid and must mean if real that pre-existing (but undiagnosed) lung cancers had had their growth accelerated by the regimen.
- We knew of no mechanism of the action of beta-carotene that could have induced such an effect.
- There were other chemoprevention trials using beta carotene ongoing, to stop CARET now would have an undesirable adverse effect on these trials.
- We owed it to science to be absolutely certain of the adverse effect before stopping the trial.

In favor of immediately stopping the trial the following views were expressed:

- This was the second trial to show an adverse effect of beta-carotene chemoprevention; it was extremely unlikely to be due to chance.
- We owed it to the participants to prevent possible further harm to them. It was perhaps particularly unfortunate that the adverse effect appeared to be present in asbestos workers as well as current smokers.
- The adverse effects appeared not to be restricted to lung cancer; there appeared to be an adverse effect on cardiovascular disease as well.

Given the lack of agreement among the SEMC, it was agreed that the following actions were required:

1. The outcome events should be allowed to continue to accumulate for another 6 months; it would then be possible to determine if an apparent adverse effect was continuing.
2. The statistical center was requested to compute the possibility that if the excess of lung cancer in the active treatment arm ceased to occur, a benefit might eventually occur that could be detected given the size of the population in the trial.

3. To allow time for the additional endpoints to be determined, we decided that a second interim analysis would be performed in June 1995, and that we would meet again as soon as possible to review the status of the trial.

We recognized that this meant that we had effectively postponed a decision to stop the trial (if we then decided that was necessary) for more than a year after the ATBC results were released. However, we knew that very shortly after the publication of the ATBC results, the principal investigator had written to all CARET participants informing them of the ATBC results and reminding them of their right to stop the trial medication immediately if they were concerned.

We met again in September 1995. At that time it was clear that the excess of lung cancer had continued to accumulate in the intervention regimen at about the same rate during the time since the first interim analysis. Further, the cardiovascular disease excess persisted. The conditional power calculations showed that it was extremely unlikely that the trial could show a beneficial effect of the intervention, even if the adverse effect ceased to occur and a delayed protective effect began to appear. Therefore the SEMC voted unanimously to recommend to NCI that the trial regimen should be stopped but the follow-up should continue.

NCI decided, given the importance of the decision, that it would convene an *ad hoc* group of three biostatistician advisors, with the principal task of reviewing the biostatistical aspects related to our recommendation to them. All three were experienced with cancer trials and one had been on the data monitoring board for the ATBC trial. The *ad hoc* group reviewed the most recent SEMC report for the CARET trial as well as the published results of the ATBC trial. This group concurred with our recommendation, and the steering committee of the trial voted unanimously to terminate the trial regimen in January 1996.

LESSONS LEARNED

Taking a decision to stop a major trial is difficult, and there is no question that having done so for CARET has had a major impact on the perception of the potential value of chemoprevention for cancer. However, the research which followed fairly soon led to the elucidation of a possible mechanism for the adverse effect,[1] and this in itself has advanced the field.

The ethical aspects related to participant safety have to be paramount for a Safety and Endpoint Monitoring committee. However, ethical issues are perceived differently by different individuals, and the initial disagreement within our committee effectively demonstrated this. Even though the relative lung cancer risk was increased, the absolute risk of an adverse effect was small, and this influenced some committee members more than others. Further, the adverse effect did not at that time seem to have a rational biological basis; thus it was relatively easy to assume that some sort of bias had created what we were seeing. It was also relevant that one of our members was an investigator in the Physicians Health Trial,[5] and it was known to her that no adverse effect of beta-carotene had so far been seen in that trial. However, there was a much smaller proportion of smokers in that trial than the ATBC and CARET trials, and we knew that the adverse effect in CARET was seen in smokers, rather than non-smokers, while ATBC had only enrolled smokers. Nevertheless, for some time, in personal discussions with the chair of the committee, the external expert that had participated in the April 1994 tele-conference maintained that our eventual decision to stop the trial regimen was completely unjustified. He maintained that there was still a possibility that the adverse effect was due to chance, and that it was critical to ensure that the possibility of a protective effect from beta-carotene was not due to chance.

In practice, two circumstances made it possible for the committee members that had initially not favored the trial regimen is being stopped to change their mind. One was the continuation of the accumulation of excess adverse events in the active intervention arm between the two interim analyses. The other was the apparent impossibility of the trial's showing a beneficial effect even if this began to appear. In practice by the time the decision to terminate the trial regimen was taken, about half of the anticipated endpoints had already occurred.

Bowen et al.[3] have documented the processes the investigators had to go through to inform the participants of the decision to terminate the trial regimen in a manner that did not cause undue alarm among them. The approaches they adopted seem to have been very successful, a reflection of the fact that the initial informed consent process had imparted the necessary information that an experimental regimen was being evaluated. The importance of an even-handed approach to informed consent is highlighted by the circumstances surrounding this trial. A similar experience occurred in the Canadian trial of mammography screening which failed to demonstrate the anticipated benefit from the screen.[6] Because under the conditions of scientific equipoise needed to initiate a trial we cannot know in advance that there will either be a benefit, or even a detriment from the experimental regimen, it is in our view essential that both those allocated to the active treatment and those allocated to the control group provide informed consent. Thus what is called by some "randomized consent" (the subjects are identified, randomized, and then those allocated to the active intervention are asked for their consent, with the controls not approached but followed through available data bases such as cancer registries and vital statistics files) is not ethically valid, as it is the right of controls to know they are being considered for a trial, and to refuse (or agree) to participate in the light of their own circumstances and beliefs about possibilities of benefit and harm.

The SEMC was blinded on a "need-to-know" basis; that is, the SEMC could choose to unblind itself when it determined it was important to know the treatment arm codes. This facilitated an unbiased approach to the first (advanced) interim analyses. Although concern with potential toxicity of a regimen (as we were in the early years of our deliberations) may result in one making inferences as to which coded arm is which, when toxicity is minimal, as it was in CARET, the placebo effect will usually result in committees remaining unblinded. This was in effect what happened during all our deliberations, until we took our unanimous decision that we should be unblinded in August 1994, when it became apparent that we needed to know whether CARET was showing early indications of a benefit from the intervention, in which case continuation of the trial to the defined endpoint was essential, or whether the adverse effect seen in ATBC had been replicated in CARET.

There seems little doubt now, with the benefit of hindsight, that we made the correct recommendation in September 1995. Also with the benefit of hindsight, given that the adverse effect has not gone away, it does not seem likely that we could have prevented many, if any, adverse events occurring if we had taken that decision one year earlier. Although the decision was delayed for a year, this has to be placed in the perspective of the state of the art of chemoprevention at that time, and the strong belief, largely derived from observational epidemiology data, that beta-carotene in physiological doses is beneficial. Indeed, reports are still appearing of diet and cancer studies that are interpreted to show a beneficial effect of such consumption. This suggests that it was the high, non-physiological doses of beta-carotene that caused the adverse effect, with unusual metabolic functions coming into play, a hypothesis that seems to be confirmed by mechanistic studies that have been performed.[1]

REFERENCES

1. IARC Handbooks on Cancer Prevention. Volume 2 Carotenoids. 1998. Lyon, International Agency for Research on Cancer.
2. O'Brien PC, Fleming TR. 1979. A multiple testing procedure for clinical trials. *Biometrics* 35:549-556.
3. Bowen DJ, Thornqvist M, Anderson K, Barnett M, Powell C, Goodman G, Omenn G. 2003. Stopping the active intervention: CARET. *Control Clin Trials* 24:39-50.

4. The Alpha-Tocopherol Beta Carotene Prevention Study Group. 1994. The effect of vitamin E and beta carotene on the incidence of lung cancer and other cancers in male smokers. *N Engl J Med* 330:1029-1035.
5. Hennekens CH Buring JE, Manson JE, Stampfer M, Rosner B, Cook NR, et al. 1996. Lack of long-term supplementation with beta carotene on the incidence of malignant neoplasms and cardiovascular disease. *N Engl J Med* 334:1145-1149.
6. Miller AB, To T, Baines CJ, Wall C. 2000. Canadian National Breast Screening Study-2: 13-year results of a randomized trial in women age 50-59 years. *J Natl Cancer Inst* 92:1490-1499.

Monitoring a Clinical Trial With Waiver of Informed Consent: Diaspirin Cross-Linked Hemoglobin for Emergency Treatment of Post–Traumatic Shock

Roger J. Lewis
Norman Fost

ABSTRACT

In 1996, the FDA and DHHS regulations were modified to allow randomized controlled trials in emergency settings with a waiver of informed consent (from patients or surrogates) under specified conditions. The first large multi-center trial under the new regulations was sponsored by Baxter Laboratories, comparing a semi-synthetic hemoglobin to standard care in the initial resuscitation of adults presenting with post-hemorrhagic shock. In addition to the familiar problems that the Data Monitoring Committee had to face, there were new issues, such as reviewing procedures for community disclosure and community consultation, and a heightened sense of scrutiny because of the waiver of traditional consent. The trial was terminated because of higher than expected mortality in the group receiving the experimental treatment. The number of trials initiated under the regulations seems to be less than anticipated, perhaps because the regulatory burden is seens as too onerous.

INTRODUCTION AND BACKGROUND

Death and disability can occur suddenly and without warning, for example, following cardiac arrest or major trauma. Clinical research in these settings has been limited by the requirement to obtain prospective informed consent from the patient or an appropriate representative. The patient is typically incapacitated, and next of kin are commonly not available in the short interval during which the intervention is most likely to be effective.

These facts have resulted in two unfortunate consequences: first, a paucity of well-designed clinical trials in emergency settings and, second, increasing use of untested "innovative" therapies. Because the use of innovative therapies is largely unregulated, physicians in non-research emergency settings have been free to use untested interventions, while paradoxically restricted in their ability to test the same interventions under well designed, controlled clinical trial.[1,2] There are both theoretical and empirical arguments supporting the view that a preference for innovative therapy over explicit research is neither in the interests of the patient nor society.[3] As Smithells asked plaintively, "Why is that I can give a new drug to all of my patients but not to half of my patients?"[4] Lietman put it even more provocatively, "As long as you promise not to learn anything from what you're doing, you don't have to go through an IRB."[5]

Prior to 1996, the regulations of the U.S. Department of Health and Human Services (DHHS), known as the Common Rule, allowed consent to be waived only if the research presented no more than minimal risk.[6] This excluded the testing of most drugs that would be used in emergency settings. The Food and Drug Administration (FDA) allowed unapproved drugs to be used in emergency settings without consent but only if, in the opinion of the physician, the treatment was necessary to save the life of the patient.[7] Since a placebo is rarely if ever necessary to save a patient's life, this rule seemed to prohibit placebo-controlled trials in the absence of consent.

In November 1996 the FDA and DHHS, in response to outside concerns,[1] changed the rules, allowing an exception to the requirement for informed consent if certain requirements were met.[7,8] These requirements included review of the trial by the FDA when the trial involved a drug or device, public disclosure and consultation with the community in which the trial would be conducted, and creation of an independent Data Monitoring Committee (DMC). The first large-scale, multi-center trial to be conducted under this rule, sponsored by Baxter Healthcare Corporation, was designed to compare the addition of a semi-synthetic hemoglobin—diaspirin cross-linked hemoglobin (DCLHb)—to standard care in the initial resuscitation of adults experiencing post-traumatic hemorrhagic shock.[9,10] In addition to its oxygen-carrying capacity, DCLHb was thought to have a direct pharmacologic effect that would increase the blood pressure of patients in shock.

Earlier trials had been conducted, using a process termed "deferred consent," based on arguments that the research intervention did not involve more than minimal risk, either because standard treatments were being used in both arms and the only added risk was randomization,[11] because the intervention was medically of low risk,[12] or because the differential risk of receiving the study agent, compared to standard care, was low.[13]

For the DCLHb trial, a sample size of 850 subjects was estimated to yield an 85% power with an alpha of .05% to detect a reduction in 28-day mortality from 40% to 30%. The design included plans for four interim analyses based on data available from 10%, 25%, 50%, and 75% of the planned 850 patients. The trial's DMC was scheduled to meet approximately three months after each enrollment milestone to allow time for data acquisition, processing, and analysis by the statistical center. In addition to being charged with monitoring for safety and efficacy, the DMC was specifically given responsibility for recommending early termination if there were "no reasonable chance of demonstrating benefit;" i.e., futility.

DATA MONITORING EXPERIENCE

At an organizational meeting in April 1997, the DMC requested and received ongoing access to reports from the monitoring committee for a similar Baxter trial already underway in Europe. The DMC met by conference call in October 1997 and agreed to add a minority representative, partly in response to comments by the FDA regarding inadequate representation of minorities in the development of the waived consent regulations. The next scheduled meeting was planned for March 1998, at which time complete data from the first 85 patients were expected to be available. At the suggestion of the sponsor, an additional face to face meeting was called for December 8-9, 1997, concurrent with a meeting of the study investigators, for the purpose of updating the DMC on a variety of issues.

At a closed session of the DMC on December 8, the statistical center disclosed a disturbing asymmetry in the mortality rate between the two arms of the trial: 6 versus 17 out of a total of 74 patients enrolled (the number of patients in each treatment group was unknown). Based on an assumption of equal enrollment in the two arms, the p-value was <0.006. The members agreed that the identity of the treatments would affect their judgment about how to respond to this information and voted to unblind themselves. The apparent excess in deaths had occurred in the group that received DCLHb.

After extensive discussion, the DMC concluded they needed additional information to interpret this observation, including additional data regarding the reported deaths, enrollment by treatment group, and baseline characteristics of patients who had received the experimental therapy. These requests were discussed with a senior representative from Baxter and the needed information was collected over the next three days and transmitted to the statistical center. For the purpose of this expedited data collection, standard data verification methodologies were suspended.

The DMC met by conference call on December 11. The adjusted data showed a mortality rate of 21% in the saline infusion group, and 38% in the DCLHb group (p < 0.098). The change in the p-value was due to an imbalance in assignment to the two groups, and the ascertainment of two additional deaths in the saline group. Preliminary data from the European study was also reviewed, and the DMC recommended that the trial continue, with an accelerated schedule of data collection and analysis over the next two weeks, when higher enrollment was anticipated due to motor vehicle crashes during the holiday season.

On December 19, the DMC again met by conference call and learned that there now appeared to be excess mortality in the DCLHb group with a p-value of 0.018. There were reasons to suspect possible confounding factors in the assignment of patients to the two groups, so further analysis of baseline characteristics of enrolled subjects was requested. On January 1, 1998 the DMC reviewed this additional information. There was still a higher mortality in the DCLHb group (p < 0.010) and, although the cause of this differential mortality was unclear, the DMC recommended an immediate moratorium on new enrollment. This recommendation was accepted and implemented by the sponsor immediately and no further patients were enrolled.

Subsequent analyses and conference calls on February 20th and March 17th identified complex questions, reviewed in detail by Lewis,[9] and the DMC recommended termination of the trial. Although extensive data analyses were unable to substantiate an alternative explanation for the increased mortality in patients receiving DCLHb, members of the DMC were reluctant to make any conclusive statements regarding causality. The final recommendation to terminate the trial relied heavily on futility considerations.

Later analyses by Sloan[10,14,15] raised further questions about whether the differential mortality was due to DCLHb or baseline differences in enrolled subjects. Nonetheless, based on the American and European trials it seems unlikely that DCLHb confers benefit as an initial resuscitation fluid in the treatment of acute hemorrhagic shock.

In the U.S. study, 94% of patients were enrolled with a waiver of consent, and consent to continue was granted by 98% of patients or their families.[15] This is similar to the high acceptance found in an earlier study using waiver of consent, before the change in the regulations.[13]

LESSONS LEARNED

1. The decision about whether to recommend early termination of this trial was not fundamentally different from similar decisions faced by other DMCs, but the stakes seemed higher to some committee members

because of the waiver of consent. Because informed consent had not been obtained, and would not be obtained from future patients, the DMC may have felt a special obligation to protect potential and future subjects.

2. In addition to the traditional roles of reviewing trial design and reviewing interim data for efficacy, toxicity, and futility, the DMC, with the FDA, was given the added responsibility of reviewing and commenting on each of the 20 sites' methods for community disclosure and consultation. Since this requirement was unprecedented, there were no standards or benchmarks by which to judge the adequacy of each institution's approach. The DMC found all but one of these plans acceptable. That site conducted additional disclosure and consultation activities.

In the ensuing years, some additional trials have been conducted with a waiver of consent provision, and there is now more experience and analysis of the effectiveness and acceptability of alternative approaches to fulfilling the requirements of the regulations.[16-20]

3. The 1996 revisions facilitated clinical trials that had previously been prohibited, or whose legal status was sufficiently unclear as to inhibit sponsors, investigators, and IRBs. On the other hand, the difficulties in defining and implementing the requirements for community disclosure and consultation seem to be inhibiting sponsors, so that the number of trials using the waiver in emergency settings has been less than originally anticipated. The requirements for community consultation may need to be more detailed and explicit, or their necessity may need to be reconsidered. The FDA has published a "guidance document" to clarify these issues.[21]

4. The political risks of conducting a trial using the emergency exception were demonstrated when then Baxter trial was terminated due to apparent excess mortality in the treatment group. Some ethicists ridiculed the new rules.[22] This also illustrated the ambiguity about which participants in a clinical trial are the "guinea pigs." Critics are divided about whether those in the placebo group are being unfairly deprived of an effective treatment[23] or those in the treatment group are being exposed to unreasonable risks. The answer, of course, is that there is no way of knowing until a well-designed study is conducted.

5. The Baxter trial demonstrates again the utility of well-designed research studies with careful data monitoring by independent data monitoring committees. If DCLHb had been an approved drug, emergency physicians could have used it as a resuscitation fluid under the rubric of "innovative therapy." If the increased mortality in the Baxter trial was, in fact, caused by the DCLHb (a conjecture that is irrevocably unclear), it is unlikely that this would have been discovered as promptly as occurred in the closely monitored trial, if at all.

6. Despite the continued recognition of the importance of developing and testing therapies for acute, incapacitating, and life-threatening illnesses, there still remains relatively little experience with conducting clinical trials under the existing exception to informed consent regulations.[17,20] Further, it is difficult to ascertain the exact number or types of trials being planned, initiated, or completed that utilize the exception. It is likely that some of these trials are initiated by single investigators or small groups of investigators and conducted at only one or a few institutions. Furthermore, if the trials do not utilize an FDA-regulated product (e.g., a trial comparing methods of cardiopulmonary resuscitation) they may not be formally registered with the FDA or other regulatory authorities. Industry-initiated studies that utilize the regulations are generally only widely publicized when they reach the stage of community consultation and public disclosure, so relatively little is known about the number of such studies that have been planned but not initiated, or are currently being planned.

Interestingly, two of the more widely publicized trials currently being initiated and to be conducted under the waiver involve the evaluation of "next-generation" blood substitutes for victims of trauma. Two companies, Northfield Laboratories and Biopure Corporation are both initiating trauma studies of blood substitute products utilizing the exception of informed consent provisions in the FDA regulations. In the latter case, the planned study is a collaboration between Biopure and the US Navy.[24,25]

FINAL COMMENTS

It is widely believed, but difficult to prove, that the limited conduct of studies utilizing the emergency exception from informed consent is due, at least in part, to the perceived difficulty in successfully initiating a trial using the waiver. The processes of community consultation and public disclosure are potentially onerous, expensive, and extend the time necessary to initiate a study. In some cases, industrial sponsors may choose instead to test their products in non-emergency situations, which are more easily controlled and in which informed consent may be obtained from the patient or a legally-authorized surrogate, with the hope of obtaining FDA approval for the non-emergency indication. As often occurs, products approved for non-emergency indications may be utilized in emergency situations based on physician judgment; i.e. under the rubric of "innovative therapy."[3] Unfortunately, with this approach to gaining regulatory and marketing approval, objective data are difficult to obtain on the true effectiveness of the medications in emergency situations. As illustrated by the DCLHb trauma trial, the outcome of patients treated with investigational products in the emergency setting may be widely disparate from the outcomes of patients treated in a more controlled setting, such as elective surgery.

The current regulations allowing an emergency exception to the general requirement for informed consent provide a fundamental opportunity to determine the true effectiveness of new products for the treatment of sudden, incapacitating, and life-threatening illness. While the unique ethical challenges associated with conducting medical research on patients who face life-threatening situations and are unable to provide informed consent underscore the importance of careful data and safety monitoring, not performing such research will condemn future generations of patients suffering the same illnesses to receive unproven and potentially harmful therapies, albeit administered by well-meaning caregivers.

ACKNOWLEDGMENTS

Much of the description of the study and the deliberations of the Data Monitoring Committee is adapted from Lewis.[9] We are grateful to the publishers, Mosby/Elsevier, for permission to use that article in this way.

REFERENCES

1. Biros MH, Lewis RJ, Olson CM, Runge JW, Cummins RO, Fost N. 1995. Informed Consent in Emergency Research: Consensus statement from the Coalition Conference of Acute Resuscitation and Critical Care Researchers. *JAMA* 273:1283-1287.
2. Fost N. 1998. Waived consent for emergency research. *Am J Law Med* 24:163-183.
3. Fost N. 1998. Ethical dilemmas in medical innovation and research: Distinguishing experimentation from practice. *Seminars in Perinatology* 22:223-232.
4. Smithells R. 1975. Iatrogenic hazards and their effects. *Postgraduate Medicine* 51(supp 2):39.
5. Lietman P. Personal communication. 1972.
6. Protection of Human Subjects. 45 CFR 46:116(d).
7. Exception from general requirements. 21CFR 50.23(a)(1), 45 CFR 46:116(f).
8. Protection of Human Subjects: Informed consent and waiver of informed consent requirements in certain emergency research. 61 Federal Register 51498-51533, 1966. Codified at 21 CFR 545, 46, 50.24.
9. Lewis RJ, Berry DA, Cryer H 3rd, Fost N, Krome R, Washington GR, et al. 2001. Monitoring a clinical trial conducted under the Food and Drug Administration Regulations allowing a waiver of prospective informed consent: The diaspirin cross-linked hemoglobin traumatic hemorrhagic shock efficacy trial. *Ann Emerg Med* 28:397-404.
10. Sloan EP, Koenigsberg M, Gens D, Cipolle M, Runge J, Mallory MN, Rodman G Jr. 1999. Diaspirin cross-linked hemoglobin (DCLHb) in the treatment of severe traumatic hemorrhagic shock: a randomized controlled efficacy trial. *JAMA* 282:1857-1864.
11. Prentice ED, Antonson DL, Leibrock LG, Kelso TK, Sears TD. 1993. IRB review of a Phase II randomized clinical trial involving incompetent patients suffering from severe closed head injury. *IRB: A Review of Human Subjects Research* 15:1-7.
12. Fost NC, Robertson JA. 1980. Deferring consent with incompetent patients in an intensive care unit. *Irb: A Review of Human Subjects Research* 2:5-6.
13. Abramson NS, Meisel A, Safar P. 1986. Deferred consent: a new approach for resuscitation research on comatose patients. *JAMA* 255:2466-2471.

14. Sloan EP, Koenigsberg M, Brunett PH, Bynoe RP, Morris JA, Tinkoff G, Dalsey WC, Ochsner MG. DCLHb Traumatic Hemorrhagic Shock Study Group. 2002. Post hoc mortality analysis of the efficacy trial of diaspirin cross-linked hemoglobin in the treatment of severe traumatic hemorrhagic shock. *J Trauma-Injury Infect Crit Care* 52:887–895.
15. Sloan EP. The clinical trials of diaspirin cross-linked hemoglobin (DCLHb) in severe traumatic hemorrhagic shock: the tale of two continents. *Intens Care Med.* 29:347–349, 2003.
16. Baren AM, Anicetti JP, Ledesma S, Biros MH, Mahabee-Gittens M, Lewis RJ, et al. 1999. An approach to community consultation prior to initiating an emergency research study incorporating a waiver of informed consent. *Acad Emerg Med* 6:1210–1215.
17. Biros MH. 2003. Research Without Consent: Current Status, 2003. *Ann of Emerg Med* 42:550–564.
18. Dix ES, Esposito D, Spinosa F, Olson N, Chapman S. 2004. Implementation of Community Consultation for Waiver of Informed Consent in Emergency Research: One Institutional Review Board's Experience. *J Invest Med* 52:109–112.
19. Raju TN. 2004. Waiver of Informed Consent in Emergency Research and Community Disclosures and Consultations. *J Invest Med* 52:113–116.
20. Shah AN, Sugarman J. 2003. Protecting Research Subjects Under the Waiver of Informed Consent for Emergency Research: Experiences with Efforts to Inform the Community. *Ann Emerg Med* 41:72–78.
21. FDA Guidance for Institutional Review Boards, Clinical Investigators, and Sponsors: Exception from Informed Consent Requirements for Emergency Research [Draft Guidance dated March 30, 2000]. Available at http://www.fda.gov
22. Kolata G. Ban on Medical Experiments Without Consent Is Relaxed. 1996. *NY Times,* Nov 5, Section A, page 1, column 3.
23. Rothman KJ. Michels KB. 1994. The continuing unethical use of placebo controls. *N Engl J Med* 331:394–398.
24. Northfield Laboratories Inc. to Receive Defense Appropriation for PolyHeme(R) Development. http://www.northfieldlabs.com (Accessed Oct 3, 2004).
25. U.S. Navy to Help Fund and Conduct Biopure's Pivotal Clinical Trial of Hemopure(R) in Trauma. http://www.biopure.com (Accessed Oct 4, 2004).

Consideration of Early Stopping and Other Challenges in Monitoring the Heart and Estrogen/Progestin Replacement Study

Stephen B. Hulley
Deborah Grady
Eric Vittinghoff
O. Dale Williams

ABSTRACT

The Heart and Estrogen-progestin Replacement Study (HERS) was the first major randomized blinded trial to test the widespread belief that hormone therapy would prevent fatal and non-fatal coronary heart disease (CHD). The main findings—CHD events were not prevented and thromboembolic events were increased—illustrates in a powerful way the evidence-based medicine principle that well-designed and executed randomized blinded trials are a necessary basis for drug treatments. The HERS Data and Safety Monitoring Board played an important role in a number of difficult decisions that led to more definitive conclusions, notably the decisions not to stop the trial early in the face of adverse experience in both primary and secondary disease outcomes. HERS, with its complex and unexpected findings, illustrates the value of designing flexible interim monitoring guidelines that allow for decisions based on the judgment of a diverse group of experts as to benefits and harms, ethical implications for participants, and the social obligation to have an optimal impact on policy and practice guidelines.

INTRODUCTION AND BACKGROUND

HERS began in a climate of widespread belief that "replacing" the estrogen lost at menopause would prevent many of the manifestations of aging, including coronary heart disease (CHD), osteoporotic fractures, and a decline

236

in cognitive and sexual function. This attractive and plausible view led to extensive use of estrogens after menopause in the era before randomized trials with disease endpoints were required for testing new drugs. Clinicians were drawn in by other accumulating lines of evidence—observational studies that showed less heart disease among women taking estrogen,[1] pathophysiologic mechanisms that provided biologic plausibility,[2] and clinical trials that revealed improvements in blood lipids and other surrogate measures.[3]

In the 1980s, estrogen treatment after menopause was found to be causing endometrial cancer.[4] Although uncommon and usually curable, this cancer could be prevented by antagonizing the estrogen with a progestin,[4] and several estrogen plus progestin (E+P) combinations were explored in the search for one that preserved the benefits of estrogen. In the 1990s, after finding that lipid effects remained largely favorable when conjugated estrogens were combined with medroxyprogesterone acetate (MPA),[3] this particular E+P regimen became the most widely used in the United States for women with a uterus.

PROTOCOL DESIGN

The Heart and Estrogen/progestin Replacement Study (HERS), financed by Wyeth-Ayerst but under the scientific control of the Steering Committee of investigators and the Coordinating Center at UCSF, was the first major trial of the effects of hormone therapy on CHD outcomes.[5,6] It was a secondary prevention trial of women with established coronary disease who were recruited beginning early in 1993. A total of 2,763 women were randomized to either a combination of conjugated equine estrogen (0.625 mg/day) and medroxyprogesterone acetate (2.5 mg/day), or to a placebo. The primary outcome was the incidence of CHD events, defined as non-fatal MI or CHD death.

Participants and Randomization

Participants were post-menopausal women ≤80 years of age with known coronary disease defined as prior myocardial infarction, coronary artery bypass surgery, percutaneous transluminal coronary angioplasty, or angiographic evidence of ≥50% narrowing of one or more major coronary arteries. Women were excluded for a number of reasons, including prior hysterectomy, a coronary event within the six months before randomization, serum triglyceride level greater than 300 mg/dl, hormone use within three months, or a history of conditions that would contraindicate estrogen therapy. The women were randomly assigned within clinical centers to

0.625 mg of conjugated equine estrogen plus 2.5 mg of medroxyproges-terone acetate in one tablet daily (n = 1,380) or a placebo of identical appear-ance (n = 1,383).

Outcome Ascertainment

Suspected outcome events were either reported by participants to the clinical center staff or were identified via participant interviews that were conducted every four months. Records of all hospitalizations were reviewed, and an independent morbidity and mortality subcommittee that was blinded to treatment assignment adjudicated all suspected outcome events. Non-fatal myocardial infarctions were diagnosed using an algorithm based on ischemic symptoms, new electrocardiographic abnormalities, and elevated cardiac enzymes levels, or evidence of fresh myocardial infarction at autopsy.[5] Although power was limited, secondary cardiovascular outcomes included coronary artery bypass surgery, percutaneous coronary revascularization, hospitalization for unstable angina, resuscitated cardiac arrest, congestive heart failure, stroke or transient ischemic attack, and peripheral arterial disease. Other pre-specified secondary outcomes were total mortality; cancer death; non-CHD/non-cancer death; breast, endometrial, and other cancer; deep vein thrombosis; pulmonary embolism; hip and other fracture; and gall-bladder disease.

Sample Size and Power

We estimated that we needed to enroll 2,340 women, assuming a primary CHD event rate in the placebo group of 5% per year, a combined non-CHD death and loss to follow-up rate of 2% per year; crossovers from active to placebo of 5%, 4%, and 3%, in the first three years and 2% per year thereafter; crossovers from placebo to active of 1% each year, and average follow-up of 4.15 years.[6] We assumed that half the reduction in primary CHD events would operate through non-lipid mechanisms (and therefore be immediate) and half would operate through lipid changes (and therefore begin after a two-year lag period). These assumptions resulted in 90% power at a two-tailed alpha of 5% to detect an intention-to-treat effect size of 24%. In the actual study, the annual event rate was only 3.3%, compliance was less than expected, and treatment duration was only 4.2 years. (The reason for the shorter than expected treatment duration, despite ending the study at the planned calendar time, was the fact that most women were enrolled toward the end of the intake period as we became more successful at recruitment.) The reduction in power caused by these deviations from pre-study assump-tions was partially offset by recruiting 2,763 women, 18% more than planned.[6]

Statistical Analyses

The primary analysis compared the rate of CHD events among women assigned to active medication with the rate among women assigned to placebo using an unadjusted Cox proportional hazards model for time to first CHD event (equivalent to the log rank test). The analysis was by intention-to-treat, categorizing participants according to randomized treatment assignment regardless of compliance. Participants who asked to drop out of the study were censored for morbidity outcomes at their last visit (this occurred for 31 women in the hormone group and 38 women in the placebo group); however, vital status was assessed at the end of the trial for 100% of the entire cohort.

Main Findings

Overall, there were no significant differences between groups in the primary or in any of the secondary cardiovascular outcomes: during the average 4.1 years of follow-up, 172 women in the estrogen plus progestin group and 176 women in the placebo group had myocardial infarction or CHD death (relative hazard [RH] 0.99; 95% CI 0.80–1.22).[6] Within the overall null effect there was a statistically significant time trend, with more CHD events in the hormone group than in the placebo group in year 1, and fewer in years 4 and 5 (Table 1). More women in the estrogen-plus-progestin group than in the placebo group experienced venous thromboembolic events (34 vs. 12; RH 2.89; 95% CI 1.50–5.58) and gallbladder disease (84 vs. 62; RH 1.38; 95% CI 1.00–1.92).[6] There were no statistically significant differences between the estrogen-plus-progestin group and the placebo group in several other endpoints for which power was limited, including fracture, cancer, and total mortality.

Table 1 Early Harm and Later Benefit? (MI/CHD death by year in HERS)

Year	E + P	Placebo	RH	95%CI
1	57	38	1.5*	1.0–2.3
2	47	48	1.0*	0.7–1.5
3	35	41	0.8*	0.5–1.3
4 + 5	33	49	0.7*	0.5–1.1
Overall	172	176	1.0	0.8–1.2

* p for trend = 0.03.

DATA AND SAFETY MONITORING EXPERIENCE

An independent DSMB was established during the design phase of HERS. DSMB members included experts in cardiology, epidemiology, gynecology, statistics, clinical trials, and ethics. Representatives of the sponsor (Wyeth-Ayerst, Inc.) were present at open meetings of the DSMB but did not attend closed meetings at which outcome data were reviewed and were not privy to these data (held at the UCSF Coordinating Center). Representatives of the Coordinating Center (including Drs. Hulley, Vittinghoff, and Grady) were non-voting members of the board and attended both open and closed meetings. All members of the board were required to disclose potential conflicts of interest (stock options or employment by the sponsor, and consultation, honoraria or speaking fees).

An initial meeting to review and approve the protocol and the interim monitoring procedures was held before the first participant was randomized. We planned to conduct interim analyses every 6–12 months using the method of Lan and DeMets.[7] However, at an early meeting, evidence of increased risk of CHD events in the hormone-treated group led the board to review the accumulating data in meetings or conference calls every 3–6 months. The Lan and DeMets plots included formal statistical stopping boundaries, but the board had wisely decided at the outset that a recommendation to modify or discontinue the trial would not be based solely on statistical grounds. Instead, the board adopted Canner's proposal[8] that "no single statistical decision rule or procedure can take the place of the well-reasoned consideration of all aspects of the data by a group of concerned, competent and experienced persons with a wide range of scientific backgrounds and points of view."

During the course of HERS, the investigators at the Coordinating Center and DSMB labored over four major design questions that each had to do with when to stop the trial:

- *Stop early because of early harmful trend in CHD outcomes?* In the early years of follow-up the board noted the finding—astonishing at the time—of adverse trends in the major CHD outcomes (Table 1). At the beginning of the trial, the board had discussed formal stopping boundaries for unexpected magnitude or rate of benefit in the primary outcome, but not for unexpected harm in this outcome. Given that trials are generally not designed to determine harm, many argue that stopping boundaries for unexpected harm should be less conservative than those for unexpected benefit. However, given the diverse and consistent prior evidence from observational and methodologic studies favoring a beneficial, rather than harmful effect on CHD events, the widespread use of conjugated estrogens in the general population and the multiplicity of endpoints being followed, the board decided to use symmetric and fairly conservative stopping boundaries for benefit or harm.

These boundaries were not crossed for the primary outcome (non-fatal MI plus CHD death) nor for any of the secondary cardiac outcomes. However for one of the important secondary outcomes—CHD deaths—the difference between treated and placebo groups reached a p-value of .02 at a DSMB meeting two-thirds of the way through follow-up, and appeared destined to cross the stopping boundary (Figure 1a). Given the prior evidence and widespread belief that hormone therapy was beneficial for prevention of CHD events, the large number of endpoints being tested, and the fact that the stopping boundary was not closely approached for any other CHD outcome, including the primary endpoint (Figure 1b), the board voted to continue the trial. (The board requested that the sponsor test a sample of the blinded medication to assure that treatment assignment had not been reversed.) As events turned out, the decision not to stop early revealed a more favorable trend in the between-group comparison of cardiac outcomes in the last third of the study (Figure 2ab) and provided more precise estimates of the overall effect of this hormone treatment over a mean of 4.1 years.

- *Stop early because of significant harm in a secondary outcome?* In the middle years of the trial, an increased risk of venous thromboembolic events in the hormone-treated group did cross the stopping boundaries. At the time HERS began, there was evidence that oral contraceptive pills increased risk for venous thromboembolic events, but little evidence that the relatively low dose of estrogen in post-menopausal hormone therapy increased risk. The possibility of this adverse effect was discussed in the informed consent, but was not stated as a known risk. After HERS began, several observational studies reported an increased risk of venous thromboembolic events among users of post-menopausal hormone therapy[9-11] but a causal basis for this risk had not been documented in a clinical trial. The board's view was that this was a serious but relatively uncommon harm (the excess risk of pulmonary embolism or deep vein thrombosis was 4/1,000/year, and the estimated risk of dying of it about 1/10 of this), and that the magnitude of the harm did not require that the trial be stopped. After discussing numerous options, the board advised HERS investigators to inform HERS women of the finding; to institute additional measures to assure that HERS treatment was stopped in any women whose risk of thromboembolism was increased by fracture, cancer, major operation, or immobility; and to publish a brief report on the findings regarding increased risk of venous thrombosis. These

a.

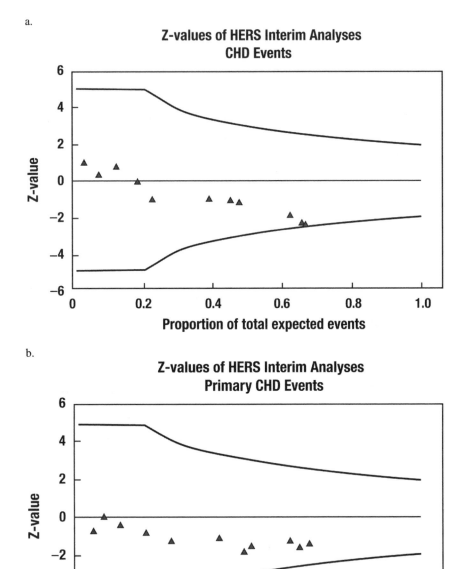

Figure 1 Lan and DeMets plots of Z-values over the first two-thirds of the study for interim looks at the relative hazard comparing hormone treatment to placebo for CHD deaths (a) and for the primary outcome CHD deaths plus non-fatal MI (b). Positive values represent lower event rates in the hormone treatment group.

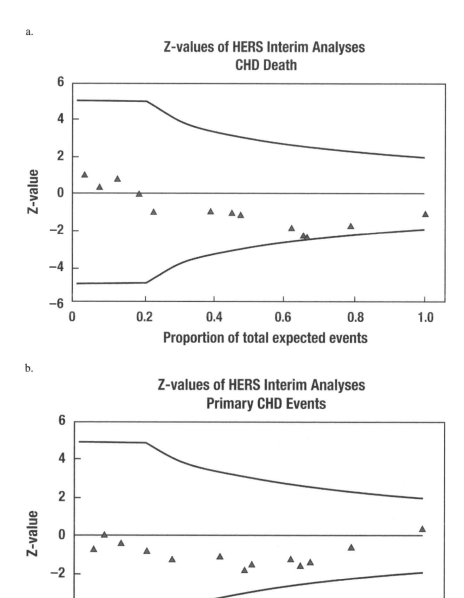

Figure 2 Same as Figure 1, but including data for entire study.

things were done, and a letter to the editor appeared in JAMA[12] one year before the final report from HERS.

- *Stop early because of the futility of seeking a benefit in CHD outcomes?* During the final year of the trial, the board discussed the possibility of stopping the trial early because the conditional power to discover an overall benefit in the primary endpoint (non-fatal MI and CHD death) over the next several years, given the adverse early trend, was nearly zero. Moreover, in addition to the significant increase in thromboembolic events in the hormone-treated group, there were non-significant trends toward increased rates of gall bladder disease, breast cancer, stroke, and total mortality, and there were no favorable trends. The question arose, is it ethical to continue a trial that has virtually no possibility of revealing a benefit, to make the estimated effects (which might include significant harm) more precise and convincing? The board adopted the view, given the widespread beliefs among physicians and the public in the benefits of hormone treatment, that it would be wrong to stop the study early in the absence of findings that were sufficiently definitive in their potential influence on clinical practice one way or the other.

- *Extend trial to confirm the late beneficial trend in CHD outcomes?* Near the end of the study, the board noted a trend toward lower rates of non-fatal MI in the hormone group (Table 1) and a nominally significant time trend of early harm and later benefit (*post hoc* p = 0.01). Given the expected delay in the effects on CHD incidence of hormone-induced lowering of LDL-cholesterol and raising of HDL-cholesterol, it seemed possible that extending the trial might eventually reveal an overall benefit. This course of action would have required that the participants be invited to give new informed consent for an additional 2–3 years of randomized treatment, and the investigators were concerned that many of these elderly women with coronary disease were weary and would not want to continue randomized treatment. Even more important, conditional power to detect delayed benefit needed to be based on the entire period of follow-up, including the early harm in the first two years, and was therefore marginal even under optimistic assumptions about a growing magnitude of benefit. In addition, the board considered the argument that a preventive intervention that causes early harm and needs to be continued for longer than four years to show benefit is not likely to be clinically useful. Therefore the Board recommended that randomized treatment end at the originally scheduled time (April–July, 1998).

As an alternative to extending the trial, the board endorsed the investigators' plan to continue disease event surveillance in an observational mode. During this further follow-up ("HERS 2"), very few of the women who had been in the placebo group chose to begin hormone therapy (after being informed of the early harm observed in the trial) and most of the women who had been in the hormone treatment group chose to continue on open label treatment (given the trial's finding of possible delayed benefit). As a result, HERS 2 served to continue the randomized trial, albeit with some increased cross-over. Three additional years of follow-up revealed no benefit in the primary endpoint[13] or any other outcome,[14] and helped to discount the possibility raised at the end of HERS that longer term treatment might have had a more favorable outcome.

In addition to these questions, the investigators and board wrestled with a number of practical and ethical considerations in closing out the trial. This led to a plan to inform participants about the results of the trial but leave decisions about subsequent open-label hormone therapy to the women and their personal physicians. This made ultra-rapid publication of the findings necessary in order to allow HERS participants to make timely informed decisions as to continuing (for those randomized to active treatment) or initiating (for those in the placebo group) hormone therapy. The timetable for accomplishing the expedited publication of a nearly complete set of HERS results was extremely challenging, requiring an acceleration of the process of reporting and adjudicating events, and of analyzing and interpreting the findings and writing and reviewing the report. This challenge was complicated by the need for confidentiality until the end when HERS scientists, staff, participants, and the public all needed to be rapidly informed of the conclusions and their implications for hormone treatment. Fortunately, close-out proceeded without major problems and the main JAMA report appeared a month after the last clinic visit, in mid-August 1998.[6]

Although the main HERS report was received with skepticism by many practicing physicians and some authorities, the results led to revised practice guidelines that were a major step toward abandoning the use of hormone therapy for prevention of coronary disease,[15,16] even before the results of the first Women's Health Initiative Trial were published in 2002. However, sales of post-menopausal hormones did not decrease appreciably until 2003,[17] after publication of the results of HERS 2[13] and the first Women's Health Initiative trial.[18] This much larger primary prevention trial confirmed the absence of a beneficial effect of estrogen plus progestin treatment on CHD outcomes and the increased risk of venous thromboembolic events and revealed serious adverse effects on other outcomes including breast cancer, stroke and dementia. It remains possible that other hormone preparations and doses in other populations (particularly earlier in menopause) might be more beneficial, but it is now clear that this must be shown to be the case with randomized blinded trials that have disease endpoints as the outcome.

LESSONS LEARNED

HERS illustrates in a powerful way the evidence-based medicine principle that well designed and executed randomized blinded trials are a necessary basis for drug treatments. It shows that a clinical trial with disease endpoints that is properly designed and carried out will trump inferences drawn from a large and consistent body of evidence, including observational epidemiology, pathophysiology, and clinical trials with surrogate outcomes. Several important Data and Safety Monitoring Board decisions contributed to the strength of the HERS conclusions.

1. One of these was the decision not to stop the trial prematurely despite strong adverse trends in an important component of the primary outcome (coronary deaths) as well as moderate adverse trends in other clinical outcomes, and extremely low conditional power for observing a benefit in the primary outcome. The board decided that the over-riding consideration, given the widespread belief that hormone treatment was beneficial and the HERS evidence to the contrary, was to continue the trial in order to produce the most definitive conclusions possible.

2. Another important decision was not stopping the trial prematurely in the face of a highly significant increase in the risk of a serious but relatively uncommon secondary outcome (thromboembolic events). The board determined that this could be managed ethically by stopping study drugs in the small group of women with particular risk factors for thromboembolism, and by informing HERS women and the public of the finding.

3. A third important decision was recommending continued disease event surveillance for several years after stopping randomized treatment (in HERS 2), rather than attempting to extend the trial beyond its scheduled ending. This was an inexpensive, ethical, and feasible approach to expanding the information available from the study.

In general, HERS illustrates the fact that trials may produce a complex set of findings, including some that are entirely unexpected. Interim monitoring guidelines should address a wide range of possible outcomes and include stopping boundaries that do not restrict the number or timing of looks at the outcome data (such as those of Lan and DeMets).[7] There should be flexibility that allows for decisions based on the judgment of a diverse group of experts as to benefits and harms, ethical implications, and the social obligation to have an optimal impact on policy and practice guidelines.

ACKNOWLEDGEMENTS

Dr. Hulley was PI of the HERS Coordinating Center at UCSF, Dr. Grady was Co-PI and Dr. Vittinghoff was the principal statistician. Dr. Williams chaired the DSMB, which also included Drs. Christine Cassel David DeMets, Judith Hochman, Susan Johnson, Genell Knatterud, and Neil Stone, who participated in the HERS decisions but were not involved in preparing this chapter.

REFERENCES

1. Barrett-Connor E, Grady D. 1998. Hormone replacement therapy, heart disease, and other considerations. *Ann Rev Pub Health* 19:55-72.
2. Mendelsohn ME, Karas RH. 1999. The protective effects of estrogen on the cardiovascular system. *N Engl J Med* 340:1801-1811.
3. PEPI Writing Group. 1995. Effects of estrogen or estrogen/progestin regimens on heart disease risk factors in postmenopausal women. *JAMA* 273:199-208.
4. Grady D, Gebretsadik T, Kerlikowske K, Ernster V, Petitti D. 1995. Hormone replacement therapy and endometrial cancer risk: A meta-analysis. *Obstet Gynecol* 85:304-313.
5. Grady D, Appgate W. Bush T, et al. 1998. Heart and Estrogen/progestin Replacement Study (HERS): design, methods, and baseline characteristics. *Control Clin Trials* 19:314-335.
6. Hulley S, Grady D, Bush T, Furberg C, Herrington D, Riggs B, et al. 1998. Randomized trial of estrogen plus progestin for secondary prevention of coronary heart disease in postmenopausal women. Heart and Estrogen/progestin Replacement Study (HERS) Research Group. *JAMA* 280:605-613.
7. Lan KKG, DeMets DL, Halperin M. 1984. More flexible sequential and non-sequential designs in long-term clinical trials. *Commun Stat Theory Method* 3:2339-2354.
8. Coronary Drug Project Research Group. 1981. Practical aspects of decision making in clinical trials: The Coronary Drug Project as a case study. *Control Clin Trials* 1:363-376.
9. Daly E, Vessey MP, Hawkins MM, Carson JL, Gough P, Marsh S. 1996. Risk of venous thromboembolism in users of hormone replacement therapy. *Lancet* 348:977-980.
10. Jick H, Derby LE, Myers MW, Vasilakis C, Newton KM. 1996. Risk of hospital admission for idiopathic venous thromboembolism among users of postmenopausal oestrogens. *Lancet* 348:981-983.
11. Grodstein F, Stampfer MJ, Goldhaber SZ, et al. 1996. Prospective study of exogenous hormones and risk of pulmonary embolism in women. *Lancet* 348:983-987.
12. Grady D, Hulley SB, Furberg CD. 1997. Venous thromboembolic events associated with hormone replacement therapy. *JAMA* 278:477.
13. Grady D, Herrington D, Bittner V, Blumenthal R, Davidson M, Hlatky M, et al. 2002. Cardiovascular outcomes during 6.8 years of hormone therapy: HERS II. *JAMA* 288:49-57.
14. Hulley S, Furberg C, Barrett-Connor E, Cauley J, Grady D, Haskell W, Knopp R, et al. 2002. Non-cardiovascular disease outcomes during 6.8 years of hormone therapy: HERS II. *JAMA* 288:58-66.
15. USPHS Task Force. 2002. Postmenopausal hormone replacement therapy for primary prevention of chronic conditions. *Ann Intern Med* 137:834-839.
16. Mosca L, Collins P, Herrington D. 2001. Hormone replacement therapy and cardiovascular disease: A statement for healthcare professionals from the American Heart Association. *Circulation* 104:499-503.
17. Hersh AL, Stefanick ML, Stafford RS. 2004. National use of postmenopausal hormone therapy: annual trends and response to recent evidence. *JAMA* 291:47-53.
18. WHI Study Group. 2002. Risks and benefits of estrogen plus progestin in health postmenopausal women. *JAMA* 288:321-333.

Data Monitoring in the Antihypertensive and Lipid-Lowering Treatment to Prevent Heart Attack Trial: Early Termination of the Doxazosin Treatment Arm

Barry R. Davis
Jeffrey A. Cutler

ABSTRACT

The Antihypertensive and Lipid-Lowering Treatment to Prevent Heart Attack Trial's (ALLHAT) hypertension component was designed to determine whether the incidence of fatal coronary heart disease or non-fatal myocardial infarction differs between diuretic (chlorthalidone) treatment and each of three other classes of antihypertensive drugs—a calcium antagonist (amlodipine), an angiotensin-converting enzyme inhibitor (lisinopril), or an alpha-adrenergic blocker (doxazosin) in high-risk hypertensive persons aged 55 years and older. A Data and Safety Monitoring Board met twice yearly to review data on participant recruitment, retention, endpoints, and other patient safety issues. The doxazosin arm of the trial was terminated earlier than planned due to the low likelihood of finding a significant difference in the primary outcome by the study's scheduled end and a significant 25% increase in cardiovascular events for doxazosin compared with chlorthalidone. This decision was made based on recommendations from an *ad hoc* review committee following a split vote of the Data and Safety Monitoring Board. This paper describes the monitoring guidelines established for ALLHAT and how they were used, the role of secondary endpoints in DSMB deliberations, advance preparations for possible closeout of a study arm, the role of a Special Review Committee, processes for closeout of the doxazosin arm, and lessons learned.

INTRODUCTION AND BACKGROUND

Coronary heart disease (CHD) is the leading cause of death in the United States.[1] Analyses of previous antihypertensive trials showed that the observed reduction in CHD was smaller than what would be expected from epidemiological overviews whereas the observed reduction in stroke was as expected.[1] A possible explanation for this might be the adverse metabolic effects (hypokalemia, dyslipidemia, hyperglycemia) seen with diuretics but not with newer antihypertensive agents. Thus ALLHAT was conceived to determine if the newer agents were superior in preventing CHD because of the absence of adverse effects on metabolism and possibly beneficial effects on other putative disease mediators. Similar blood pressure in all arms was expected to be achieved in ALLHAT so that any event differences that did occur could be explained by blood-pressure-independent effects. In addition to the aforementioned hypertensive component, ALLHAT had a lipid-lowering component involving about one-fourth of the trial's participants and designed to determine if lowering LDL-cholesterol in older, moderately hypercholesterolemic patients would reduce the incidence of all-cause mortality.[2]

PROTOCOL DESIGN

The design of ALLHAT has been described in detail.[2] Participants were assigned by a randomization schedule to one of four first-line treatments: chlorthalidone, amlodipine, lisinopril, or doxazosin, in a ratio of $1.7 : 1 : 1 : 1$, respectively. Randomization was stratified by center and blocked over time to maintain the ratio. The treatment goal in all four arms was a DBP of less than 90 mm Hg and an SBP of less than 140 mm Hg. All four drugs were encapsulated and identical in appearance, so the identity of each agent was masked at each dosage level. Dosages for doxazosin were 2, 4, and 8 mg/day; corresponding dosages for chlorthalidone were 12.5, 12.5, and 25 mg/day, respectively. If participants did not meet the BP goal while taking the maximum tolerated dose, second and third-line drugs could be added.

The primary outcome was CHD, defined as non-fatal myocardial infarction or fatal CHD. Secondary outcomes were total mortality, stroke, combined CHD (CHD, coronary revascularization procedures, hospitalized angina), and combined cardiovascular disease [CVD] (combined CHD, stroke, treated angina, treated/hospitalized/fatal heart failure, treated lower extremity arterial disease). The trial was initially designed to randomize 40,000 patients for 82.5% power to detect a 16% reduction in CHD for each of the three newer agents compared to chlorthalidone using a two-tailed 0.017 significance level (adjusted for multiple comparisons using the Dunnett procedure to provide an overall alpha = 0.05).[3] This design assumed a 12.5% cumulative rate of CHD over the five years of planned follow-up. The primary test statistic to compare time to CHD between chlorthalidone and each of the three newer agents was the logrank test.[4] ALLHAT had an independent Data and Safety Monitoring Board (DSMB) which was scheduled to meet once or twice yearly. The eight members of the DSMB were appointed by the Director, NHLBI, and included six physicians (two cardiologists) with special expertise in hypertension, other CVD risk factors, and minority health; one other CVD epidemiologist/trialist; and a biostatistician with experience running coordinating centers for multicenter trials.

Patient enrollment began in February 1994, and follow-up was scheduled to be completed in March 2002. Following data reviews on January 6, 2000 (by the DSMB) and January 21, 2000 (by an *ad hoc* Special Review Committee [SRC]), the director of the National Heart, Lung, and Blood Institute accepted a recommendation to discontinue the doxazosin treatment arm in the blood pressure (BP) component of the trial. While there were essentially no differences in the rates of the primary outcome or all-cause mortality between the two treatment groups, there was a statistically significant 25% higher incidence of major CVD events in participants assigned to the doxazosin group compared with those assigned to the chlorthalidone group. In addition, the likelihood of observing a significant difference for the primary outcome by the scheduled end of the trial was very low based on conditional power.[5] It was determined that participants assigned to the doxazosin group should be informed of their BP treatment assignment and that the major clinical findings regarding this treatment and its comparison agent, chlorthalidone, should be reported as soon as possible.[6,7] Regarding other treatment comparisons, the ALLHAT Data and Safety Monitoring Board (DSMB) emphasized the crucial importance of continuing the rest of the BP and lipid-lowering components of the trial. This paper describes the monitoring guidelines established for ALLHAT and how they were used, the role of secondary endpoints in DSMB deliberations, advance preparations for possible closeout of a study arm, the role of a Special Review Committee, processes for closeout of the doxazosin arm, and lessons learned.

DATA MONITORING EXPERIENCE

In December 1993, the Protocol Review Committee met for the first time to review and approve the protocol. After the meeting, this committee became the DSMB which met once or twice per year to review accumulating data and to monitor the trial for either superiority or inferiority of the three agents compared with chlorthalidone. A specific charge to the DSMB was to evaluate the unblinded data for emergence of clinically important treatment differences that might warrant alteration of the protocol or early termination of one or more arms or the entire trial. The Lan–DeMets version of the O'Brien–Fleming group sequential boundaries was used to assess treatment group differences for the primary endpoint (CHD) and conditional power was used to assess futility.[5,8,9] The sequential boundaries for the logrank test statistic are shown in Figure 1 and in Table 1. No formal monitoring procedures were established for secondary endpoints.

Information time was to be calculated as proportion of expected primary outcome events in the diuretic arm (estimated to be 1,000). Official looks at the unblinded outcome data were to occur whenever each increment of 100 primary events had occurred in the diuretic group beginning with an initial occurrence of 200 events. Meetings were held in June 1994, January 1995, August 1995, February 1996, May 1996, September 1996, March 1997, March 1998 (22% information time or the first official look), December 1998 (37% information time), July 1999 (50% information time), and January 2000 (59% information time). The Special Review Committee also met in January 2000 to resolve ambiguities in the recommendations of the DSMB.

At the March 1998 and December 1998 meetings, the board voted to continue the trial. No differences were noted for any of three comparisons with

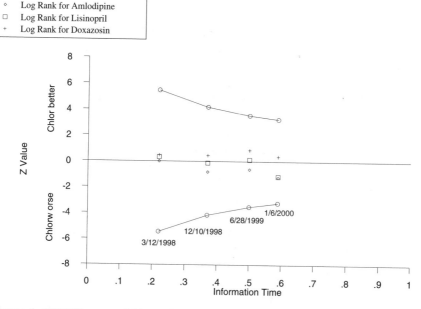

Figure 1 ALLHAT sequential boundaries for the primary endpoint.

Table 1 ALLHAT Interim Data (Primary outcome)

| Meeting date | Information time | CHD Events— n, rate per 100 (SE) | | Log rank | Sequential boundaries | |
		Chlorthalidone (N = 15,255)	Doxazosin (N = 9,061)		Z_L	Z_U
3/12/98	0.22	224	140	0.46	−5.46	5.46
		2.9 (0.2)*	2.8 (0.3)			
12/10/98	0.37	366	226	0.45	−4.16	4.16
		3.4 (0.2)**	3.5 (0.3)			
6/28/99	0.50	498	310	0.86	−3.53	3.53
		6.4 (0.4)**	6.3 (0.5)			
1/6/00	0.59	608	365	0.38	−3.24	3.24
		6.3 (0.4)**	6.3 (0.3)			

* Year 3 rate
** Year 4 rate

regard to the primary outcome. At the July 1999 DSMB meeting (50% information time), the board noted that compared with doxazosin, chlorthalidone yielded an essentially equal risk of CHD (the primary endpoint) but reduced the risk of combined CVD events (a specified secondary endpoint), particularly heart failure (HF). Because HF is not necessarily a straightforward diagnosis, at the board's request, additional data analyses were to be conducted by the time of the next meeting.

The ALLHAT Endpoints Subcommittee had not previously reviewed HF cases. However, in accordance with the board's request, 50 cases were randomly selected and reviewed for consistency with the study's definition of HF. Individual signs and symptoms were evaluated as well as the overall diagnosis. All of the cases reviewed were hospitalized, since detailed sign and symptom data were not collected for nonhospitalized cases. This review did not require additional data collection from the sites, as only available discharge summaries were used. Thirty-nine (78%) of the 50 case records contained sufficient data for review of ALLHAT criteria signs and symptoms. The subcommittee agreed with the diagnosis of HF in 90% of the reviewed chlorthalidone cases and 90% of the reviewed doxazosin cases. Ejection fractions were also reviewed to gain further insight. They had been performed in about half of all hospitalized HF cases (n = 629) in both groups. Among cases with reported ejection fraction results, the data were similar in the chlorthalidone and doxazosin groups. The post-case prescription of open-label diuretics, ACE inhibitors, and beta-blockers was about the same in cases in both treatment groups. Two additional points to be made regarding all of the HF cases are that (1) for the harder outcome of hospitalized plus fatal HF, the results for doxazosin versus chlorthalidone were similar to the broader endpoint of hospitalized plus fatal plus treated HF, and (2) two-year total mortality rates subsequent to HF diagnosis were high (as expected) and similar in both treatment groups (19% in the chlorthalidone group and 22% in the doxazosin group, p = 0.83). Further details on these results have been provided.[10]

All the aforementioned analyses supported the validity of HF diagnoses in ALLHAT. This information, plus the knowledge that the likelihood of observing a significant difference for the primary outcome by the scheduled end of the trial was only 2% for the protocol-specified reduction of 16%, prompted meetings by representatives of the ALLHAT NHLBI Project Office, the Clinical Trials Center, and the Steering Committee chair several months prior to the January 2000 DSMB meeting. These trends were discussed and a timetable was prepared for possible closeout if the DSMB decided to discontinue the doxazosin arm. Discussions began regarding the required materials, including a letter notifying the investigators, letters to the participants, and a short paper describing the pertinent results, as well as other materials.

Also, three individuals from the ALLHAT regional teams were nominated to participate as members of the closeout team with the Steering Committee chair and representatives from the NHLBI and Clinical Trials Center. Since the nominees previously had been blinded to the data, they were not notified of their selection prior to the decision to terminate the doxazosin arm. By the time of the January 2000 DSMB meeting, letters to the principal investigators and the participants, as well as a short paper describing the comparison of doxazosin and chlorthalidone, had been drafted.

The DSMB met on January 6, 2000 to discuss the data and the requested confirmatory analyses regarding HF diagnoses. The outcomes data table, three key graphs—the doxazosin versus chlorthalidone comparisons for the primary outcome, combined CVD, and HF (Table 2 and Figure 2) and the sequential boundaries results (Table 1 and Figure 1) were important to making a decision. For the comparison of doxazosin to chlorthalidone, the relative risk (D/C) for the primary endpoint was 1.03 (not significant). The conditional power to detect a difference, assuming an actual 16% risk reduction, was 2%. Secondary outcome relative risks and p-values were total mortality, 1.03 (p = 0.56); stroke, 1.19 (p = 0.04); combined CHD, 1.10 (p = 0.046); combined CVD, 1.25 (p < 0.001); and HF, 2.04 (p < 0.001). The board unanimously voted to continue the lisinopril and amlodipine arms, but there was a closely split decision as to whether to continue the doxazosin arm. The key issues for those who voted for continuation were (1) continuing uncertainties about the validity of HF diagnoses and the possibility of bias favoring the chlorthalidone arm, despite the results of the special analyses; (2) a general reluctance to stop an arm; and (3) suspicion that data lags in endpoint reporting, which could make conditional power higher than it

Table 2 Major CV Events in ALLHAT as of January 6, 2000 DSMB Meeting, According to Treatment Group

OUTCOME	Treatment group (n, 4-year rate per 100 [SE])		z	p-value
	Chlorthalidone	Doxazosin		
Patients in group	15,255	9,061		
CHD	608	365	0.38	0.71
	6.30 (0.38)	6.26 (0.30)		
All-cause mortality	851	514	0.58	0.56
	9.08 (0.35)	9.62 (0.49)		
Combined CHD	1,211	775	2.00	0.05
	11.97 (0.38)	13.06 (0.53)		
Stroke	351	244	2.05	0.04
	3.61 (0.22)	4.23 (0.32)		
Combined CVD	2,245	1,592	6.77	<0.001
	21.76 (0.49)	25.45 (0.68)		
Heart failure	420	491	10.95	<0.001
	4.45 (0.26)	8.13 (0.43)		
Coronary revascularization	502	337	2.00	0.05
	5.20 (0.27)	6.21 (0.39)		
Angina	1,082	725	3.01	<0.001
	10.19 (0.35)	11.54 (0.48)		
Peripheral arterial disease	264	165	0.67	0.50
	2.87 (0.21)	2.89 (0.26)		

seemed. (The lisinopril and amlodipine results seen in Figure 1 were quite different than doxazosin in having better prospects of reaching a significant finding for the primary outcome—43% and 47%, respectively, to detect a protocol-specified 16% difference in CHD.)

Since there was such a close vote on an important matter, NHLBI, with the concurrence and support of the board's chair, decided to convene a Special Review Committee (SRC) to seek an additional opinion. Specifically, the panel was asked to review the data and reach a consensus recommendation for the NHLBI Director regarding continuation of the doxazosin arm of ALLHAT's antihypertensive component.

The SRC met on January 21, 2000. It was composed of two physicians, both very experienced in leading and monitoring CVD trials and one with special expertise in HF, and a biostatistician highly experienced in CVD trials. Key elements in this review were, again, validity of HF diagnoses and the weight that this condition should have in a decision to stop the doxazosin arm. Although the SRC would have preferred to see analyses based on a subset of HF cases with the strongest diagnostic data, such as a positive chest x-ray, they judged the diagnoses to be accurate and unbiased. Also, they thought that continuing the doxazosin arm would have been acceptable in

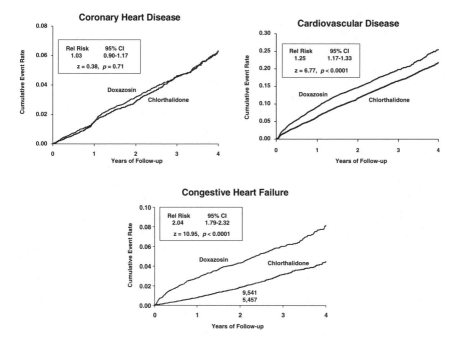

Figure 2 Kaplan–Meier curves for coronary heart disease, combined cardiovascular disease, and heart failure—doxazosin vs. chlorthalidone.[6]

the absence of an effect on total mortality, but they concluded that with such low conditional power, it was not justified, given that HF is a serious outcome.

After the SRC review, a recommendation was issued for termination of the doxazosin arm based on the observations previously described. The NHLBI director accepted that recommendation on January 24, 2000, setting in motion a series of activities including release of information to the Steering Committee and Regional teams (February 3, 2000), press release from NHLBI (March 8, 2000), and a presentation at the American College of Cardiology meeting (March 15, 2000).

Upon the acceptance of the recommendation, the NHLBI Project Office notified the Clinical Trials Center. The ALLHAT Steering Committee was scheduled to meet on February 3–4, 2000, for a routine face-to-face meeting. Two agendas were prepared: one for distribution in advance of the meeting that did not mention the closeout of the doxazosin arm, and another agenda that included details on the data, the decision, the activities, and a timeline for closeout.

Because chlorthalidone was found to be better at preventing combined cardiovascular disease events (a specified secondary endpoint), particularly heart failure, compared with doxazosin, open-label chlorthalidone was provided for use in participants who would be discontinuing doxazosin. However, use of the open-label chlorthalidone was not mandatory, and investigators could prescribe alternative antihypertensive therapy at their discretion. Treatment could include the open-label chlorthalidone and/or any of the step 2 and step 3 medications provided by ALLHAT (atenolol, clonidine, reserpine, hydralazine); other antihypertensive medications could be prescribed but would be paid for by the participant. These treatment recommendations followed those of the Sixth Report of the Joint National Committee on Hypertension,[11] although the final treatment decision was up to the investigator. Guidelines were also provided in a document, "Frequently Asked Questions (FAQ) for Regional and Study Coordinators," regarding what to advise participants on open-label alpha-blockers for benign prostatic hypertrophy.

Participants assigned to doxazosin and not enrolled in the lipid trial (i.e., participants discontinuing their ALLHAT participation) who were recruited from among patients in ALLHAT investigators' practices were provided a four-month supply of antihypertensive medication and continued their antihypertensive treatment with the physician investigator outside of the study. Other participants who were assigned to doxazosin and not enrolled in the lipid trial could receive a four-month supply of antihypertensive medication from ALLHAT and returned to other primary caregivers for subsequent antihypertensive treatment and usual routine follow-up. Participants assigned to doxazosin and enrolled in the lipid trial continued follow-up for that trial component, and were able to receive ALLHAT open-label medications as described previously for the duration of the study.

Pfizer, Inc. provided doxazosin for ALLHAT. A few days prior to the Steering Committee meeting, NHLBI representatives informed Pfizer and the Food and Drug Administration of the decision to terminate the doxazosin arm.

Several factors came into play regarding the release of the doxazosin/chlorthalidone comparison results. Considerations included the importance of quickly getting new and important scientific information into the hands of clinicians, as well as the need to have this information presented in a balanced way with a proper interpretation of the study data as a result of a peer-review process. The manuscript of the results was approved by the Steering Committee during a conference call on February 14, 2000, and submitted to the *Journal of the American Medical Association (JAMA)*. *JAMA* accepted the request for expedited peer review; and the paper was reviewed, revised, and received final approval by March 10. The NHLBI issued a press release on March 8, and the data were presented at the American College of Cardiology meeting on March 15. The paper was published on the web in *JAMA Express* on April 5 and was in print in the April 19, 2000, issue.

The published analyses were based on the data as of December 3, 1999,[6] and not on data from the doxazosin closeout forms. Censoring dates were based on the last known follow-up prior to this date. This information formed the basis of the review committee's recommendation to discontinue the doxazosin arm. A final paper was published on the doxazosin / chlorthalidone comparison, that included all events occurring on or before February 15, 2000, when the results were released to the clinical sites.[12]

LESSONS LEARNED

The ALLHAT experience has provided the cardiology and clinical trial communities some valuable lessons. One is that accepted beliefs can be wrong. Prior to ALLHAT, the consensus was that antihypertensive pressure agents that improved lipid and glucose levels along with lowering high blood pressure would provide added benefit to the patient with hypertension in terms of reducing clinical outcomes compared to agents without these properties. The fact that elevated hyperglycemia and dyslipidemia are predictive of subsequent risk of CHD, stroke, and other forms of CVD led many to argue that the newer drugs would be superior to the older agent, diuretic. ALLHAT proved that this is not true. ALLHAT participants randomized to doxazosin did have modestly improved lipid and glucose levels compared to those randomized to chlorthalidone, but those randomized to chlorthalidone had more favorable results with respect to cardiovascular outcomes. Lowering glucose and lipid levels is important, but is clearly not sufficient to offset differences in effects on BP or the superiority of diuretics for preventing HF. This trial is one of many that have demonstrated the challenges and dangers of using surrogate outcomes.

The issue of stopping a trial based on a secondary outcome also arises in ALLHAT. A similar experience occurred in the Physician's Health Study.[13] There was no observed difference in the primary outcome, and based on conditional power calculations, it was highly unlikely that there would be any seen by the trial's scheduled end. However, there was a highly statistically significant result for a secondary outcome. The driving force behind this outcome was a serious medical condition (heart failure) that increases the incidence of subsequent mortality. This was noted from both external and internal evidence.

Regardless of how detailed a DSMB's charter and monitoring plan are, DSMBs often have to react to unexpected events and situations. A DSMB has to have flexibility and wisdom to respond to changing circumstances and to do so in a timely fashion. In the case of ALLHAT, the DSMB recognized the potential problem with the emerging treatment differences in HF. A review of cases by the Endpoint Subcommittee and a series of analyses by the CTC helped to clarify the situation.

Finally, the ALLHAT DSMB had to weigh the balance between obtaining more persuasive evidence and an ethical responsibility to current and future patients. If a trial is not allowed to continue until the data become convincing, then belief and practice may not change, which would have put even more patients at risk. However, continuing the trial beyond the point where the data have become convincing would be placing current patients at unnecessary risk. The point at which this happens is largely based on the DSMB's best judgment. The doxazosin arm of the ALLHAT trial was stopped at a time when the data were convincing, and as a result the trend toward increased use of alpha-blockers for hypertension treatment has been reversed.[14] Statistical methods such as sequential monitoring boundaries and conditional power can be very useful for the primary outcome (or secondary outcomes), but the totality of evidence must be considered in any DSMB recommendation.

REFERENCES

1. Collins R, Peto R, Godwin J, MacMahon S. 1990. Blood pressure and coronary heart disease. *Lancet.* 336:370–371.
2. Davis BR, Cutler JA, Gordon D, et al. for the ALLHAT Research Group. 1996. Rationale and design of the Antihypertensive and Lipid-Lowering Treatment to Prevent Heart Attack Trial (ALLHAT). *Am J Hypertens* 9:342–360.
3. Dunnett CW. 1955. A multiple comparison procedure for comparing several treatments with a control. *J Am Stat Assoc* 60:573–583.
4. Klein JP, Moeschberger ML. 1977. Survival Analysis: Techniques for Censored and Truncated Regression. Springer-Verlag, New York.
5. Davis BR, Hardy RJ. 1990. Upper bounds for type I and type II error rates in conditional power calculations. *Comm Stat* A19:3571–3584.
6. ALLHAT Investigators. 2000. Major cardiovascular events in hypertensive patients randomized to doxazosin vs. chlorthalidone: The Antihypertensive and Lipid-Lowering Treatment to Prevent Heart Attack Trial (ALLHAT). *JAMA* 283:1967–1975.
7. Pressel SL , Davis BR, Wright JT, Jr. et al. for the ALLHAT Collaborative Research Group. 2001. Operational Aspects of Terminating the Doxazosin Arm of the Antihypertensive and Lipid Lowering Treatment to Prevent Heart Attack Trial (ALLHAT). *Control Clin Trials* 22:29–41.
8. Jennison C, Turnbull BW. 2000. Group Sequential Methods With Applications to Clinical Trials. Chapman & Hall/CRC Press, Boca Raton, FL.
9. Lan KKG, DeMets DL. 1983. Discrete sequential boundaries for clinical trials. *Biometrika* 70:659–663.
10. Piller LB, Davis BR, Cutler JA, Cushman WC, Wright Jr JT, Williamson JD, et al. for the ALLHAT Collaborative Research Group. 2002. Validation of heart failure events in ALLHAT participants assigned to doxazosin. *Curr Control Trials Cardiovasc Med* 3:10.
11. The sixth report of the Joint National Committee on Prevention, Detection, Evaluation, and Treatment of High Blood Pressure. 1997. *Arch Intern Med* 157:2413–2446.

12. ALLHAT Officers and Coordinators for the ALLHAT Collaborative Research Group. 2003. Diuretic Versus α-Blocker as First-Step Antihypertensive Therapy—Final Results From the Antihypertensive and Lipid-Lowering Treatment to Prevent Heart Attack Trial (ALLHAT). *Hypertension* 42:239-246.
13. The Steering Committee of the Physicians' Health Study Research Group. 1989. Final report on the aspirin component of the ongoing Physicians' Health Study. *N Engl J Med* 321:129-135.
14. Stafford RS, Furberg CD, Findelstein SN, Cockburn IM, Alahegn T, Ma J. 2004. Impact of clinical trial results on national trends in α-blocker prescribing, 1996-2002. *JAMA*. 291:54-62.

Data Monitoring Experience in the Moxonidine Congestive Heart Failure Trial*

Stuart Pocock
Lars Wilhelmsen
Kenneth Dickstein
Gary Francis
Janet Wittes

ABSTRACT

The MOXonidine CONgestive Heart Failure Trial was a randomized placebo-controlled trial designed to evaluate reliably the effects of moxonidine, a central sympathetic inhibitor, on mortality and major morbid events in patients with heart failure.

The primary endpoint was all-cause mortality, and the trial was intended to follow around 4,500 patients for an average of around 2.5 years until 724 deaths had occurred. Within a few months of study starting, the Data Monitoring Board (DMB) observed an emerging trend of an excess of death on moxonidine compared with placebo. Ten months after the first patient was randomized the study was stopped based on 46 versus 25 deaths in 990 moxonidine and 943 placebo patients respectively, p = 0.01. The final published evidence had 54 versus 32 deaths, p = 0.012.

This study illustrates the problems faced by a DMB, and subsequently the trial Executive Committee and sponsor, in deciding how to act in the face of an emerging (and agonizing) negative trend for mortality in a major international trial. The paper also points to the difficulty of publishing results of such negative trials.

INTRODUCTION AND BACKGROUND

The MOXonidine CONgestive Heart Failure Trial (MOXCON)[1] was undertaken to evaluate the long-term efficacy of sustained-release moxonidine (a central sympathetic nervous system inhibitor) on fatal and non-fatal outcomes in patients with chronic heart failure being treated with other relevant background therapy.

---

* This paper first published in *Eur Heart J* 2004; 25:1974–1978.

Moxonidine reduces plasma norepinephrine (NE) levels, known to be elevated in heart failure, and a prognostic factor for mortality. A shorter-acting version is a well-tolerated and effective anti-hypertensive agent. Previous short-term trials of related drugs had revealed reductions in plasma NE, favorable hemodynamic effects, and symptomatic improvement.

MOXCON was designed as a randomized double-blind placebo controlled trial in patients with NYHA class II–IV heart failure, with ejection fraction ≤35%. Moxonidine SR or matching placebo was given in a forced titration in four stages, from an initial low dose to a dose of 1.5 mg BID, unless symptomatic hypotension, worsening renal function, or other severe side effects were noted.

The primary endpoint was all-cause mortality, and the main secondary endpoints were (1) hospitalisation due to worsening heart failure, (2) the combination of such hospitalisation or death, and (3) cardiovascular mortality.

The study was powered to detect a 20% reduction in mortality relative to an anticipated 2.5-year all-cause mortality rate in the placebo arm of 22.75%, using a logrank test, two-sided 5% type 1 error, and 80% power. This required around 4,500 patients to be recruited and then followed until 724 deaths occurred. Patient recruitment was at 425 centers in 17 countries. The study was sponsored by Eli Lilly and Company and Solvay Pharmaceuticals. Executive and Steering Committees (chair Jay Cohn) oversaw study conduct, a Clinical Endpoint Committee (chair Marc Pfeffer) adjudicated events, and a Data Monitoring Board (DMB) monitored the interim results, as explained below. The DMB had five members: three clinicians—Lars Wilhelmsen (Chair), Kenneth Dickstein, Gary Francis—and two statisticians—Stuart Pocock and Janet Wittes. All interim reports were prepared by Larry Meinert.

The DMB were also to monitor patient safety in an ongoing phase II trial (MOXSE) which was comparing five different dose levels of moxonidine with placebo in heart failure patients.[2] The prime purpose of MOXSE was to determine the relation of plasma NE levels with dose, a key issue in deciding the dose of moxonidine for the MOXCON trial.

The DMB had a planning meeting with sponsor representatives present on March 28, 1998, at which point the MOXSE trial was already underway. Some concerns were expressed about the complexity of starting MOXCON before MOXSE was completed, especially as regards the difficulty of selecting the moxonidine dose for MOXCON so soon.

Statistical Stopping Guidelines

The primary efficacy results for all-cause mortality were to be monitored four times over the course of the study, when 25%, 50%, 75%, and 100% of the expected 724 deaths had occurred. The nominal two-sided p-values for early stopping for efficacy (i.e., fewer deaths on moxonide compared with placebo) were 0.0001 at the 25% analysis and 0.001 at the 50% and 75% analyses.

The DMB was also to conduct safety monitoring reviews at least every six months throughout the course of the study. A safety stopping criterion for all cause mortality was one-sided $P < 0.05$, with at least a 20% observed increase in all cause mortality for moxonidine versus placebo.

DATA MONITORING EXPERIENCE

Randomization began in May 1998, and since there was quite rapidly accelerating recruitment, the DMB's first face-to-face meeting to inspect interim data was on October 20, 1998. The DMB also inspected near-final results of the MOXSE trial. There were no discernible safety concerns and the DMB recommended that the MOXCON study continue as planned.

The DMB next met by teleconference on February 2, 1999, by which time 1,469 patients had been randomized. The main concern was that there were 25 deaths in the moxonidine group and 14 in the placebo group, $p = 0.08$. The DMB consensus was that the total number of deaths was too small to allow a definitive assessment. While a face-to-face DMB meeting had been provisionally planned for March 9, 1999, the DMB concluded it would be inadvisable to wait until then, and that a teleconference be held in the interim.

Accordingly the DMB's next meeting (by teleconference) was on February 16, 1999. By then 1,639 patients had been recruited (839 moxonidine, 800 placebo). The unfavourable trend in mortality had increased further, with 37 deaths reported in the moxonidine group compared with 20 deaths in the placebo group, logrank $P = 0.02$.

The DMB were faced with the disconcerting observation of almost twice as many deaths on moxonidine compared with placebo; this difference was in excess of the pre-defined statistical stopping boundary.

Additional data pertinent to the DMB's decision making was:

1. Causes of death were studied, though for some recent deaths such information was not yet available. No discernible pattern of causes was revealed that might explain the excess mortality, most known causes being typical of such a heart failure population.

2. Data on the time from randomization to death and the dose of moxonidine being received prior to death did not reveal any additional insights. For most patients follow-up was short, median time between three and four months, and the excess of deaths increased steadily over this limited time period.

3. There were no unexpected treatment differences in the incidence of non-fatal serious adverse events (SAE), which incidentally required the same speed of reporting as for deaths.

4. Data on patient baseline characteristics, hospitalizations for heart failure and patient symptoms were much less complete, since as planned these were being reported and processed more slowly than the priority data on deaths and SAEs. The available data showed no evidence of any treatment difference.

5. The earlier phase II trial of moxonidine (MOXSE) had compared five different dose levels with placebo[2] and was now completed. MOXCON had gone on to use the highest of these five doses, on the basis of the plasma norepinephrine level reduction achieved, and there was concern that this might have been an inappropriate choice of dose for safety reasons. Substantial rebound effect has been reported following abrupt cessation of chronic, sustained-release moxonidine.[3] Deaths observed in this phase II trial were 10 out of 230 patients on moxonidine (all five dose groups combined) versus 0 out of 38 patients on placebo. There was no discernible trend in death rates across doses. This phase II trial provided the only additional mortality data for sustained-release moxonidine, and though limited, it added slightly to concern that moxonidine might be causing excess mortality.

The DMB decided, on the basis of this totality of available evidence, to recommend to the Executive Committee that the trial be stopped immediately. The principal argument was that since all-cause mortality was the primary endpoint of the study, the observed negative trend in mortality suggested that a true reduction in mortality due to moxonidine was highly unlikely to be present and detectable with more data. On the other hand, continuing MOXCON's recruitment and follow-up of patients might confer a real risk of further excess deaths attributable to moxonidine, an ethically highly undesirable prospect.

Decision-Making Following the DMB Recommendation

On transmitting this recommendation to the Executive Committee, which included the essential data on which it was based, the chairman of the DMB proposed a joint meeting of the DMB, Executive Committee, and sponsor representatives as soon as possible. Any additional data that accrued in the interim would be available at that meeting. Fortunately, many involved were attending the upcoming American College of Cardiology annual conference, so this meeting took place on March 9, 1999, less that three weeks after the DMB recommendation, a short period of trial continuation that both the DMB and Executive Committee thought appropriate.

At the time of the meeting, 46 deaths had been reported in the moxonidine group and 25 deaths in the placebo group. That is, a further 15 deaths had occurred (9 moxonidine, 5 placebo), making the difference slightly more significant than earlier, P = 0.01.

The members of the Executive Committee debated extensively regarding whether (1) the DMB's recommendation be accepted at this point or (2) additional follow-up and recruitment be sought, i.e., the study continue as planned for the time being with a view to reviewing the situation again a few weeks later. This type of occasion often highlights the inevitable divergence of roles, and hence views, from the two committees. Both committees have ethical and scientific responsibilities, but the two emphases differ. The DMB's remit is primarily ethical: based on all the available evidence, taking account of all patient interests (i.e., those already randomized, those due to be randomized, those in the broader community of similar patients requiring treatment in future), is it ethical for the study to continue as planned. The Executive Committee's remit also concerns scientific and organizational issues: having established the study operations, they wished the study's design and conduct to be of the highest possible standards so that it gives the most reliable evidence regarding the efficacy and safety of the randomized active treatment, thus enhancing scientific knowledge and the care of future patients.

Such full achievement of scientific understanding may be inhibited by the early termination of a study for ethical reasons, since fewer patients followed for less time inevitably means that estimates of treatment effect have poorer precision. Thus, there is a scientific basis for the Executive Committee to want the study to continue longer:

1. Arguments for continuing follow-up were strongly based on the fact that the number of deaths so far amounted to less than 10% of the study's planned total deaths (724) until completion, so this was a very early point at which to stop such an extensive international collaboration, which in organizational terms was proceeding very satisfactorily.

2. There was widespread expert scientific interest in the hypothesis that a central sympathetic inhibitor could prolong survival, improve symptoms, and reduce hospitalizations in patients with chronic heart failure. MOXCON was uniquely placed to be the definitive study of this hypothesis. Thus stopping the study early would prevent studying the hypothesis further in any future randomized trials.

3. It was envisaged that moxonidine treatment in heart failure should to be given over a substantial period. Indeed, in MOXCON the average follow-up was planned to be over two years if the trial continued to its intended conclusion. In contrast, the average patient follow-up in this interim analysis was under four months. Those who urged continuation of the trial argued that the limited follow-up in the current data could give little insight into the

true eventual mortality treatment difference after several years. The data could not rule out the hypothesis that excess mortality on moxonidine (if genuine) in the short-term might be reversed into a longer term reduction. Examples do exist of survival curves crossing (e.g., surgery often carries immediate risks followed by longer-term benefit), but they are rare in drug versus placebo trials. More commonly, a treatment has little or no real effect on survival initially, but a substantial benefit accrues subsequently (e.g., statins appear in some trials to take a year or more to reduce coronary mortality).

An additional factor is that many individuals have devoted considerable collaborative effort in MOXCON with the plausible hope of contributing to a therapeutic advance of major importance. Hence there was considerable collective disappointment at the prospect of such early trial termination for safety reasons, which understandably provoked some reluctance by Executive Committee members to accept the DMB's recommendation. It is also important to recognize that the ultimate decision-making responsibility rests with the sponsor's Senior Management.

After a lengthy discussion the DMB and Executive Committee reached the following consensus:

- Stop the study in its present form.
- Suspend randomization into the trial until the Executive Committee modifies the protocol.
- For patients currently at the target dose, reduce the dosage to a level to be determined by the Executive Committee.
- For patients currently in the dose optimization phase, maintain their current dose until the protocol is modified.
- The DMB would continue to follow and assess mortality every 2 weeks for approximately 6 weeks.
- The sponsor representatives and Executive Committee will remain unblinded until the final protocol decisions are reached.
- The sponsor's Senior Management will make their assessment and decide whether to accept the Joint Meeting consensus on Thursday, March 11, 1999.

In fact, the sponsor's Senior Management decided on 11 March to stop the MOXCON trial. Patient recruitment stopped that day. All investigators were immediately informed of the reason and need to terminate the trial and were advised that patients already in the study should visit them as soon as possible so that their randomized treatment could be stopped. Within a few days the sponsor issued a press release explaining how and why the study was stopped early.

Published Results

Follow-up for analysis had ceased immediately on March 12, so that the final results included all deaths that occurred on or before that date. Compared with data available on the March 9 meeting there were 15 additional deaths (8 moxonidine, 7 placebo). The final results were based on 1,934 randomised patients (990 moxonidine, 943 placebo). There were 54 deaths on moxonidine compared with 34 on placebo, logrank p = 0.012. The survival plot (Figure 1) revealed a steadily diverging treatment difference in the risk of dying.

The Clinical Endpoint Committee adjudicated causes of death. The excess deaths in the moxonidine group appeared to be related to both sudden deaths (26 moxonidine, 11 placebo) and deaths classified as pump failure (15 moxonidine, 10 placebo). Other adjudicated endpoints also were more common in the moxonidine group, including hospitalization for worsening heart failure (75 moxonidine, 54 placebo) and acute myocardial infarction (16 moxonidine, 8 placebo). Discontinuation from the trial related to an adverse event occurred in 27 moxonidine patients and 10 placebo patients.

These results were presented at the next available international cardiology meetings, the European Society of Cardiology and the American Heart Association in August and November 1999, respectively. Achieving publica-

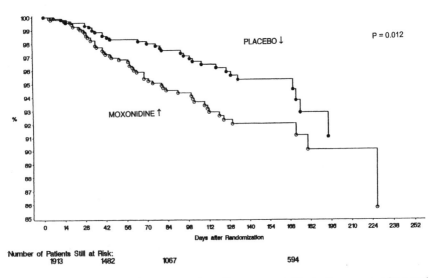

Figure 1 Kaplan–Meier plots comparing all-cause mortality in the moxonidine and placebo groups.

tion in a major medical journal was less straightforward. Despite substantial effort by the trial executive, acceptance in one of the major general medical journals could not be obtained. Hence, to ensure that the detailed results were publicly available in a peer-reviewed journal without further delay, MOXCON appeared in a specialist journal[1] over three years after attempts were begun to publish. We suspect this reflects a common trend, whereby important results of major trials which have not shown a therapeutic advance have difficulty in gaining publication in the leading journals.

So for some years the only publicly accessibly MOXCON results were brief accounts in the magazine SCRIP[4] and a European Society of Cardiology meeting report.[5] Such publication issues were primarily the responsibility of the Executive Committee. The DMB had fulfilled its data monitoring role and had no further pre-defined function, although individual DMB members expressed concern about the need for peer-reviewed publication.

Concluding Remarks

The MOXCON trial is an informative example of the difficulties in deciding whether and when to stop a major trial when emerging data suggest a major hazard of a new treatment. This problem has been referred to as "the agonizing negative trend" in data monitoring, by DeMets, Pocock, and Julian,[6] who present several previous examples.

There is a clear tension between two conflicting undesirable outcomes to be avoided:

1. Stopping too soon on only modest evidence of potential harm, thereby risks the abandonment of a treatment that could potentially have proved beneficial had substantial additional trial data been allowed to accrue.
2. Allowing a trial to continue in the face of growing evidence of harm, thereby risking exposure of more patients over a longer period to a hazardous treatment.

The statistical stopping guideline for harm in MOXCON was rather non-stringent: one-sided $P < 0.05$ with no correction for multiple testing. In hindsight, one might prefer a more stringent rule to reduce the risk of stopping too soon. Note that in practice the evidence for a mortality excess at the point of deciding to stop MOXCON had reached two-sided $p = 0.01$.

LESSONS LEARNED

1. The MOXCON experience illustrates that the collaborative process leading to the decision to stop a trial for harm requires substantially more

insight into data, their interpretation, and the consequences of one's actions than just a helpful statistical guideline.

2. This study illustrates the difficulties, delays and ethical concerns in getting the results of trials that do not show benefit of the experimental treatment published in a peer-reviewed journal. Though a DMB has no formal role in publication, DMB members should actively encourage timely reporting of results.

ACKNOWLEDGMENTS

We are grateful to members of the MOXCON trial Executive Committee and representatives of the sponsors, Eli Lilly and Company and Solvay Pharmaceuticals, for their helpful comments in the development of this article.

REFERENCES

1. Cohn JN, Pfeffer MA, Rouleau J, Sharpe N, Swedberg K, Straub M, et al. 2003. Adverse mortality effect of central sympathetic inhibition with sustained-release moxonidine in patients with heart failure (MOXCON). *Eur J Heart Failure* 5:659–667.
2. Swedberg K, Bristow MR, Cohn JN, Dargie H, Straub M, Wiltse C, Wright TJ. 2002. Effects of sustained-release moxonidine, an imidazoline agonist, on plasma norepinephrine in patients with chronic heart failure. *Circulation* 105:1797–1803.
3. Dickstein K, Manhenke C, Aarsland T, NcNay J, Wiltse C, Wright T. 2000. The effects of chronic, sustained-release moxonidine therapy on clinical and neurohumoral status in patients with heart failure. *Int J Cardiol* 75:167–176.
4. SCRIP. Moxonidine ups mortality in heart failure. SCRIP No. 2421, March 19, 1999:18.
5. Jones CG, Cleland JGF. 1999. Meeting report: the LIDO, HOPE, MOXCON and WASH studies. *Eur J Heart Failure* 1:425–431.
6. DeMets DL, Pocock SJ, Julian DG. 1999. The agonising negative trend in monitoring of clinical trials. *Lancet* 354:1983–1988.

Data Monitoring of a Placebo-Controlled Trial of Daclizumab in Acute Graft-Versus-Host Disease

David Zahrieh
Stephanie J. Lee
David Harrington

ABSTRACT

This trial was undertaken to test the hypothesis that two-drug initial therapy for acute graft-versus-host disease (GVHD) would produce better control of GVHD and less exposure to corticosteroids than the standard treatment of corticosteroids alone. All participants had undergone allogeneic hematopoietic stem cell transplantation (HSCT) and developed acute GVHD. Subjects were randomized to treatment with corticosteroids plus placebo or corticosteroids plus daclizumab. The trial was continued past its first interim analysis (~30% evaluable subjects) but was stopped after the second interim analysis (~50% evaluable subjects) when the two-drug arm was associated with worse overall survival.

INTRODUCTION AND BACKGROUND

Allogeneic HSCT is an established treatment for hematologic malignancies such as leukemia, lymphoma, multiple myeloma, myelodysplastic syndrome, and other blood disorders. In allogeneic HSCT, a patient's bone marrow and immune system are replaced by donor-derived blood cells, hopefully destroying the hematologic cancer in the process. Patients are first treated with chemotherapy, with or without radiation, followed by an infusion of donor stem cells. These stem cells may come from another person's blood, bone marrow, or in some instances, be isolated from umbilical cord blood. The donor stem cells repopulate the patient's bone marrow and produce red blood cells, platelets, and immune cells.

One of the major complications of allogeneic HSCT is acute GVHD. Approximately 30–70% of people undergoing allogeneic HSCT develop some amount of GVHD,[1,2] thought to be caused by recognition of the patient's tissues as "foreign" by the new immune system. This syndrome may be associated with skin rashes, diarrhea, and liver failure and can result in death. The standard treatment for GVHD is moderate-dose corticosteroids, and with this therapy alone, approximately 30–50% of acute GVHD can be controlled.[3,4] If a person fails to respond to steroids, a number of salvage therapies are available, including daclizumab. However, the need to use salvage regimens after failing initial therapy with corticosteroids is associated with a high mortality rate, up to 80% in some reports.[5] One of the major research efforts in the field of allogeneic HSCT is prevention and control of GVHD. However, complete elimination of GVHD is not necessarily the goal, as the presence of GVHD is also associated with a graft's ability to eradicate cancer.

Daclizumab is a humanized monoclonal antibody directed against the interleukin-2 receptor found on activated T lymphocytes. Phase II trials suggest that daclizumab is effective in treating steroid-refractory GVHD. As the side effect profile was reported to be mild in other populations (notably, kidney and heart transplantation)[6-8] and in other HSCT settings (when used to try to prevent GVHD),[9] we initiated a randomized, multicenter, double-blinded, phase III trial to test the efficacy of corticosteroids plus placebo versus corticosteroids plus daclizumab for initial therapy of acute GVHD.

PROTOCOL DESIGN

The study was designed as a randomized, multi-center, placebo-controlled, double-blinded study of daclizumab versus placebo added to corticosteroids as initial therapy for acute GVHD. The primary endpoint of the study was the proportion of patients in each treatment arm who experienced a decrease of acute GVHD overall severity by at least one grade on study day 42 without failing treatment (death, unblinding of study medication because of worsening acute GVHD, or initiation of any secondary treatment for acute GVHD before study day 42). Pre-specified secondary endpoints included mortality by day 100 post-HSCT, proportion of complete responses (resolution of acute GVHD by study day 42), total days of antibiotics and antifungal agents administered within the first 100 days post-HSCT, total steroid dose administered, and incidence of steroid-related complications. Patients were followed for at least one year to assess the incidence of chronic GVHD, overall survival, and disease-free survival. Randomization was 1 : 1 and stratified to ensure balance of key clinical characteristics. All analyses were based on intention-to-treat.

For the response-rate endpoint, we assumed that on either treatment arm, 35% of patients would remain at a stable acute GVHD level (neither worsening nor improving by study day 42). We also assumed that on the placebo arm, 30% of patients would experience an improvement of at least one grade in their GVHD severity, compared to 50% of people on the daclizumab arm. This corresponds to an odds ratio of 1 under the null hypothesis and an odds ratio of 2.3 (daclizumab/placebo) under the alternative hypothesis. Using a Fisher exact test and testing at a 0.05 one-sided significance level, we would have 80% power to detect this difference if we randomized 166 eligible and evaluable patients on the study. The number of patients targeted for accrual was inflated 15% to account for patients becoming ineligible or unevaluable for outcome assessment within 7 days of enrollment. A one-sided trial was felt to be justified based on the presumed mechanism of action, the substantial literature showing safe administration to solid organ transplant recipients, and several studies in HSCT. The trial had somewhat lower power than many national multicenter trials, in part because the use of this agent in the past in uncontrolled studies had suggested it would be effective and because conducting a much larger study in a small number of participating cites would not be feasible.

The independent Dana-Farber/Harvard Cancer Center Data and Safety Monitoring Board (DSMB), composed of internal and external content and methodology experts, assumed responsibility for monitoring the trial as it approached its first interim analysis. It was pre-specified in the protocol that the DSMB would review the results when outcome data, as described above, were available on 30%, 50%, 75%, and 100% of patients. Interim efficacy monitoring used the O'Brien–Fleming boundary.[10] The nominal significance levels for these tests, using a one-sided Fisher exact test, were 0.00035, 0.0054, 0.0217, and 0.0424. Lack of efficacy was assessed using the method of repeated confidence intervals of Jennison and Turnbull.[11]

The study was activated on January 3, 2001. At the time of the first interim analysis on October 28, 2002, there was no evidence to suggest that the trial be stopped in favor of corticosteroids plus daclizumab or for lack of efficacy. However, at the time of the second interim analysis, approximately one year later, the DSMB recommended that the study be terminated due to the unexpected finding of a significantly worse survival in the group receiving corticosteroids plus daclizumab.

DATA MONITORING EXPERIENCE

The DSMB met on October 28, 2002, and reviewed data on the first 28% of 166 eligible and evaluable patients. The nominal significance level for the first interim analysis was changed from 0.00035 to 0.0002 to reflect that only 28% of information was available as opposed to 30% information under the original study design. The treatment arms remained blinded during DSMB review and were labeled as X and Y. The Dana-Farber/Harvard Cancer Center

(DF/HCC) DSMB has specified in its standard operating procedures that it does not want to be aware of the identity of treatment arms in initial analyses. Although this is a matter of some debate among trialists, our DSMB felt it could provide a more objective review of trial data by remaining blinded, largely to prevent the DSMB members from speculating about treatment mechanisms and effects based on early data. The DF/HCC DSMB has the option to ask for blinding codes at any time, and did so for this trial after initial review. The response rates in both arms were similar, failing to meet the stopping rules for both efficacy and lack of efficacy. After review of the biostatistical report, the DSMB requested 100-day mortality results according to randomized treatment arm. Of the 13 deaths on arm Y, five died on or before 100 days following HSCT. Of the seven deaths on arm X, two patients died on or before day 100. The percent alive at 100 days post-HSCT was lower for patients randomized to arm Y (78% $\pm$ 9) in comparison with patients randomized to arm X (90% $\pm$ 7); however, the result was not statistically significant ($p = 0.22$). The DSMB elected not to unblind the trial at the time of the first interim analysis, and planned to review the trial again when it reached its second interim analysis.

The DSMB was scheduled to convene on October 23, 2003, one year later, to review blinded results from the second interim analysis. Of the 95 patients enrolled, 92 were eligible and evaluable. Of the 92 patients, 87 patients (52% of the targeted enrollment) had complete overall acute GVHD follow-up information by study day 42. The recalculated nominal significance level corresponding to 52% of total information as opposed to 50% information was changed to 0.0064.

In order to prepare for the second interim analysis, the deadline for data submission was August 13, 2003. By September 10, 2003, all data were to be entered, cleaned, and submitted to the biostatistician for review. As the data were beginning to be analyzed for the second interim analysis, the results showed a statistically significant worse survival for patients randomized to treatment arm Y (data given below). The study statistician asked a second statistician on the Dana Farber Cancer Institute (DFCI) faculty to review the data, then notified the DSMB internal statistician, who reviewed the data, then notified other DSMB members. A telephone conference occurred on October 1, 2003, approximately three weeks before the scheduled DSMB meeting. As a general practice, all DSMB reports in the DF/HCC are reviewed by a statistician not directly involved in preparing the report and by the DSMB internal statistician member before distribution.

The GVHD response rate for patients randomized to treatment arm X was 50% and the response rate for patients randomized to treatment arm Y was 49%. The calculated one-sided Fisher exact p-value for the observed data was 0.63. There was not strong evidence for the alternative hypothesis for the main endpoint. In addition, the method of repeated confidence intervals did not provide evidence to stop the trial for lack of efficacy. Again, the odds ratio under the alternative hypothesis, namely, 2.3 (daclizumab/placebo), did not fall outside the upper limit of the confidence interval calculated from the observed data. The calculated confidence interval for the second interim analysis was [0.4, 3.1].

Survival status was known for all 92 eligible and evaluable patients at the time of the second interim analysis. The median follow-up for alive patients on arm X was 340 days (range 98–923 days) and the median follow-up for alive patients on arm Y was 350 days (range 96–862 days). Of the 31 deaths on arm Y, 11 died on or before 100 days post-HSCT. Of the 16 deaths on arm X, 3 died on or before 100 days post-HSCT. Table 1 presents 100-day Kaplan–Meier survival estimates and the respective point-wise 95% confidence intervals according to the blinded randomized treatment arms. The percent alive at 100 days post-HSCT was significantly lower for patients randomized to treatment arm Y compared with patients randomized to treatment arm X (77% vs. 93%, p = 0.05). Figure 1 displays the Kaplan–Meier survival curves according to treatment arm and the logrank p-value. There was a statistically significant difference in overall survival between the two randomized treatment arms (p = 0.003). The hazards ratio comparing treatment arm Y to treatment arm X was 2.4 [95% CI: 1.3, 4.4]. In other words, the risk of death for patients randomized to treatment arm Y was more than two times higher than for patients randomized to treatment arm X.

Following this telephone conference, the DSMB requested that the results be unblinded. This revealed that patients randomized to combination therapy had a statistically inferior overall survival than patients randomized to receive corticosteroids plus placebo. The DSMB immediately recommended that the study be suspended to accrual until further review of the data and requested additional data including updated follow-up on some subjects and analysis of causes of death prior to day 100 post-HSCT. That same day the Institutional Review Board (IRB), Food and Drug Administration (FDA), sponsoring company, and the Principal Investigators at each participating site were notified. Further data collection and analysis confirmed the preliminary findings, and on October 23, 2003, during the scheduled DSMB meeting, three weeks

Table 1 100-Day Survival at second interim analysis

Arm	Total patients	Deaths	No. at risk	100 Day OS % ± SE	95% CI	p-Value
X	45	3	41	93 ± 4	[85, 100]	0.05
Y	47	11	35	77 ± 6	[65, 89]	

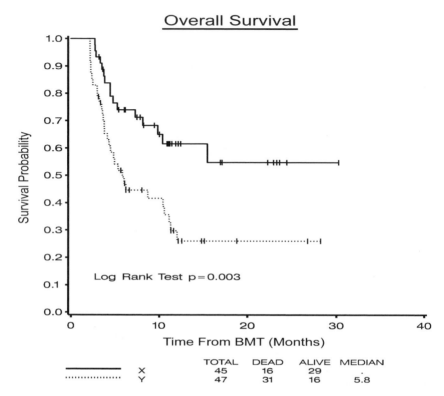

		TOTAL	DEAD	ALIVE	MEDIAN
———	X	45	16	29	.
··············	Y	47	31	16	5.8

Figure 1 Overall survival is better for treatment arm X at 100 days (93% vs. 77%, p = 0.05).

after the conference call, there was a unanimous recommendation for termination of the study and immediate publication of the results.

Regulatory Responsibilities

This trial was conducted under an IND (Investigational New Drug Application) held by the Principal Investigator. When the trial was closed to enrollment as a result of the DSMB recommendation, the Principal Investigator was responsible for notifying the primary site IRB, FDA, the sponsoring company, and other-site-responsible Principal Investigators so that they could immediately notify their local IRBs. This was accomplished by personal phone calls on the day of the closure, followed up by express mailed documentation. When the trial was officially terminated, the overall Principal Investigator was again responsible for notification of all the parties, as well as reporting back to the DSMB that all communications had successfully taken place.

The final responsibility of the Principal Investigator, once all participating institutions, IRBs, and regulatory bodies were notified of trial termination, was to disseminate the information quickly to practicing physicians. This was accomplished by presenting the preliminary results at a well-attended workshop at a subspecialty meeting and rapid final analysis of the data and submission of the manuscript for publication. This dissemination effort was also reported back to the DSMB.

LESSONS LEARNED

This trial did not meet any of the pre-specified stopping criteria based on acute GVHD control. In fact, rates of acute GVHD control and resolution were similar in the two arms. Early toxicity profiles were evaluated by the DSMB at each interim analysis, and were similar. The trial was terminated based on the difference in overall survival, despite the fact that overall survival at one year was only intended as a secondary endpoint based on prior experience in other populations and data in HSCT. One lesson learned is that the DSMB should look at both early and late endpoints (including survival) if data are available, especially if the underlying disease or treatment is associated with high mortality.

After the second interim analysis, the DSMB had requested additional data and analyses to help better understand the findings. However, while this detailed analysis was ongoing, it was important that sites and IRBs be notified of enrollment closure, but not be told of the trial results until they were confirmed. If after further analysis the DSMB had allowed the trial to continue, future enrollment could have been compromised by loss of equipoise. Thus, discussion with sites and the subsequent enrollment closure memo from the DSMB emphasized the need for further data, but gave no indication of the issues involved. No participating investigator or local IRB demanded immediate access to the data, apparently accepting the DSMB's oversight and promise to communicate recommendations clearly once they were available. The DSMB was also able to negotiate with the responsible IRB to keep details of the deliberations confidential until the recommendation to close permanently the trial. This was aided by the knowledge that no subjects were undergoing protocol-directed therapy, and would have been more contentious if any subjects were actively being treated.

Although it is impossible for the study statistician to anticipate all the possible scenarios the DSMB may consider, unexpected or statistically significant findings on interim analysis should prompt the study statistician to be proactive about gathering data needed by the DSMB to make appropriate recommendations. At the time the trial was suspended, by chance alone no patients were being treated with protocol agents. If any subjects had been on active treatment, the DSMB would have to determine whether their study participation should be ended pending further analysis, effectively indicating the DSMB's concern about the trial to local sites. Another lesson learned is that in any situation where a study statistician anticipates that a major decision will be made about discontinuing some or all of the treatments in a trial, the statistician should prepare (before the meeting) a list of all patients currently being treated, how long they have been on protocol therapy, and their expected remaining time on therapy.

It is common for the independent DSMBs for NCI-sponsored Cancer Centers and Cancer Cooperative Groups to monitor several phase III trials at the same time. This approach is both cost efficient and provides an opportunity for a single group to monitor the portfolio of an organization's studies consistently. These organizationally based DSMBs are generally made up of representatives from the major subdisciplines of cancer treatment. In this case, the DSMB representative for hematologic malignancies (one of the two internal Dana-Farber/Harvard Cancer Center members of the DSMB), was also the study Principal Investigator. Consequently, the DSMB expert on the content of the trial had to be recused for much of the discussion and deliberation about the trial. DSMBs constructed this way should have a roster of ad hoc reviewers who can step in if a current DSMB member has a conflict of interest with the trial under review.

ACKNOWLEDGMENTS

This research was originally published in *Blood*.[12]

REFERENCES

1. Weisdorf D, Haake R, Blazar B, Miller W, McGlave P, Ramsay N, et al. 1990. Treatment of moderate/severe acute graft-versus-host disease after allogeneic bone marrow transplantation: an analysis of clinical risk features and outcome. *Blood* 75:1024–1030.
2. Hansen JA, Gooley TA, Martin PJ, Appelbaum F, Chauncey TR, Clift RA, et al. 1998. Bone marrow transplants from unrelated donors for patients with chronic myeloid leukemia. *N Engl J Med* 338:962–968.
3. Martin PJ, Schoch G, Fisher L, Byers V, Anasetti C, Appelbaum FR, et al. 1990. A retrospective analysis of therapy for acute graft-versus-host disease: initial treatment. *Blood* 76:1464–1472.
4. MacMillan ML, Weisdorf DJ, Wagner JE, DeFor TE, Burns LJ, Ramsay NK, et al. 2002. Response of 443 patients to steroids as primary therapy for acute graft-versus-host disease: comparison of grading systems. *Biol Blood Marrow Transplant* 8:387–394.
5. Przepiorka D, Weisdorf D, Martin P, Klingemann HG, Beatty P, Hows J, Thomas ED. 1995. 1994 Consensus Conference on Acute GVHD Grading. *Bone Marrow Transplant* 15:825–828.
6. Beniaminovitz A, Itescu S, Lietz K, Donovan M, Burke EM, Groff BD, Edwards N, Mancini DM. 2000. Prevention of rejection in cardiac transplantation by blockade of the interleukin-2 receptor with a monoclonal antibody [comment]. *N Engl J Med* 342:613–619.

7. Bumgardner GL, Hardie I, Johnson RW, Lin A, Nashan B, Pescovitz MD, Ramos E, Vincenti F. Phase III Daclizumab Study Group. 2001. Results of 3-year phase III clinical trials with daclizumab prophylaxis for prevention of acute rejection after renal transplantation. *Transplantation* 72:839–845.
8. Adu D, Cockwell P, Ives NJ, Shaw J, Wheatley K. 2003. Interleukin-2 receptor monoclonal antibodies in renal transplantation: meta-analysis of randomised trials. *BMJ* 326:789.
9. Przepiorka D, Kernan NA, Ippoliti C, Papadopoulos EB, Giralt S, Khouri I, et al. 2000. Daclizumab, a humanized anti-interleukin-2 receptor alpha chain antibody, for treatment of acute graft-versus-host disease. *Blood* 95:83–89.
10. O'Brien PC, Fleming TR. 1979. A multiple testing procedure for clinical trials. *Biometrics* 35:549–556.
11. Jennison C, Turnbull BW. 1989. The repeated confidence interval approach. *J Royal Stat Soc* 51:305–334.
12. Lee SJ, Zahrieh D, Agura E, MacMillan ML, Maziarz RT, McCarthy PL Jr, et al. 2004. Effect of up-front daclizumab when combined with steroids for the treatment of acute graft-versus-host disease: Results of a randomized trial. *Blood* 104:1559–1564.

Special Issues

Introduction to Case Studies With Special Issues

David L. DeMets
Curt D. Furberg
Lawrence M. Friedman

In the two previous sections, case studies were presented which described monitoring issues for emerging trends which were either beneficial or harmful. In this section, we consider cases that have issues that are beyond emerging beneficial or harmful trends. For these cases, the issues would most likely not have been anticipated. No single rule or algorithm could resolve these challenges. Instead, the monitoring committees that were involved in each case had to rely on first principles of clinical trials, their experience and their wisdom. The issues raised range from data flow problems, changing endpoints, and changing relevance of the question posed to resolution of differing views on the role of the monitoring committee and recommendations made.

In the Nocturnal Oxygen Therapy Trial (NOTT) described in Case 22, the monitoring committee was confronted with apparent emerging statistically significant trends in mortality in a subgroup of the most severe chronic obstructive lung disease patient, favoring the continuous use of oxygen supplementation over nocturnal use. However, due to their own instincts and astute observation, the statistical center discovered a substantial lag in reporting of the mortality results from one or two clinics in the study. The apparent trend in mortality at that time was strictly due to the reporting lag. The monitoring committee for this trial was fortunately able to avoid making an incorrect recommendation to terminate the trial early in that high risk subgroup. As the trial progressed, the mortality results became significant for the overall comparison to the two treatment arms.

One of the fundamental principles of clinical trial design and analysis is that interim unblinded results should not be used to modify the protocol. The concern is that such knowledge could bias the results of the trial. Monitoring committees should generally not be involved in making protocol modifications, especially in changing the primary outcome of the trial, even if they are partially blinded as to the identity of the interventions. In the CAPRICORN trial (Case 27) evaluating a new intervention for chronic heart failure, the monitoring committee recognized that the mortality rate was lower than expected in the design as the primary outcome. They alerted the trial steering committee to this fact. The steering committee decided to change the primary outcome from mortality alone to a composite outcome of death plus hospitalization. When the trial was completed, the comparison of the two treatment arms using the new composite primary outcome did not achieve statistical significance, whereas the comparison using mortality was significant. However, the mortality outcome now played the role as the leading secondary outcome, leading to a dilemma for the investigators and sponsor.

In some cases, the monitoring committee can provide important guidance to the trial, especially if the discipline conducting the trial is not familiar with interim analysis methods and data monitoring committee practices. A herpes trial (Case 21) illustrates how monitoring committees can provide key leadership and contribute to the integrity of the trial.

In general, monitoring committees do not release information during the course of a trial unless the results are convincing. A breast cancer study (Case 28) illustrates the problems and challenges that arise when a monitoring committee releases information during the course of a trial. This same case also utilized hypothetical scenarios to aid the monitoring committee in preparing for their ultimate task. While these scenarios may not be realized, the process can sometimes be useful. In addition, this case also illustrates the principle that a monitoring committee must be flexible and reacts to the data as presented, adhering to the generally agreed upon principles while applying them to specific issues being faced.

The Toxoplasmosis Encephalitis (TE) Trial, or the TOXO trial (Case 25), was designed to evaluate the effect of drugs in preventing toxoplasmosis encephalitis in patients with HIV infection which had progressed to AIDS. During the course of the trial, ancillary treatment reduced the incidence of TE such that the original question was no longer of the same relevance. In addition, due to delays in reporting of data, the pipeline effect had a notable impact on the final results compared to the interim results reviewed by the monitoring committee. For trials where the question under study is affected by other non study factors such as changing background treatment, the monitoring committee and their interim reports had to be flexible to respond to these changes.

One issue described by the bevacizumab trial (Case 29) is whether a monitoring committee can in fact operate with considerable independence from investigators or sponsors. In this colorectal cancer trial with mortality as an outcome, the monitoring had considerable challenges to work through while respecting the needs and the constraints of the sponsor, and yet maintaining the blind for both sponsor and investigators.

The warfarin trial (Case 24) is also an illustration of how the window of opportunity to evaluate a new therapeutic strategy can be narrowed or even closed due to changes in medical practice and external information. There are several reasons why the evaluation of a new intervention, or a class of interventions, often must be completed in a window of time. One may be that certain interventions may become part of accepted medical practice before the evidence is in. Another is that multiple trials are sometimes launched within a similar time frame. The trials which get completed first, especially with a positive benefit, may affect the ability of the later starting trials to finish. This is the situation described in Case 24 where warfarin is being compared to placebo for the treatment of atrial fibrillation. Five trials were initiated and the early completion of three of them indicating a positive benefit affected the ability of the other two to be completed.

RESOLVD (Case 26) illustrates the challenges in decision-making when a monitoring committee makes a recommendation to the sponsor and trial steering committee. This trial deals with cardiovascular disease, a field where considerable experience in monitoring trials previously existed. Nevertheless, the process became complicated, resulting in the need for second committees to resolve differences. In RESOLVD, the monitoring committee recommendation to the steering committee to terminate early was not accepted immediately. Rather, a second-opinion committee was formed by the steering committee.

Finally, in CONSENSUS II (Case 23), the monitoring committee recommended that the steering committee terminate early due to futility. That is, negative trends favoring the control were substantial enough to make the likelihood of demonstrating a therapeutic benefit remote. Early termination for futility can be controversial, but in this case the steering committee and monitoring committee had agreed to this in advance. CONSENSUS-II is also an example where the independent statistician is internal to the sponsor but must not share information with colleagues or superiors.

These trials are but a sample of the unanticipated and nonconventional issues that a monitoring committee may face in fulfilling their role. We hope that these examples will be useful to monitoring committees who must react to these challenges when no rules or charters cover the contingencies presented by the trial.

Clinical Trials of Herpes Simplex Encephalitis: The Role of the Data Monitoring Committee

Richard J. Whitley

ABSTRACT

Herpes simplex encephalitis (HSE) is the most frequent cause of focal necrotizing encephalitis, accounting for approximately 2,500 cases annually in the United States. Studies initiated in the early 1970s have continuously evaluated promising antiviral drugs for the treatment of this disease, utilizing randomized, blinded, controlled clinical trial designs. Fundamental to the early studies was the requirement for brain biopsy in order to establish a diagnosis of HSE unequivocally by isolation of herpes simplex virus (HSV) from brain tissue in cell culture. From the outset of these studies in 1973, Data Monitoring Committees (DMCs) were established by the program sponsor, the National Institute of Allergy and Infectious Diseases (NIAID), to assess clinical trial performance, data quality, and outcome. With several iterations over a period of 30 years, these DMCs have terminated one trial because of excessive drug toxicity and two trials because of significantly reduced mortality in recipients of an active therapeutic. These studies represented the first clinical trials sponsored by NIAID that utilized a DMC. The role of the DMC in the monitoring of these trials is described.

INTRODUCTION AND BACKGROUND

Herpes simplex encephalitis (HSE) is the most common cause of sporadic fatal encephalitis in the Western world.[1] While West Nile Virus (WNV) encephalitis has become the most common cause of epidemic encephalitis in the United States today, HSE is the most significant cause of severe and devastating infections of the brain in spite of licensed antiviral therapeutics. Herpes simplex encephalitis accounts for approximately 2,500 cases of disease annually in the United States, occurring at an incidence of about

285

$1:250,000.^{2,3}$ In the absence of therapy, 70% of patients succumb and only one of ten survivors returns to normal function.[4] Even with effective therapy, the mortality remains approximately 30% six months after treatment. Of those individuals who survive, nearly two out of three have significant neurological sequelae, being unable to return to prior employment.[9] Thus, significant research efforts have been and continue to be devoted to the development of improved therapeutic measures for this disease.

In the early 1970s, antiviral therapy was just emerging as a reality for the medical community, particularly in the management of HSV infections. Because of the recognized severity of HSE, this entity has always been a prime target for therapeutic intervention. At that time, two medications were purported to be effective in the treatment of this entity, idoxuridine and cytosine arabinoside. However, the trials evaluating these medications suffered from two fundamental flaws. First, and most importantly, none of the clinical trials for either of these medications was placebo controlled. Second, and equally important, the trials did not use standard diagnostic methodology. As a consequence, the clinical presumption of disease supported by less than rigorous serologic evaluations led to unjustified conclusions regarding potential efficacy of both of these compounds.[5-8]

PROTOCOL DESIGN

In 1973, the NIAID established the Collaborative Antiviral Study Group (CASG). As a component of the initial work plan, a clinical trial comparing a then-promising antiviral agent, adenine arabinoside (vidarabine), was instituted for treatment of HSE. In this clinical trial, brain biopsy was utilized to establish diagnosis unequivocally and a placebo-controlled design was employed. Furthermore, because the literature was replete with suggestions that idoxuridine was beneficial in the management of HSE, a third arm randomized patients to this medication. The randomization was balanced at $1:1:1$. Patients were randomized at the time of brain biopsy and not after the results of brain biopsy became available some five days later. Cerebrospinal fluid and sera specimens were collected from all patients to determine the etiology of central nervous system disease if HSV was not isolated in cell culture from brain tissue.

At the time of randomization, therapy was immediately instituted for a period of ten days if the biopsy revealed evidence of HSV. If the brain biopsy was negative for HSV, administration of the therapeutic agent was discontinued on day 5. The primary endpoint for the clinical trial was survival 30 days after the onset of disease, a time interval considered standard for such studies at the time. Secondary endpoints were the mean duration of survival and neurologic outcome, according to randomization group. Serial evaluations of blood and urine were performed to assess potential toxicity.

A Data Monitoring Committee (DMC) was established at the Division of Microbiology and Infectious Diseases (DMID), NIAID, consisting of two medical officers from that division, a statistician affiliated with the Institute and an infectious diseases physician from the Clinical Center at the National Institutes of Health (NIH) who was familiar with HSE. According to the design of the clinical trial, data summaries and coded outcome events were to be provided to the DMC by the biostatistical section of the Central Unit at the University of Alabama at Birmingham. These summaries were not available to the Principal Investigators at that institution. Because of the concern for potential toxicity of the study medications, data were provided to the DMC after every 20 confirmed patients were entered into the clinical trial, irrespective of biopsy status (proven HSE or not).

This initial clinical trial was subsequently followed by an additional controlled study that compared the proven active agent from the first study, vidarabine, with a promising new agent with greater potential for efficacy, acyclovir. This second trial utilized a double-blind, randomized design. For this clinical trial, a second DMC was established consisting of two independent biostatisticians, not involved at the NIAID, and physicians familiar with HSE from the greater Metropolitan Washington, D.C., area but not employed by either the NIH or Food and Drug Administration. Field monitors verified data in the field and transferred it to the Central Biostatistical Unit at the University of Alabama at Birmingham. Data were submitted to the project officer at the NIAID at pre-specified intervals with attached appropriate analyses (coded).

DATA MONITORING EXPERIENCE

The first clinical trial led to two interventions by the DMC. In 1974, the DMC terminated one arm of the clinical trial as all idoxuridine recipients, irrespective of biopsy proof of HSV or with other established diseases, experienced unexpected either high mortality or morbidity that was directly attributed to toxicity induced by the medication. Specifically, idoxuridine resulted in significant depression of white blood cell and platelets counts, resulting in secondary bacterial infection, bleeding diatheses and demise. A total of 7 of the 12 randomized patients died following idoxuridine administration.[9] The remaining five patients experienced inordinate laboratory toxicities. Of note, none of these toxicities had been reported in the prior experience with this medication in treating HSE; however, the same had been noted in clinical trials of other diseases. As a consequence, the idoxuridine arm of the study was deleted, leaving a 1 : 1 randomization of vidarabine to placebo recipients.

In 1976, with data available on 38 biopsy-proven patients, the DMC recommended termination of trial because of the significant reduction in mortality for the vidarabine recipients at one month (28%) as compared to the placebo recipients (70%), p = 0.03.[4]

For this trial, no statistical criteria were defined for trial termination; however, the DMC judged the clinical events so striking that nominal significance should result in its closure. In order to verify the results of the placebo-controlled study, an open clinical trial of vidarabine under identical circumstances, namely, brain biopsy proof of HSE, was performed with the additional component of long term follow-up in order to define mortality at six months with subsequent extent of morbidity. In this subsequent trial, 75 patients[3] were proven to have HSE. The mortality at 28 days was 33%, virtually identical to that reported in the first study. However, as these patients were followed longer, the six-month mortality increased to 39%, a finding not unanticipated from the natural history descriptions of this disease. The increased mortality was attributed to the neurologic complications experienced by a proportion of the 30-day survivors.

The second controlled clinical trial compared acyclovir, a second-generation selective inhibitor of HSV replication, with vidarabine in a blinded-controlled study, again utilizing biopsy evidence of HSE. As with the first clinical trial, if the brain biopsy was negative for HSV, administration of the therapeutic intervention was discontinued on day 5.

A DMC, as defined above, had been established by the project officers at the NIAID. Three interim analyses were specified according to the termination boundaries of O'Brien and Fleming.[10] At the second interim analysis, the mortality for the acyclovir recipients was significantly less than that for the counterpart vidarabine recipients (54% vs. 28%), p = 0.008.[11] Furthermore, the frequency of adverse events, particularly Grade III or higher laboratory abnormalities, was higher in those patients who received vidarabine as compared to the counterpart acyclovir recipients.

Importantly, from this clinical trial, factors that influenced clinical outcome were identified utilizing logistic regression analyses. Level of consciousness at the time of initiation of therapy and the age of the patient predicted both mortality and morbidity.

Taken together, this series of clinical trials led to the first medication licensed for the treatment of HSE, namely, adenine arabinoside, and to the second drug that remains, even to this day, the standard treatment for the disease entity, namely, acyclovir.

LESSONS LEARNED

These clinical trials provided several lessons on the historical evolution of DMCs for life-threatening infectious diseases, such as HSE, as well as medical insight into this disease. First as it relates to DMC, when these studies were initiated, the utilization of DMC was non-existent in the infectious diseases community. NIAID, as one Institute at the NIH, began a tradition in the use of DMCs, as was becoming routine for such other institutes as National Institute of Heart, Lung, and Blood or the National Cancer Institute. As was evident in the evolution of studies of HSE, the initial DMC was composed of personnel employed by the NIH, as recognized today, this created a potential bias in the monitoring of the clinical trial. Subsequently, the second DMC consisted of members independent of the NIH, representing members of the Infectious Diseases and Biostatistical communities. From the perspective of the academic infectious diseases community, DMCs were an unknown and poorly understood component of clinical trials. As AIDS appeared on the scene, with its myriad of complex clinical trials, the DMC became both better understood and warmly accepted.

Second, the importance of DMC reviews was obvious because of the need to monitor the collected and edited data rigorously to ensure proper clinical trial conduct. The DMC must assure the quality of the performance of the clinical trial as well as protect volunteers who participated in the study in order to avoid either undue toxicity (idoxuridine trial) or early evidence of efficacy (acyclovir trial). In the performance of both HSE clinical trials, data were provided in a timely fashion for nearly instantaneous review by the DMC.

Third, the climate that surrounded the performance of these studies was electric both for the DMC and the investigators. On one side of the ethical community, investigators condemned the use of a placebo control.[12] The critics of the NIH studies felt that there was enough evidence to establish the value of idoxuridine such that a placebo was unjustified. Specifically, the critics of placebo controls believed that the mortality of HSE was so high that any reduction provided by an intervention would indicate efficacy. Such a conclusion could hardly have been further from the truth. Indeed, the use of a placebo control in the first study actually accelerated the proof of toxicity for idoxuridine and in the second the efficacy of vidarabine. Without the unitization of placebo controls in these early studies, an increased number of patients would have been exposed to a potentially lethal medication, namely, idoxuridine. Furthermore, with a placebo-controlled study of vidarabine, efficacy could be established in a reasonable and propitious fashion.

From a medical perspective, lessons regarding the diagnosis and natural history of infection were as important as those relating to the efficacy and toxicity of acyclovir and idoxuridine, respectively. Ironically, the same critics of the placebo-controlled design also criticized the use of brain biopsy for the purposes of diagnosis.[12] Without utilizing brain biopsy, it would have been impossible to diagnose these patients accurately and analyze the efficacy of the interventions, since no other diagnostic intervention was available at that time. Further, as we learned, the diseases that occurred in patients who did not have HSE were associated with a significantly lower mortality and improved morbidity. To mix HSV-proven patients and patients with other diseases predicated upon clinical diagnosis or flawed serologic assays would have resulted in erroneous conclusions.

Because specimens of cerebrospinal fluid were collected prospectively from all patients entered into the trial, opportunities to develop noninvasive diagnostics arose. As a consequence, in 1995 polymerase chain reaction (PCR) detection of viral DNA was proven of value and has subsequently been established as the diagnostic method of choice, replacing brain biopsy in the evaluation of these patients.

The conduct of these studies allowed for the precise definition of the natural history of HSE, not just from the prospective of mortality but also from the factors that influence outcome and events which occur well after a patient is enrolled on therapeutic intervention of short duration. As it relates to the former, factors that influenced outcome included the age of the patient and the level of consciousness at the time of the initiation of treatment, as noted above. As it relates to the latter, historical studies had only used follow-up of one month to determine mortality for patients with HSE. However, long-term studies indicate that mortality increases because of complications related to the primary infection itself. Stated more simply, many surviving patients at one month were left with severe neurologic impairment requiring continued hospitalization. Subsequent secondary nosocomial infection contributed to the demise of these individuals.

As with other clinical trials, the role of the DMC in the conduct of a study is of paramount importance in contemporary medicine today. Judgments of a DMC go well beyond simply assessing outcome and potential toxicity but include ensuring the rigor of a trial and assisting the investigators in taking a clinical trial to conclusion in an appropriate and ethical fashion. In the current medical research climate which is focusing on the safety, efficacy and ehtical use of drugs, the collegial relationship between the DMC and the clinical trialists ensures the well-being of the volunteers who participate in these studies.

ACKNOWLEDGMENTS

This project was funded in whole or in part with federal funds from the National Institute of Allergy and Infectious Diseases; National Institutes of Health, Department of Health and Human Services, under contract (NO1-AI-30025, NO1-AI -65306, NO1-AI -15113, NO1-AI-62554, N01-AI-30025); the General Clinical Research Unit (RR-032); and the State of Alabama.

REFERENCES

1. Meyers HM Jr, Johnson RT, Crawford IP, Dascomb HE, Rogers NG. 1960. Central nervous system syndromes of "viral" etiology: A study of 713 cases. *Am J Med* 29:334-347.

2. Longson M. The general nature of viral encephalitis in the United Kingdom. *Viral Diseases of the Central Nervous System*, pp. 19-31. Ellis LS. (ed.), 1984. Bailliere Tindall, London.

3. Whitley, RJ, Soong SJ, Hirsch MS, Karchmer AW, Dolin R, Galasso G, et al. 1981. Herpes simplex encephalitis: Vidarabine therapy and diagnostic problems. *N Engl J Med* 304:313-318.

4. Whitley RJ, Soong SJ, Dolin R, Galasso GJ, Chien LT, Alford CA. 1977. Adenine arabinoside therapy of biopsy-proved herpes simplex encephalitis: National Institute of Allergy and Infectious Diseases Collaborative Antiviral Study. *N Engl J Med* 297:289-294.

5. Lerner AM, Bailey EJ. 1973. Concentrations of idoxuridine in serum, urine, and cerebrospinal fluid of patients with suspected diagnosis of herpesvirus hominis encephalitis. *J Clin Invest* 51:45-49.

6. Lerner AM, Lauter CB, Nolan DC, Shippey MJ. 1972. Passive hemagglutinating antibodies in cerebrospinal fluids in herpes virus hominis encephalitis. *Proc Soc Exp Biol Med* 140:1460-1466.

7. Wilfert CM, Huang ES, Stagno S. 1982. Restriction endonuclease analysis of cytomegalovirus deoxyribonucleic acid as an epidemiologic tool. *Pediatrics* 70:717-721.

8. Wilfert CM, Lehrman SN, Katz SL. 1983. Enteroviruses and meningitis. *Pediatr Infect Dis J* 2:333-341.

9. Boston Interhospital Virus Study Group and the NIAID Sponsored Cooperative Antiviral Clinical Study. Alford CA, Chien LT, Whitley R, et al. 1975. Failure of high dose 5-deoxyuridine in the therapy of herpes simplex virus encephalitis: Evidence of unacceptable toxicity. *N Engl J Med* 292:600-603.

10. O'Brien PC, Fleming TR. 1979. A multiple testing procedure for clinical trials. *Biometrics* 35:549-556.

11. Whitley RJ, Alford CA, Hirsch MS, Schooley RT, Luby JP, Aoki FY, et al. 1986. Vidarabine versus acyclovir therapy of herpes simplex encephalitis. *N Engl J Med* 314:144-149, 1986.

12. McCartney JJ. 1978. Encephalitis and ara-A: An ethical case study. *Hastings Cent Rep* 8:5-7.

The Nocturnal Oxygen Therapy Trial Data Monitoring Experience: Problem With Reporting Lags

David L. DeMets
George W. Williams
Byron W. Brown, Jr.

ABSTRACT

The Nocturnal Oxygen Therapy Trial (NOTT) was a randomized controlled trial designed to evaluate the role of continuous oxygen compared to only nocturnal use for patients with advanced chronic obstructive pulmonary disease. The data monitoring committee for the NOTT had to consider issues of multiple outcomes, extension of patient recruitment, and problems with reporting lags in key outcome data. While statistical methods are very useful, they do not address all of the issues that must be considered. The data monitoring committee had to be alert to unanticipated problems and react accordingly.

INTRODUCTION AND BACKGROUND

Patients with advanced chronic obstructive pulmonary disease (COPD) in general have a poor prognosis due to the diminished mechanical functioning and gas exchange in their lungs.[1-5] During the 1970s, these patients were often treated with supplemental oxygen as outpatients. Chronic use of oxygen supplementation resulted in improved exercise tolerance and decreased pulmonary hypertension as well as improved neuropsychological function.[4-6] Long-term continuous oxygen supplementation is an expensive form of therapy, since typically patients must have portable units. COPD patients are most hypoxemic while they are sleeping.[3] Given the expense of continuous oxygen supplementation and that the most severe hypoxemia was during sleep, the hypothesis was put forward that supplemental oxygen could be reduced from continuous use to just nocturnal use, including the hours of sleep. The Nocturnal Oxygen Therapy Trial (NOTT) was designed and sponsored by the National Heart, Lung, and Blood Institute (NHLBI) to test this hypothesis.[7] A Policy Advisory Board (PAB) was formed for NOTT, which had responsibility for monitoring the progress of the trial and for examining interim data for evidence of benefit or harm. The data monitoring experience for the NOTT has been described in detail previously.[8]

PROTOCOL DESIGN

The NOTT was a randomized trial comparing continuous oxygen supplementation with nocturnal use, conducted in six clinical sites in North America. Continuous oxygen was the standard of care (control), and nocturnal oxygen (approximately 12 hours) was the experimental treatment strategy. The primary outcome variables used to assess effectiveness were pulmonary and cardiac function, quality of life, neuropsychological function, and survival. In current nomenclature, the NOTT might be described as a non-inferiority trial in that the goal was to demonstrate that nocturnal oxygen use was "just about as good" as continuous oxygen and certainly no worse by some tolerable amount. At the time NOTT was designed, the margins of non-inferiority were not defined for the many outcome variables. However, an alternative treatment effect was specified for one of the outcome variables, FEV1, which might be viewed loosely as the margin of difference that was to be ruled out. If nocturnal oxygen therapy (NOT) was similar in treatment effect to continuous oxygen therapy (COT), the NOT would be less expensive, more convenient, and thus most likely the recommended treatment. It was not expected that NOT would be superior to the standard COT treatment. Patients were to be followed for a minimum of one year and evaluated periodically, depending on the outcome variable, with the major evaluation time points being at 6 and 12 months.

The design called for a sample size of 300 COPD patients to be randomized equally between the two arms, with a two-sided 0.05 significance level and 0.90 power.[8] The sample-size estimation was a complex process. The annual mortality for these COPD patients was estimated to be approximately 20%. While mortality was the outcome of most interest, the sample-size estimates based on the assumed mortality rate would have required 1,000 or more patients, unless the difference between the groups was 50% or greater. Sample sizes of this magnitude were beyond the resources of the trial. Since such substantial differences were not anticipated, mortality was designated as a secondary outcome. The original plan was for the 300 patients to be recruited over two years with a total of three years for follow-up.

However, the many morbidity outcome variables, (listed in Table 1), measured different functionality of COPD patients. None was considered to be adequate alone to evaluate the potential differences in the two oxygen treat-

Table 1 Baseline Characteristics*

General and cardiopulmonary characteristics
    Patients, no[†]
    Age, *yrs*
    Male, %[†]
    White, %[†]
    Pa_{O_2}, *mm Hg*
    Pa_{CO2}, *mm Hg*
    pH
    Hematocrit, %
    FEV_1, % *predicted*
    FVC, % *predicted*
    FRC, % *predicted*
    Mean sleep Sa_{O2}, air, %
    Mean sleep Sa_{O2}, O_2, %
    Maximum workload, air, *W*
    Heart rate, *min⁻¹*
    Mean pulmonary artery pressure, *mm Hg*
    Cardiac index, *L/min-m²*
    Pulmonary vascular resistance, *dyne/s-cm²*
Neuropsychiatric characteristics[ʲ]
    Overall rating (3.5)
    Halstead impairment index (0.63)
    Russell Neuringer average impairment index (1.8)
    Brain age quotient (89)
Quality of life[ʲ]
    MMPI, average scales 0.9 (54.5)
    SIP
        Physical scale (0.6)
        Psychosocial scale (1.6)
    POMS—mood disturbance (26.4)

* FEV_1 = forced expiratory volume in 1 second. FVC = forced
vital capacity; FRC = = functional residual capacity; MMPI =
Minnesota Multipasic Personality Inventory; SIP = Sickness
Impact Profile; POMS = Profile of Mood States.
[†] All values reported for the two groups are mean values except
numbers of subjects.
[ʲ] Normal values are shown in parentheses.
Source: Nocturnal Oxygen Therapy Trial Group.[7]

ment strategies, so sample-size calculations were determined for several of these. It was estimated that 250–300 patients would provide 80–90% power to detect differences of clinical interest. Thus, a long list of outcome variables were designated as "primary," a feature not desirable but seemingly unavoidable in this trial context.

DATA MONITORING EXPERIENCE

Recruitment for NOTT began in 1977. Despite best efforts by the participating clinical centers after two years, the initial goal of 300 patients was not achievable during the two years of recruitment. As described below, the sample size was adjusted downward to 220 patients at 1.5 years of recruitment. At the time the NOTT trial terminated, the investigators had recruited 203 patients, 102 to nocturnal oxygen therapy and 101 to continuous oxygen therapy. As discussed further below, the NOTT was terminated before the target of 220 patients was attained due to an impressive reduction in mortality in the COT arm compared to the NOT arm.[7]

The two treatment arms were balanced with respect to all measured demographic, pulmonary, and neuropsychological and quality of life baseline variables shown in Table 1. Compliance to the two treatment strategies was excellent, with the COT arm patients averaging 18 hours per day and the NOT arm averaging 12 hours per day. Only two patients were lost to follow-up, both in the COT group but within two months of the trial closeout. Thus, baseline comparability and compliance were not issues for the PAB.

Of all of the primary outcome variables, only two demonstrated a significant difference. These were hematocrit and pulmonary vascular resistance. In general, the results indicated that these COPD patients were sick and getting worse over time. However, they also indicated that the two treatment arms appeared similar overall, conditional on the differences that NOTT was powered to detect.

However, the NOTT mortality results showed a significant difference $(p = 0.01)$ based on the logrank test, indicating a survival advantage for the continuous oxygen treatment strategy over the nocturnal oxygen treatment strategy. Survival curves are shown in Figure 1. At 12 months, for example,

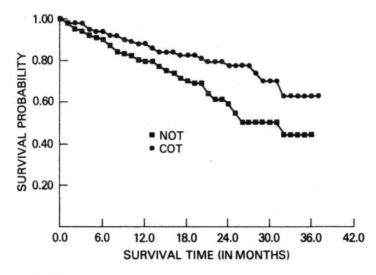

Figure 1 NOTT survival experience for 102 patients on nocturnal oxygen therapy (NOT) and 101 patients on continuous oxygen therapy (COT). From DeMets et al.[8]

mortality was reduced from 20.6% to 11.9%, and by 24 months, the mortality was reduced from 40.2% to 22.4%.

The NOTT PAB Experience

The PAB had to deal with three main issues during the interim analyses. These were (1) the multiplicity of outcomes, (2) slow recruitment, and (3) a lag in reporting outcome data, especially mortality data.

Repeated Analysis of Multiple Outcomes

Three general classes of outcomes were designated as "primary." There were pulmonary and cardiac function, neuropsychological function, and quality of life. Mortality was specified as a secondary outcome. These three classes of primary outcomes generated over 100 potential different outcome variables, several of which are shown in Table 1. Analysis of multiple variables is known to increase the false-positive error or Type 1 error rate.[9] The PAB discussed reducing this number and after some effort, a smaller list of 34 variables shown in Table 1 was selected. This of course still made the multiple comparison issue a monitoring problem for NOTT.

In addition, repeated analysis of a single outcome also increases the type 1 error for that outcome.[10] Canner had demonstrated using the Coronary Drug Project[11] the hazards of using nominal p-values for interim analysis of accumulating data in a clinical trial. The NOTT PAB adopted a more conservative standard of a nominal p-value of 0.01 (corresponding to a standardized test statistic of 2.58) as minimal evidence before considering early termination. This was similar to criteria used in other previous trials at that time, such as the Coronary Drug Project.[11] In addition, to deal with the multiplicity of outcomes, more than one of the 34 designated "primary" outcomes listed would have to meet this criteria. The PAB, therefore, also decided to evaluate consistency across outcome variables and subgroups. During the course of the trial, publications on group sequential boundaries appeared.[12,13] These were not adopted midstream, but the PAB understood that interpretation of interim analyses needed to be more conservative than simply reacting to nominal p-values. As stated by Armitage, informed judgment is a necessary although not a well-defined complement to any body of statistical methods available.[14] The message from this previous experience a trial should not stop based on "nominal statistical significance alone."

As it turned out, except for hematocrit and pulmonary vascular resistance, none of the functionality, neuropsychological, and quality of life outcomes shown in Table 1 were nominally significantly different between the NOT and COT arms; and these comparisons never came close to the interim critical value of 2.58 or a corresponding nominal pvalue of 0.01. However, the NOT versus COT mortality comparison met that criterion and the survival cures are shown in Figure 1.

As in many trials, the recruitment rate for NOTT was not as high as expected. For the planned two-year recruitment period, the observed rate at 1.5 years would project a total of 220 patients at the scheduled end of the trial, short of the 300 targeted in the protocol. The PAB was asked to consider whether recruitment should be extended to reach the target of 300 as planned. Given that NOTT was essentially a non-inferiority trial, having adequate power to detect differences of clinical importance was essential.

The initial sample-size calculations, ranging from 250 to 300, for the extensive list of primary outcome variables, were based on data from small studies. Thus estimates of variability used in these calculations for these outcome variables, for example, were not very precise or specific to this COPD population. The PAB examined new power calculations with updated estimates of variability from the interim NOTT data, using both 220 and 300 patient sample sizes for many of the 34 designated variables. It is important to emphasize that the PAB did not take current trends in treatment group differences into account in these calculations. Of course, increasing the sample size from 220 to 300 does not increase the power substantially. Of the 34 designated variables, 13 had less than 50% power to detect the pre-specified clinical differences of interest for both sample sizes. The PAB believed that to increase the power to 80% or better would require a sample size not achievable with the NOTT sites. However, most of the rest of the designated variables had 70% or greater power to detect the pre-specified differences with the smaller projected sample size of 220. The estimates of variability used in these calculations for these outcome measures were very close to the variability estimates observed when the trial was terminated.

After evaluating this matrix of power calculations for many variables and two sample sizes, the PAB determined that a sample size of 220 would be adequate and thus recommended that recruitment stop after two years.

Mortality Monitoring

While mortality was one of the secondary outcome variables of interest in the design phase, the sample size to detect minimal differences of clinical importance was unachievable for the NOTT sites. Furthermore, major differences in mortality were not expected. However, mortality differences between NOT and COT did in fact emerge. In Table 2, the overall mortality data for each treatment arm are presented as seen at the PAB meetings during the last year of the conduct of the trial and for those participants with low FEV1 (Forced Expiratory Volume at 1 second) percent predicted who are at high risk. At the PAB meeting in March of 1979, the mortality was 18 versus

Table 2 Mortality Results at Various Policy Advisory Board Meetings, as Originally Presented, for the Total Group and for the Low FEV_1 Subgroup

| Meeting date | Total group | | | Low FEV1 subgroup | | | |
	12 hr	24 hr	p[a]	Cutpoint	12 hr	24 hr	p
June, 1979[b]	18/101	9/100	0.07	0.8[c]	12/41	5/36	0.01
August, 1979[b]	20/102	12/101	0.11	0.53[d]	7/29	0/23	0.01
September, 1979	21/102	12/101	0.09	0.53	8/29	0/23	0.008
October, 1979[b]	21/102	18/101	0.52	0.53	8/29	3/23	0.25
January, 1980	27/102	19/101	0.15	0.53	12/29	4/23	0.05
March, 1980	32/102	20/101	0.06	0.53	13/29	4/23	0.05
June, 1980	41/102	23/101	0.01				

[a] Obtained from Cox model.
[b] Formal Interim analyses.
[c] 0.8 represents the median value.
[d] 0.53 represents the lower quartile.
Source: DeMets et al.[8]

9 in favor of COT. The PAB was concerned that this mortality trend could be largely in the low-FEV1 subgroup of COPD patients who are at higher risk. The low-FEV1 subgroup was defined as those participants below the then observed value of 80% percent predicted.

The mortality results seen at the June 1979 PAB meeting are presented in Table 2. The overall mortality comparison for NOT versus COT treatment arms had a p-value of 0.07 with the low-FEV1 subgroup having a p-value of 0.01; the more severely ill patient appeared to have a lower mortality rate on COT compared to NOT. While the PAB recognized that the number of events was small so that trends could easily change, and that many outcome variables had been considered which could lead more likely to chance results, the PAB was still concerned with this mortality difference in the low-FEV1 subgroup. If the trial were terminated for the low-FEV1 subgroup, this value could become part of clinical practice in deciding when to use NOT. In addition, a U.S. federal agency was evaluating the existing guidelines for usage and payment of continuous oxygen. Thus, early termination might have a profound implication for the care of these patients. The overall mortality results were not nominally significant, much less meeting the 0.01 p-value interim criteria the NOTT PAB had set earlier. The 34 designated outcome variables were very similar between the two groups, except for pulmonary vascular resistance, which favored continuous oxygen. The PAB wanted to be ethically responsible to the recruited NOTT patients as well as other COPD patients, but also wanted to avoid over-reaction.

The PAB decided to recommend continuation of the NOTT but to review these issues again carefully at the next meeting, scheduled for September of

1979. The NOTT statisticians would conduct additional analyses in the interim. In addition, if the overall mortality comparison were to result in a p-value less than 0.01 before the next PAB, the statisticians would notify the PAB chair who should then confer with a PAB subcommittee as to whether to then call for an emergency meeting of the entire PAB. The initial definition of the low-FEV1 subgroup was also redefined for future analyses as being less than 0.53 FEV1, which was the 25th percentile. That is, the PAB wanted to focus on the most severe patients in the NOTT.

During August, in preparation for the September meeting, the statistical center sent a preliminary report to the PAB subcommittee using the new FEV1 cutoff. The results for the new, more severely ill, FEV1 subgroup were still favoring continuous oxygen, with seven versus no deaths but were less severe than in the June for that low subgroup (p = 0.11). At the September 1979 meeting of the full PAB, the mortality results were slightly less in favor of continuous oxygen overall (p = 0.09) and for the low-FEV1 subgroup (8 versus 0 deaths, p = 0.008). Still the PAB was concerned about the implications of this low-FEV1 subgroup, particularly given that the overall comparison was not even nominally significant. The PAB considered whether to recommend early termination or wait until the next scheduled meeting in January of 1980. In preparation for the September meeting, the NOTT statistical center had polled sites for mortality updates on all patients. The statisticians were concerned that there may have been delays in reporting deaths, especially from sites in large metropolitan areas. Thus, the PAB could not even be sure that the data they were reviewing were reasonably current.

The PAB asked the NOTT statistical center to proceed as quickly as possible to update the mortality data and prepare a new report. The October 1979 results, shown in Table 2, indicate that neither the overall trial mortality comparisons between NOT and COT nor the low-FEV1 subgroup comparisons were even close to nominal significance. While the trends were still in the same direction, the large difference seen in previous PAB interim reports was due to the reporting lag. Because of the astute observation at the statistical center, the PAB had avoided making an inappropriate and unfortunate recommendation.

The NOTT continued as scheduled. As shown in Table 2, when the NOTT trial finally closed follow-up on schedule in June of 1980, the overall mortality comparison had achieved a p-value of 0.01, less than the 0.05 alpha level set forth in the design. It also met the interim analysis p-value of 0.01 so that the PAB might have closed the trial at that point, even if it had not been the close-out of follow-up.[7] The implication of the complete NOTT results was that continuous oxygen provided a survival benefit to all advanced COPD patients, not just for those in the low-FEV1 subgroup. Another trial conducted in the United Kingdom[15] demonstrated that continuous oxygen was superior to no oxygen supplementation, which was consistent with results seen in NOTT.

LESSONS LEARNED

1. One of the lessons is that monitoring committees should expect the unexpected. Of all the 34 designated "primary" outcomes shown in Table 1, none demonstrated any treatment difference between continuous oxygen and nocturnal oxygen therapy, except for hematocrit and pulmonary vascular resistance. In spite of failure to see a nominal 0.05 significant comparison with almost all of the surrogate measures, mortality emerged with convincing evidence of treatment benefit for continuous oxygen therapy strategy, showing a nearly 50% reduction over two years of follow-up (p = 0.01). Had the NOTT only measured the short-term pulmonary function and neuropsychological outcomes, the conclusion from NOTT might well have been that the COT was just as effective as NOT.

2. A second lesson is that data must be reasonably up-to-date for a data monitoring committee to make appropriate recommendations. This is especially true for mortality or serious morbidity outcomes. As technology improves, reporting of these types of events can be within a day of being detected. No monitoring committee wants to make decisions on data that is several months old. The NOTT PAB could have avoided several anxious months if the data had been more current. Had the PAB made the recommendation to terminate the low FEV1 subgroup, they would more than likely have been extremely embarrassed, as the database was finally updated and analyzed. Interim decisions on the trial might well have damaged the study and led too serious errors in clinical conclusions. Results for high-FEV1 subgroup may have been inconclusive as well. COPD patients and federal agencies would have been denied the very data needed to ascertain whether this therapy was beneficial and cost effective. Perhaps another trial would have been required to answer this clinically important question.

3. A third lesson is to be cautious in the interpretation of subgroups, especially during interim analyses. Subgroups can be arbitrarily defined and are usually subject to small numbers, which can vary and easily change the strength of any interpretation. Even if the mortality reporting lag had not been an issue, early trends favoring continuous oxygen, largely in the low-FEV1 subgroup, became statistically significant in the overall combined (low- and high-FEV1) cohort at the end of the trial. An early decision on the low-FEV1 subgroup would have been misleading for the overall use of continuous oxygen therapy. Extreme caution is required in evaluating subgroups for anything beyond a general sense of consistency.

REFERENCES

1. Burrows B, Earle RH. 1969. Course and prognosis of chronic obstructive lung disease, a prospective study of 200 patients. *N Engl J Med* 280:397-404.
2. Flenley DC, Douglas NJ, Lamb D. 1980. Nocturnal hypoxemia and long term domiciliary oxygen in blue and bloated bronchitics. *Chest* 77:305-307.
3. Koo KW, Sax DS, Snider GL. 1975. Arterial blood gases and pH during sleep in chronic obstructive lung disease. *Amer J Med* 58:663-670.
4. Krop HD, Block AJ, Cohen E. 1973. Neuropsychologic effects of continuous oxygen therapy in chronic obstructive pulmonary disease. *Chest* 64:317-322.
5. Levine BE, Bigelow DB, Hamstra RD, Beckwitt HJ, Mitchell RS, Nett LM, Stephen TA, Petty TL. 1967. The role of long-term continuous oxygen administration in patients with chronic airway obstruction with hypoxemia. *Ann Intern Med* 66:639-650.
6. Petty TL, Finigan MM. 1968. The clinical evaluation of prolonged ambulatory oxygen therapy in patients with chronic airway obstruction. *Am J Med* 45:242-252.
7. Nocturnal Oxygen Therapy Trial Group. 1980. Continuous or nocturnal oxygen therapy in hypoxemic chronic obstructive lung disease. A clinical trial. *Ann Intern Med* 93:391-398.
8. DeMets DL, Williams GW, Brown BW Jr., and the NOTT Research Group. 1982. A case report of data monitoring experience: The Nocturnal Oxygen Therapy Trial. *Control Clin Trials* 3:113-124.
9. Miller RG. 1966. *Simultaneous Statistical Inference.* McGraw Hill, New York:
10. Armitage P, McPherson CK, Rowe BC. 1969. Repeated significance tests on accumulating data. *J Roy Stat Soc A* 132:235-244.
11. The Coronary Drug Project Research Group. 1981. Practical aspects of decision making in clinical trials. The Coronary Drug Project as a case study. *Control Clin Trials* 1:363-376.
12. O'Brien PC, Fleming TR. 1979. A multiple testing procedure for clinical trials. *Biometrics* 35:549-556.
13. Pocock SJ. 1977. Group sequential methods in the design and analysis of clinical trials. *Biometrika* 64:191-199.
14. Armitage P. 1979. The analysis of data from clinical trials. *The Statistician* 28:171-183.
15. Flenley DC, Douglas NJ, Lamb D. 1980. Nocturnal hypoxemia and long term domiciliary oxygen in blue and bloated bronchitics. *Chest* 77:305-307.

Stopping a Trial for Futility: The Cooperative New Scandinavian Enalapril Survival Study II

Steven Snapinn
Curt D. Furberg

ABSTRACT

The Cooperative New Scandinavian Enalapril Survival Study II (CON-SENSUS II) trial was designed to test the hypothesis that enalapril, an angiotensin-converting enzyme inhibitor, would reduce the risk of death in patients with an acute myocardial infarction. A sequential stopping rule that allowed for both early acceptance and early rejection of the null hypothesis, in the spirit of stochastic curtailment, was developed specifically for this trial. Very early in the trial the Data and Safety Monitoring Committee noticed an excess of mortality in the enalapril group. When this trend persisted, the committee first recommended protocol modifications, then termination of recruitment, and finally termination of the trial. The main reason was futility, as well as the possibility of harm, particularly in certain subgroups. This trial provides useful lessons regarding futility analyses, flexible monitoring rules, and the sponsor's role on both the Data Monitoring Committee and the Steering Committee.

INTRODUCTION AND BACKGROUND

Angiotensin-converting enzyme (ACE) inhibitors act on the renin-angiotensin system, a hormonal regulatory system that helps maintain the body's blood pressure. One step in the process is conversion of angiotensin I to angiotensin II, an extremely potent vasoconstrictor. By inhibiting the enzyme that facilitates this conversion, treatment with an ACE inhibitor results in vasodilation and reduction in blood pressure. Enalapril, a member of this class, was approved for the treatment of hypertension in the 1980's.

The CONSENSUS trial, published in 1987, established that treatment with enalapril also reduces the risk of death in patients with severe heart failure.[1]

The SOLVD trials later extended this result to patients with milder forms of heart failure.[2,3] Heart failure is a syndrome where symptoms, mainly shortness of breath and fatigue, are due to abnormal cardiac function. In its most severe form these symptoms are present even at rest, and the patient's prognosis is extremely poor. In the CONSENSUS, double-blind enalapril or placebo was randomly added to each patient's current therapy, and six-month mortality from all causes was 44% with placebo compared to only 26% with enalapril (p = 0.002).

Studies done in the late 1980s suggested a marked increase in angiotensin II and other cardiovascular hormones during acute myocardial infarction, with a beneficial effect on myocardial remodeling by ACE inhibition added to beta blockers. Therefore, it was hypothesized that, if given very early after the onset of an acute myocardial infarction, enalapril would limit the amount of damage to heart tissue, resulting in reduced mortality, less likelihood of development of heart failure, and fewer reinfarctions.

PROTOCOL DESIGN

The CONSENSUS II was designed and planned during 1989 and early 1990, and has been previously described.[4-6] All patients admitted to a participating coronary care unit experiencing an acute myocardial infarction were screened for eligibility in the trial. The myocardial infarction needed to be documented by chest pain lasting more than 20 minutes and confirmed by either electrocardiographic evidence or elevated cardiac enzyme levels. Exclusion criteria included patients with blood pressure below 100 mm Hg systolic or 60 mm Hg diastolic, patients in cardiogenic shock, and patients with a clear indication for ACE inhibitors. Randomization and initial therapy were within 24 hours of the onset of chest pain.

Patients enrolled in the trial continued to receive any necessary medication to treat their myocardial infarction or any other condition, with the exception that ACE inhibitors were not permitted. The initial dose of the study drug (enalapril or placebo) was an intravenous formulation, administered by an infusion lasting 2 hours. The reasons were that an intravenous infusion would ensure a rapid effect, and a concern that the first dose of an ACE inhibitor could cause the blood pressure to drop dangerously low—a slow infusion gave the clinician much greater control over the patient's blood pressure than would an oral dose. After the initial intravenous infusion, patients switched to oral study drug and remained on this for the six-month duration of the trial. Following discharge from the hospital (approximately 10–14 days after randomization), patients returned for follow-up visits at one month, three months, and six months after randomization. Patients were not followed beyond their six-month visit.

The primary objective of this trial was to demonstrate a reduction in all-cause six-month mortality due to enalapril. Based on prior studies in acute myocardial infarction the six-month mortality rate in the placebo group was predicted to be 12%. A reduction due to enalapril of 20% (to 9.6%) was deemed to be both clinically important and reasonable to expect. The sample size of 9,000 patients (4,500 per group) was based on 95% power to detect a 20% difference in six-month mortality at the 5% significance level.

The major statistical analysis was to be based on survival analysis procedures. In particular, the Kaplan–Meier mortality curves were to be presented, and the differences between the groups assessed with the logrank statistic. There were to be analyses of the primary endpoint (all-cause six-month mortality) as well as many secondary analyses, including one-month mortality, specific causes of death, time to first reinfarction, and time to first hospitalization for heart failure. Major subgroups of interest included patients who had had one or more prior infarcts, patients who experienced an anterior infarction, and patients 70 years of age or older. All analyses were to be based on an intent-to-treat approach, which included follow-up of all randomized patients, regardless of adherence to the protocol.

DATA MONITORING EXPERIENCE

CONSENSUS II was sponsored by Merck and run under the auspices of two independent committees: The Steering Committee and the Data and Safety Monitoring Committee. The Steering Committee was responsible for the scientific integrity of the trial, including development and approval of the protocol, monitoring adherence to the protocol, decisions on all scientific questions arising during the trial, and publication of the results. This group consisted of three clinicians from each of the four participating Scandinavian countries (Denmark, Finland, Norway, Sweden), one statistician, and one official representative from the sponsor, although additional sponsor representatives typically attended the meetings.

The Data and Safety Monitoring Committee was responsible for the safety of the patients participating in the trial. This committee, which consisted of three clinicians and a statistician, was to meet periodically to review unblinded statistical analyses of the data prepared by a Merck statistician. During the course of the trial, this statistician and the Data and Safety Monitoring Committee were the only ones unblinded to the results. In the case of a safety concern or of convincing evidence of drug efficacy, the Data and Safety Monitoring Committee was charged with making an appropriate recommendation to the Steering Committee. The recommendation might be to stop the trial or it might be a protocol amendment, but in either case the ultimate decision was to be made by the Steering Committee.

The Statistical Stopping Rule

The Data and Safety Monitoring Committee met prior to the start of the trial to discuss their plans. Due to the high expected recruitment rate (actual enrolment took place between March 1990 and March 1991, and at its peak averaged approximately 700 patients per month) and the large number of expected deaths (approximately 1,000), they felt that they would need to review the data frequently. The committee also discussed the issue of futility: Due to their concern for patient safety, the committee felt strongly that the trial should terminate prematurely in the event that the interim results clearly suggested that the final result would not be significantly positive in favor of enalapril.

These two features guided the choice of a sequential stopping rule. The tentative plan was for an initial analysis after the first 50 deaths and approximately monthly analyses thereafter, resulting in approximately 10 to 20 interim analyses. Because of the frequency of the interim analyses and their potentially irregular schedule, the primary consideration in planning the sequential analysis procedure was flexibility. Accordingly, the procedure used was one based on conditional probabilities, in the spirit of stochastic curtailment.[7]

The basic idea behind this type of procedure is to stop the trial early if the data collected at an interim analysis determine the outcome at the planned conclusion of the trial with high probability. The specific procedure used was developed expressly for CONSENSUS II,[8] and is summarized below.

Let p_A and p_B represent the hypothesized event rates in groups A and B upon which the power calculations are based, and let p_{null} represent the common event rate in the two groups under the null hypothesis. Now suppose that an interim analysis has been performed after n_1 patients out of a planned total of n ($n_1/2$ in each group), and the observed event rates in the two groups are q_A and q_B. Also suppose that the one-sided alternative hypothesis is that $p_A > p_B$. For the purpose of calculating the probability of eventual rejection of the null hypothesis, the future event rates in the two groups, r_A and r_B, are predicted to be weighted averages of the observed rates and the null rates, with the weights based on the observed and future sample sizes:

$$r_A = \frac{n_1 q_A + n_2 p_{null}}{n} \quad \text{and} \quad r_B = \frac{n_1 q_B + n_2 p_{null}}{n}$$

where $n_2 = n - n_1$. Notice that early in the trial the predicted future rates are nearly equal to the null rate in both groups, but that later in the trial the predicted future rate in each group becomes closer to that group's observed rate.

Using the observed data and the predictions above for the future event rates, and making normal-theory assumptions, the predicted probability of rejecting the null hypothesis at the end of the trial can be calculated as

$$\Phi\left(\frac{n_1(q_A - q_B)/2 + n_2(r_A - r_B)/2 + z_{1-\alpha}[n_1q(1-q) + n_2r(1-r)]^{1/2}}{[n_2r(1-r)]^{1/2}}\right)$$

where $q = (q_A + q_B)/2$ and $r = (r_A + r_B)/2$. The predicted probability of rejection is compared to a pre-specified cutpoint, p_{rej}, and if greater than p_{rej} the trial is stopped early with the conclusion that the event rate in group A is greater than in group B. Clearly, the possibility of early rejection of the null hypothesis tends to inflate the significance level of the test. Conversely, if early acceptance of the null hypothesis were also possible, this would tend to deflate the significance level, due to the possibility of false early acceptance. The goal of the procedure used in CONSENSUS II was to balance the probabilities of false early rejection and false early acceptance, thereby maintaining the overall significance level of the test.

The future event rates in the two groups for the purpose of calculating the probability of early acceptance were assumed to be

$$r_A = \frac{n_1q_A + n_2p_A}{n} \quad \text{and} \quad r_B = \frac{n_1q_B + n_2p_B}{n}.$$

Notice that early in the trial these predicted future rates are nearly equal to the rates under the alternative hypothesis, but that later in the trial the predicted future rate in each group becomes closer to that group's observed rate. These predicted future rates are used to determine the probability of eventual acceptance of the null hypothesis, and this value is compared to a predetermined cutoff point, p_{acc}, to determine whether to stop the trial for early acceptance.

The significance level of the overall procedure was maintained by an appropriate choice of p_{rej} and p_{acc}. Based on simulation results, the values $p_{re} = 0.95$ and $p_{acc} = 0.90$ appeared to work well and were the values used in CONSENSUS II. Simulation studies showed that with these constants the effect on the significance level of the procedure is negligible, and in addition, the cost in terms of a reduction in power is small. While a valid statistical stopping rule is essential, in practice this was to be used only as a guideline by the Data and Safety Monitoring Committee. The committee had to consider many issues besides the primary efficacy analysis when making its decisions, including analyses of secondary endpoints and safety issues.

Interim Results and Recommendations

Hypotension following intravenous infusion of a loading dose of enalaprilat ("first-dose" hypotension) was identified early as a safety concern in the CONSENSUS II population of acute myocardial infarction patients. As shown in Table 1, at the initial meeting of the Data and Safety Monitoring Committee, there were 40 deaths among 672 enalapril patients versus 31 among 633 placebo patients. None of the patients had been followed for six months. Most striking was that 11 of 60 enalapril patients with first-dose hypotension (SBP < 90 mm Hg) had died compared to none of 16 placebo patients. When this observation was confirmed weeks later, the committee unanimously recommended protocol modifications (exclusion of patients with low entry blood pressure, reduction in rate of infusion, and termination of infusion if blood pressure dropped below 100 mm Hg systolic or 55 mm Hg diastolic).

At the sixth-monthly interim analysis with 4,161 of the planned enrolment of 9,000 patients, total mortality was still higher in the enalapril group (178/2,079 versus placebo 159/2,082). Disappointingly, the troublesome association of enalapril use, first-dose hypotension, and mortality persisted in patients enrolled after the protocol amendments (although at a reduced level). Since the initial meeting, 26 additional placebo patients had developed first-dose hypotension (2 deaths) compared to 165 additional enalapril patients (25 deaths). The importance of complete adherence to the protocol amendments was raised with the Steering Committee chair.

At the committee meeting following the seventh interim analysis one month later, mortality at any time was 9.0% (242/2,690) for enalapril and 8.0% (215/2,693) for placebo (2-tailed p-value = 0.18). Although this negative trend clearly suggested that the trial was unlikely to achieve a signifi-

Table 1 Total Mortality at Selected Interim Analyses and the Final Analysis

Analysis	All randomized patients		Patients with 6 months of follow-up		Predicted probability (%)*	
	Enalapril	Placebo	Enalapril	Placebo	Rejection	Acceptance
1st interim	40/672 (5.9%)	31/633 (4.9%)	None	none	—	—
6th interim	178/2,079 (8.6%)	159/2,082 (7.6%)	38/356 (10.7%)	34/351 (9.7%)	1.1	16.5
7th interim	242/2,690 (9.0%)	215/2,693 (8.0%)	89/744 (12.0%)	74/724 (10.2%)	0.1	58.4
Final	312/3,044 (10.2%)	286/3,046 (9.4%)	164/1,475 (11.1%)	146/1,477 (9.9%)	0.01	94.8

* Based only on patients with 6 months of follow-up. Criterion for early rejection is a predicted probability of rejection of 95%. Criterion for early acceptance is a predicted probability of acceptance of 90%.

cantly positive outcome, it had not crossed the futility boundary. However, there was a difficulty in applying the sequential method: It was designed to calculate probabilities of ultimate acceptance and rejection of the null hypothesis based only on patients who had completed the six-month follow-up. Therefore, based on the overall negative trend in mortality and on safety concerns about first-dose hypotension, the committee recommended recruitment be terminated.

When a *post hoc* subgroup analysis in patients aged 70 years or older showed a continued negative trend for mortality at any time (enalapril 198/1,246 vs. placebo 168/1,210; p = 0.06), the committee weighed all the evidence and unanimously recommended termination of CONSENSUS II. In addition, overwhelming evidence indicated that the formal boundary for stopping the trial would be crossed within weeks. While early discontinuation of a major trial such as CONSENSUS II should not be undertaken lightly, the committee recommended termination for safety concerns that took precedence over continuing the trial only to obtain a more precise estimate of a negative trend.

By the end of the trial 598 patients had died—286 in the placebo group and 312 in the enalapril group (9.4% and 10.2%, respectively; p = 0.26). The relative risk associated with enalapril treatment and based on a Cox regression analysis was 1.10 (95% CI 0.93-1.29). Kaplan-Meier curves illustrating the final results are displayed in Figure 1. The results among patients who

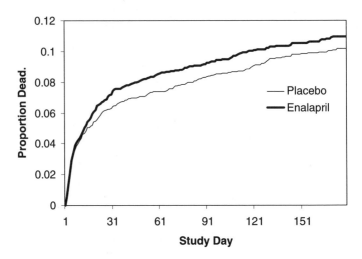

Figure 1 Kaplan-Meier curves of CONSENSUS II final results.

had completed the six-month follow-up the mortality rates were 146/1,477 (9.9%) in the placebo group versus 164/1,475 (11.1%) in the enalapril group. Based on these data and the sequential method described above, the probability of ultimate rejection of the null hypothesis in favor of enalapril was only 0.01%, and the probability of ultimate acceptance of the null hypothesis was 94.8%. Therefore, the final result had crossed the prespecified acceptance boundary of 90%.

More recent studies have demonstrated benefit with ACE inhibitors started within day 1 of an acute myocardial infarction.[9,10] However, the effect appeared to be much smaller than anticipated for CONSENSUS II, and mostly restricted to the patients with anterior location of the infarct, heart rate above 80 beats per minute, and age less than 75 years. CONSENSUS II differs from other trials in that all patients were started on an intravenous version of enalapril, and a larger proportion of patients were older than 75 years and more often had a history of myocardial infarction.

LESSONS LEARNED

The decision to recommend terminating a major clinical trial is extremely difficult to make, and in CONSENSUS II this was no exception. Stopping for futility posed a particularly difficult problem, since this can be somewhat controversial. On one side there is the opinion that without a clear trend toward efficacy or harm there is no ethical imperative to stop the trial; since stopping the trial early will prevent achievement of a clear answer and may damage ongoing substudies, this side believes that stopping for futility is inappropriate. On the other side there's the opinion that randomizing patients to an experimental therapy entails certain risks, and that patients should not be subjected to these risks once it becomes clear that any benefit is unlikely. Fortunately, the CONSENSUS II Data and Safety Monitoring Committee discussed this issue before to the start of the trial and came to a prior agreement. Not only should future Data Monitoring Committees come to a prior agreement on this issue, they should ensure that the trial leadership is also in agreement.

The stopping boundary used in CONSENSUS II had advantages and disadvantages. The advantages included flexibility in the timing and frequency of the interim analyses and the ability to stop for both overwhelming efficacy and futility. The ability of the method to balance the probabilities of false early rejection and false early acceptance, thus eliminating the need for a p-value adjustment at the end of the trial, was also a great advantage. However, basing the probabilities of ultimate rejection and acceptance only on patients who had completed the six-month follow-up was a serious disadvantage. Ultimately, the Data and Safety Monitoring Committee was forced to use its judgment in assessing the additional strength of evidence from data on patients who were still in follow-up.

As in other studies sponsored by Merck, an unblinded sponsor statistician performed the interim analyses and reported them to the Data and Safety Monitoring Committee.[11] In addition, this statistician attended the Steering Committee meetings and participated in discussions regarding the ongoing study. Although it was understood by the Steering Committee that this statistician was not to reveal any unblinded data or base any comments or suggestions on knowledge of the unblinded data, it was later recognized that this dual role poses unacceptable conflicts of interest. Subsequent to CONSENSUS II, it was acknowledged that it was necessary to implement a "firewall" between the unblinded statistician and the trial leadership.

The final lesson learned regards the role of the sponsor on the Steering Committee when the Data Monitoring Committee makes a recommendation concerning discontinuation of the trial. In order to state their case to the Steering Committee, the Data Monitoring Committee must often unblind the Steering Committee to some extent. When sponsor representatives attend the Steering Committee meeting, they will also be unblinded. This can put the sponsor in an awkward position, especially if the recommendation is to stop the trial for a safety concern, and the Steering Committee disagrees with that recommendation. Therefore, it might be in the sponsor's best interest to exclude itself from any meeting at which the Data Monitoring Committee presents a recommendation to the Steering Committee.

ACKNOWLEDGMENTS

The authors would like to thank Drs. John Kjekshus and Karl Swedberg for their careful review of this manuscript and their valuable comments.

REFERENCES

1. The CONSENSUS Trial Study Group. 1987. Effects of enalapril on mortality in severe congestive heart failure: Results of the Cooperative North Scandinavian Enalapril Survival Study (CONSENSUS). *N Engl J Med* 316:1429–1435.
2. The SOLVD Investigators. 1991. Effect of enalapril on survival in patients with reduced left ventricular ejection fraction and congestive heart failure. *N Engl J Med* 325:293–302.
3. Yusuf S, Pepine CJ, Garces C, Pouleur H, Salem D, Kostis J, et al. 1992. Effects of enalapril on myocardial infarction and unstable angina in patients with low ejection fractions. *Lancet* 340:1173–1178.
4. Kjekshus J, Swedberg K, Snapinn SM: *CONSENSUS-II*. 1999. In Nash IS, Fuster V (eds.): *Efficacy of Myocardial Infarction Therapy: An Evaluation of Clinical Trial Evidence.* Marcel Dekker, New York.
5. Snapinn, SM: *Plans for the Enalapril Post-MI Trial (CONSENSUS II).* 1992. In Peace KE (ed.): *Biopharmaceutical Sequential Statistical Applications.* Marcel Dekker, New York.
6. Swedberg K, Held P, Kjekshus J, Rasmussen K, Ryden L, Wedel H. 1992. Effects of the early administration of enalapril on mortality in patients with acute myocardial infarction.

Results of the Co-operative New Scandinavian Enalapril Survival Study (CONSENSUS-II), *N Engl J Med* 11:659-672.

7. Lan KKG, Simon R, Halperin M. 1982. Stochastically curtailed tests in long-term clinical trials. *Commun Stat C* 1:207-219.

8. Snapinn SM. 1992. Monitoring clinical trials with a conditional probability sequential stopping rule. *Stat Med* 11:659-672.

9. Gruppo Italiano per lo Studio Della Sopravivenza nell'Infarto Miocardio (GISSI-3). 1994. Effects of lisinopril and transdermal glyceryl trinitrate singly and together on 6-week mortality and ventricular function after acute myocardial infarction. *Lancet* 343:1115-1122.

10. ISIS-4 Collaborative Group. 1995. A randomized factorial trial assessing early oral captopril, oral mononitrate, and intravenous magnesium sulphate in 58,050 patients with suspected acute myocardial infarction. *Lancet* 345:686-687.

11. Snapinn S, Cook T, Shapiro D, Snavely D. 2004. The role of the unblinded sponsor statistician. *Stat Med* 23:1531-1533.

Lessons From Warfarin Trials in Atrial Fibrillation: Missing the Window of Opportunity

Charles H. Tegeler
Curt D. Furberg

ABSTRACT

Between September 1985 and June 1987, five clinical trials were initiated to evaluate the use of warfarin to prevent stroke in patients with non-rheumatic, non-valvular atrial fibrillation. They were similar in terms of study population and primary outcome, but differed in their International Normalized Ratio (INR) goals. The first three trials, all terminated early between January 1989 and November 1990, reported marked reductions in embolic complications with warfarin. As a consequence, the remaining trials were terminated ahead of schedule, primarily for ethical reasons. Publication of results from similar trials can influence ongoing trials, potentially closing the "ethical" window of opportunity by withholding proven beneficial treatment.

INTRODUCTION AND BACKGROUND

Non-valvular atrial fibrillation (AF) is a common clinical problem that represents a major etiology for embolic ischemic stroke. Up to 2.2 million Americans have intermittent or chronic AF, including up to 5.9% of those over age 65 years.[1] The prevalence of AF increases with age, and is higher among those with clinical cardiovascular disease.[2] The median age of individuals with AF is 75 years, and although more frequent in men than in women at younger ages, among those over age 75, 60% are women. This arrhythmia alone may not cause any symptoms, and up to one-third of those with AF are unaware of their condition. Without preventive treatment, the mere presence of AF confers a 5% annual risk of stroke, and a cumulative lifetime risk of about 33%.[3] AF is present in up to 75,000 strokes each year in the United States. Most strokes associated with AF are ischemic, due to cardioembolism, but other mechanisms may contribute in up to 30%. Within the cohort of people with AF, the risk factors for stroke are the presence of hypertension, prior thromboembolism, left ventricular dysfunction as evidenced by impaired fractional shortening on echocardiography or conges-tive heart failure, or female gender with age over 75 years. The absence of these factors suggests a stroke risk of less than 2% per year.

Prior to 1989, when the first of a series of clinical trials for stroke pre-vention with AF was published, no therapy had been shown safe and effec-tive for reducing the risk of stroke with non-rheumatic, non-valvular AF. Due to an accepted higher risk for stroke, anticoagulation with warfarin was the standard of care for the subset of people with AF and underlying co-morbid conditions that affect blood flow in the heart, such as mitral stenosis or pros-thetic heart valves, but there was no information documenting risk with other coexisting conditions. Besides anticoagulation with warfarin, other antithrom-botic medication options available for stroke prevention in the middle to late 1980s included aspirin, rapid-release dipyridamole, and ticlopidine. Aspirin was known to have antiplatelet activity on the arterial side and to provide modest benefit for reducing the risk of stroke after TIA or mild stroke, but the effect on cardioembolism and thrombus formation in the heart was not clear. There was no clear evidence to suggest potential benefit of rapid release dipyridamole or ticlopidine in the setting of cardioembolism.

Thus, by the mid-1980s it was clear that AF posed a substantial risk for stroke, especially among those with valvular heart disease, in whom the risk of stroke far outweighed the bleeding risks associated with chronic anti-coagulation with warfarin. There were no data regarding the safety and effec-tiveness of anticoagulation in those with non-valvular AF, nor any information regarding the use of alternative antithrombotic medications, or combinations thereof. The magnitude of the problem begged for clinical trials to identify safe and effective treatments to reduce the risk of stroke with AF. It was in this setting that investigators from Europe and North America organized five independent clinical trials to evaluate various strategies for reducing the risk of stroke with AF, focusing on the risk and benefit of anticoagulation with warfarin, and using lower doses than had been used previously in other con-ditions, to try to reduce the associated harm of treatment.[4-8] Two of the trials also included a treatment arm using aspirin.[4,5] This chapter will review the emerging evidence of benefit of warfarin over time and present the cir-cumstances that led to early termination of the last two trials, primarily for ethical reasons.

PROTOCOL DESIGN

The Copenhagen AFASAK Study

The Copenhagen AFASAK Study[4] was a single center, placebo-controlled, randomized trial to compare the effects of adjusted dose warfarin (open label), aspirin 75 mg daily, and placebo (aspirin and placebo arms double-blind) in patients with ECG-verified, non-rheumatic, chronic AF. The cohort was drawn from outpatients, identified in one of two outpatient electrocardiography laboratories in Copenhagen, Denmark, with equal randomization to each treatment group, and two years of follow up. The primary endpoint was thromboembolic complications (stroke, TIA, or systemic embolization), with death as the secondary endpoint. The target INR was 2.8–4.2. Recruitment was initiated in November 1985 (Figure 1) and all subjects were seen and examined at study entry by the lead author, who also performed an echocardiogram to measure left atrial size. Patients with cerebrovascular symptoms within the month prior to evaluation were excluded. The projected sample size was 2,000 subjects to show a 30% treatment effect for one of the active therapies. Using a group sequential approach, plans were made for five analyses at varying, predefined time points, to be done by a blinded statistician.

The fourth interim analysis, in June 1988, called for termination of the trial. There were 46 primary endpoint events, with 5 for warfarin, 20 for aspirin, and 21 for placebo, with event rates of 2.0% on warfarin, and 5.5% on both aspirin and placebo. By life-table methods the difference was significant ($p < 0.05$). There were 21 non-fatal bleeding complications on warfarin leading to drug withdrawal, compared to none on placebo. Thirty-eight percent of the warfarin group withdrew from the study, primarily from inconvenience of the blood draws or side effects. The Copenhagen AFASAK published on January 28, 1989, became the first clinical trial to show anticoagulation with adjusted dose warfarin as a safe and effective treatment for stroke prevention with chronic AF.[4]

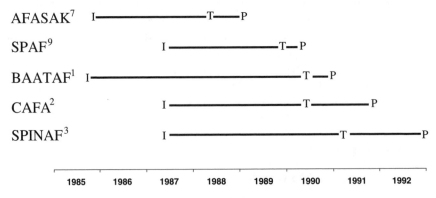

Figure 1 Time of initiation of recruitment (I), termination of follow-up and treatment (T), and publication (P) of the major results of five warfarin trials.

The Stroke Prevention in Atrial Fibrillation (SPAF) Study

The SPAF Study[5] was a multi-center, placebo-controlled trial to evaluate the safety and effectiveness of warfarin and aspirin for primary prevention of stroke and systemic embolism in patients with non-valvular AF. Carried out at 15 study centers in the United States, the cohort included patients with chronic or intermittent AF, documented within 12 months prior to enrollment. In order to accommodate concerns about the risk of treating patients with lone AF with warfarin, and the reality that some patients or physicians were not willing to be placed on warfarin, there was a two-tiered randomization scheme. Those believed eligible for warfarin (group 1) were randomized equally to adjusted-dose warfarin (open label) with a target INR of 2.0-3.5 (prothrombin time 1.3-1.8), aspirin, 325 mg daily, or placebo, while those the felt not to be candidates for anticoagulation (group 2), including those over age 75, were randomized equally to aspirin, 325 mg daily, or placebo. The aspirin and placebo regimens were double blind in both groups 1 and 2. The estimated sample size of 1,644 patients, enrolled over three years, was designed to detect differences of 50% between warfarin and placebo in group 1 and 33% between aspirin and placebo in groups 1 and 2, both separately and together. The primary endpoints were ischemic stroke or systemic embolism; and secondary endpoints were death, myocardial infarction, TIA, or unstable angina requiring hospitalization. Semi-annual group sequential interim analyses were planned for primary events in groups 1 and 2. Patients were excluded for any cerebrovascular symptoms up to 24 months prior to study evaluation.

Enrollment began in June 1987, and by the time of an interim analysis in November, 1989, a total of 1,244 patients had been enrolled: 588 to group 1 and 656 to group 2 (Figure 1). With a mean follow-up of 1.1 years, there had been 7 primary events in the combined active treatment arms in group 1 (6 warfarin and 1 aspirin), and 18 primary events in the placebo arm of group 1. Active treatment in group 1 (warfarin or aspirin) resulted in a significant reduction in event rates (8.3%/yr to 1.6%/yr), yielding an event reduction of 81% (95% CI 56-91; p < 0.00005). There were not enough events to distinguish a differential effect of warfarin or aspirin in group 1, but both treatments appeared superior to placebo. Among patients assigned to aspirin or placebo (groups 1 and 2), primary event rates were lower in those receiving aspirin (6.3%/yr vs. 3.2%/yr; p = 0.014, relative risk reduction 49%, 95% CI 15-69), but there was no apparent benefit for those over age 75 years. The annual rate of hemorrhagic events leading to hospitalization was 1.7% on warfarin and 1.2% on placebo. In November 1989, the Safety and Monitoring Committee recommended that the placebo arm of group 1 be stopped due to the benefit of active treatment (either warfarin or aspirin) as compared to placebo. In March 1990, fourteen months after the publication of Copenhagen AFASAK, SPAF became the second atrial fibrillation trial to report the benefit of warfarin in AF.[5] A major finding was that the reduction in embolic complications could be achieved with lower doses of warfarin, INR goal of 2.0-3.5 versus 2.8-4.2.

Boston Area Anticoagulation Trial for Atrial Fibrillation (BAATAF)

The BAATAF Study[5] was an unblinded, controlled trial to assess the benefit of chronic, low-dose warfarin treatment in patients with non-rheumatic, non-valvular atrial fibrillation. The cohort included patients with either chronic or intermittent atrial fibrillation, and no mitral valvular disease on echocardiography, with electrocardiogram documented AF in the 18 months prior to study entry. The target prothrombin time was 1.2-1.5 (INR 1.5-2.7), and those randomized to the control group were given the option of taking aspirin. Patients were excluded for stroke within six months, as well as previous TIA requiring ongoing treatment. Primary endpoints were ischemic stroke (intracerebral hemorrhagic was counted as a bleeding complication) and non-cerebrovascular thromboembolism. Review by an external Data Monitoring Committee was scheduled for every six months, and criteria for early termination of three standard deviations, or a two-tailed p-value of 0.0027, were established.

Active recruitment started in September 1985 and ended in June 1989, as it had exceeded the target sample size of 400 patients (212 warfarin, 208 placebo) (Figure 1). At the time of an interim analysis on April 13, 1990 (less than one month after the publication of SPAF), there were 15 definite ischemic strokes: 13 in the control group only 2 in the warfarin group, with incidence reduced from 3.0% to 0.4%, and an incidence ratio of 0.14 (95% CI, 0.04-0.49), and a relative risk reduction of 86%. A logrank test for stroke-free survival was highly significant (p = 0.0022). There were three major bleeding events (two in the warfarin group, one in control). An additional ten patients suffered hemorrhagic events that led to hospitalization (four warfarin and six placebo). Based on these findings, the Data Monitoring Committee recommended early termination of the trial and the results were published on November 29, 1990.[6] BAATF, the third trial to be completed, demonstrated that even a lower INR target, 1.5-2.7, conveyed benefit.

Canadian Atrial Fibrillation Anticoagulation (CAFA) Study

The CAFA Study[7] was the fourth multi-center, randomized, double-blind, placebo-controlled trial to evaluate warfarin for prevention of systemic thromboembolism. AF was either chronic, for a least 1 month, or intermittent, documented twice on ECG in the prior three months. Patients with stroke in the prior year were excluded. The target INR was 2.0–3.0, and the primary outcome was ischemic stroke (except lacunar), systemic embolism, and intracranial or fatal hemorrhage. The target sample size was 630 patients over four years, followed to a common endpoint at five years. Between June 1987 and April 1990, a total of 383 patients were randomized—187 to warfarin, 191 to placebo (Figure 1). Having reached 60% of the target enrollment, and about 50% of the patient-years of follow-up, and in light of the two previously published AF trials, the CAFA Steering Committee decided to terminate the study.

Intention-to-treat analysis showed 11 primary events in the placebo group (4.6%) and 8 in the warfarin group (3.4%), for a relative risk reduction of 26% (95% CI—83%, 70.4%, p = 0.25). Efficacy analysis yielded slightly better risk reduction (45%), which was still not statistically significant. Major bleeding occurred in five patients receiving warfarin and in one patient receiving placebo.

The Steering Committee did this without knowledge of the blinded study results, but with a conviction that the evidence from the recently published AFASAK and SPAF trials argued for termination of the trial since it would be unethical to withhold anticoagulation from study patients, irrespective of what CAFA might show. The window of opportunity for evaluating warfarin in AF had closed. The results were published in August 1991.[7]

Veterans Affairs Stroke Prevention in Nonrheumatic Atrial Fibrillation Study (SPINAF)

The SPINAF study was the fifth multi-center, randomized, double-blind, placebo-controlled trial to assess the benefit of low-intensity warfarin to prevent ischemic stroke in patients with AF, without evidence of rheumatic valvular heart disease. The study required AF documented on two electro-cardiograms done at least four weeks apart. Patients with prior stroke more than one month prior to study entry were eligible. Target prothrombin time was 1.2–1.5 (INR 1.4–2.8). Primary endpoint was ischemic stroke (with some deficit persisting more than 12 hours), with secondary endpoints of cerebral hemorrhage and death. Systemic embolization was not used as an endpoint. Recruitment began in June 1987, with plans for 3 years of follow-up (Figure 1). By the time of an interim analysis in January 1991, a total of 538 patients had been randomized. After randomization, 13 were judged to be ineligible, and thus 525 patients were included in the analysis. There were 23 primary endpoints, with 19 in the placebo arm and 4 in the warfarin arm, yielding a risk reduction of 79% (95% CI–0.52–0.90; p = 0.001), and a reduction in annual risk from 4.3% to 0.9%. Major bleeding occurred in seven patients in the warfarin group and four in the placebo group. When presented with these data, along with results of three published trials,[4-6] all demonstrating a significant benefit of warfarin in patients with AF, the SPINAF Data Monitoring Board recommended termination of the study, which was carried out on March 1, 1991. Results were published on November 12, 1992.[8]

LESSONS LEARNED

1. The publication of the first clinical trial demonstrating benefit (event reduction) of an intervention is rarely fully convincing to the medical community and sufficient to alter medical practice. Typically, a replication (second trial) is expected or required. Thus, not surprisingly the Copenhagen AFASAK, with a total of 26 primary events (5 warfarin vs. 21 placebo), was considered insufficient to document once and for all that warfarin reduced embolic complications in patients with AF. Additionally, the excess number of bleeding complications in patients receiving warfarin raised questions about whether lower doses would convey similar benefit, but with fewer bleeding complications.

2. The SPAF and BAATAF trials evaluated lower warfarin doses and reported a small or no increase in major bleeding complications. They also confirmed the marked benefit of warfarin in reducing the risk of embolic events and provided the replications considered essential prior to accepting a new benefit of an intervention. The completion of these trials made it difficult ethically to withhold warfarin therapy from placebo patients participating in ongoing trials. The window of opportunity closed.

3. The CAFA and SPINAF investigators responded. The CAFA Steering Committee terminated the trial without knowledge of the blinded trial results in April 1990 after the AFASAK and SPAF results were published (and the month BAATAF was terminated). The SPINAF Data Monitoring Board waited about one year to take action, but terminated the trial in March 1991. The termination of the CAFA and SPINAF trials illustrates the importance of monitoring external evidence from trials of similar interventions in similar populations and of taking responsible action. For any intervention, the proper conduct of a controlled trial has a time-limited window of opportunity.

REFERENCES

1. Feinberg WM, Blackshear JL, Laupacis A, Kronmal R, Hart RG. 1995. Prevalence, age distribution, and gender of patients with atrial fibrillation. Analysis and implications. *Arch Intern Med* 155:469–473.
2. Furberg CD, Psaty BM, Manolio TA, Gardin JM, Smith VE, Rautaharju PM. 1994. Prevalence of atrial fibrillation in elderly subjects (The Cardiovascular Health Study). *Am J Cardiol* 74:236–241.

3. Quality Standards Subcommittee of the American Academy of Neurology. 1998. Practice Parameter: Stroke Prevention in Patients with Nonvalvular Atrial Fibrillation. *Neurology* 51:671–673.
4. Petersen P, Boysen G, Godtfredsen J, Andersen ED, Andersen B. 1989. Placebo-controlled, randomised trial of warfarin and aspirin for prevention of thromboembolic complications in chronic atrial fibrillation. The Copenhagen AFASAK study. *Lancet* 1:175–179.
5. Special Report: preliminary report of the Stroke Prevention in Atrial Fibrillation study. 1990. *N Engl J Med* 322:863–868.
6. Boston Area Anticoagulation Trial for Atrial Fibrillation Investigators. 1990. The effect of low dose warfarin on the risk of stroke in non-rheumatic atrial fibrillation. *N Engl J Med* 323:1505–1511.
7. Connolly SJ, Laupacis A, Gent M, Roberts RS, Cairns JA, Joyner C. 1991. Canadian Atrial Fibrillation Anticoagulation (CAFA) Study. *J Am Coll Cardiology* 18(2):349–355.
8. Ezekowitz MD, Bridgers SL, James KE, Carliner NH, Colling CL, Gornick CC, et al. 1992. Warfarin in the prevention of stroke associated with nonrheumatic atrial fibrillation. Veterans Affairs Stroke Prevention in Nonrheumatic Atrial Fibrillation Investigators. *N Engl J Med* 327(20):1406–1412.

Data Monitoring Experience in the AIDS Toxoplasmic Encephalitis Study

James D. Neaton
Deborah N. Wentworth
Mark A. Jacobson

ABSTRACT

The toxoplasmic encephalitis (TOXO) study was designed to determine whether primary prophylaxis with pyrimethamine (25 mg thrice weekly) or clinidamycin (300 mg twice daily) would reduce the incidence of toxoplasmic encephalitis (TE) among HIV-infected patients considered at risk for the opportunistic infection. Using a modified double-blind design, patients were randomized to clindamycin or matching placbo (2 : 1) or to pyrimethamine or matching placebo (2 : 1). The clindamycin arm of the study was terminated after a median follow-up of three months due to dose-limiting toxcities; the pyrimethamine arm was terminated after a median follow-up of eight months due to a very low TE event rate in the placebo and pyrimethamine groups and a higher death rate among patients assigned pyrimethamine.

INTRODUCTION AND BACKGROUND

Prior to introduction of highly active antiretroviral therapy in 1996–97, toxoplasmic encephalitis (TE) was a major cause of morbidity and mortality among patients infected with HIV.[1,2] TE occurred primarily among patients with advanced HIV disease (CD4+ < 200) and median survival following TE was approximately six months.[3]

Most cases of TE are thought to be due to reactivation of latent *Toxoplasma (T) gondii* infection, which can be determined by testing for the presence of anti-*T. gondii* IgG antibodies. The seroprevalence of *T. gondii* varies widely around the world.[4]

At the time of the study, treatments used for TE consisted of pyrimethamine in combination with sulfadiazine or with clindamycin. To evaluate whether pyrimethamine or clindamycin were effective primary prophylaxes for TE, the Community Programs for Clinical Research on AIDS (CPCRA) initiated a placebo-controlled randomized trial (CPCRA 001 or TOXO).

PROTOCOL DESIGN

The TOXO study was initiated in September 1990. It was the first study conducted by the CPCRA. Sixteen centers enrolled patients with a positive serologic test for IgG antibody to *T. gondii*. Patients had advanced HIV disease—CD4+ cell count <200 cells/mm³ or a prior AIDS diagnosis—and were to be prescribed prophylaxis for *Pneumocystis carinii* pneumonia (PCP).

Patients were randomized to one of four groups: (1) pyrimethamine (25 mg thrice weekly); (2) placebo for pyrimethamine; (3) clindamycin (300 mg twice daily); or (4) placebo for clinidamycin. An allocation ratio of 2:1:2:1 was used and randomization was carried out within strata defined by clinical center and type of PCP prophylaxis (systemic versus aerosolized). The latter stratification was performed because systemic PCP prophylaxes were thought possibly to have activity against TE. With this design, patients and clinicians were blinded to whether patients were given active treatment or placebo, but were not blinded to whether they were in the pyrimethamine or clindamycin arm.

The planned sample size, which was estimated assuming each active treatment would be compared to the pooled placebo groups, was 750 patients. This sample size provided 80% power to detect a 50% difference in the incidence of TE at the 0.05 level of significance (two-sided), and assumed 30% of patients assigned placebo would develop TE over an average follow-up of 2.5 years. Two other important design assumptions were (1) a 25% cumulative non-adherence rate to active treatment after 2.5 years; and (2) a 33% cumulative non-TE mortality rate in each arm of the study after 2.5 years. Following randomization, patients were seen at one month and every two months thereafter.

Interim analyses for the TOXO study were reviewed by the National Institute of Allergy and Infectious Diseases (NIAID), Division of AIDS, Data and Safety Monitoring Board (DSMB). The DSMB conducted open and closed sessions for the study. A Haybittle–Peto interim analysis monitoring guideline for early termination was used. With this guideline, a 3.0 standard error difference in the TE event rate was required for early termination.[5] The chair of the study (MJ), a site investigator who also enrolled patients into the trial, was present during the open session of the DSMB but the not during the closed session, where treatment comparisons of efficacy and safety were reviewed. For interim analyses, treatments were coded (A, B, C), and treatments corresponding to the codes were available to the DSMB. The operating procedures of this DSMB have been described in some detail.[6]

DATA MONITORING EXPERIENCE

In March 1991, the clindamycin arm was stopped by the DSMB because of dose-limiting toxicities. About a year later, in March 1992, the pyrimethamine arm was stopped due to a low TE event rate and excess mortality among those assigned pyrimethamine. Data and events leading to these early termination recommendations are described in this section under two subheadings. Additional details about the findings concerning clindamycin and pyrimethamine can be found in the primary reports of the study.[7,8]

Termination of the Clindamycin Arm

The first interim analysis for the TOXO study occurred about five months after the study began. The DSMB noted a higher than expected discontinuation rate of clindamycin, primarily due to diarrhea and skin rash of mild or moderate severity (Table 1). Since the study had been open for only five months and many randomized patients had not yet attended their first follow-up visit, the DSMB requested to see updated data on a teleconference the following month. After that teleconference, the DSMB recommended termination of the clindamycin arm because of its poor tolerability. The discontinuation rates at the time of these two reviews (37.5% and 39%) after a median follow-up of only 2 and 2.5 months were higher than the non-adherence rate assumed in the design after 2.5 years (25%). With this high early intolerance rate, an increased sample size to preserve power was not considered an option. A prophylactic regimen that was to be used for a long period had to be non-toxic and clindamycin was not. In order not to unblind the pyrimethamine arm, analyses were re-done only using the clindamycin arm: clindamycin versus placebo for clindamycin. Upon review of these analyses, the study chair (MAJ) and protocol team, along with NIAID, concurred with the DSMB's recommendation.

The final results of the study, shown in the last line of Table 1, indicated that 44% of 52 patients assigned clindamycin discontinued treatment over a median follow-up of three months as compared to 9% of 32 patients on matching placebo.[7]

The TOXO study was re-designed following this closure of the clindamycin arm and the protocol was amended. The new sample size goal was set at 600 patients with twice as many patients to be assigned pyrimethamine as matching placebo. This sample size and allocation ratio provided the same power as the original design that used the pooled placebo groups as control.

Table 1 Summary of Interim Reviews that led to Termination of the Clindamycin Arm of the CPCRA Toxo Study

Interim and final analysis	Clindamycin		Pyrimethamine		Pooled Placebo		Placebo for Clindamycin	
	No.	% Discontinued treatment	No.	% Discontinued treatment	No.	% Discontinued treatment	No.	% Discontinued treatment
1st review: 10 Feb 1991	32	37.5	28	17.9	35	11.4	NP*	NP
2nd review: 19 Mar 1991	36	39.0	41	11.1	49	16.3	NP	NP
Final results Through 22 Mar 1991	52	44.0	NP	NP	NP	NP	32	9.0

* NP = Not presented at time of review.

Like the original design, sample size considered non-adherence to the treatment arms and took into account competing mortality. Patients previously in the clindamycin arm were allowed to be re-randomized and 47 chose to do so.

Termination of the Pyrimethamine Arm

Enrollment continued into the pyrimethamine arm. Two additional DSMB reviews were conducted at approximately 6 month intervals (lines 1 and 2 of Table 2). At the fourth review of the study (second after the termination of the clindamycin arm) in February 1992, the DSMB recommended stopping the study. The TE event was very low in the placebo group, and this appeared to be due, in part, to the use of systemic prophylaxis for PCP, dapsone or trimethoprim/sulfamethoxazole (TMP/SMX), instead of aerosolized pentamidine. Importantly, mortality was higher in the pyrimethamine than placebo group. The DSMB felt that pyrimethamine was unlikely to prove to be an effective primary prophylaxis given the low TE event rate and the possibly higher mortality for those taking pyrimethamine. Based on a power analysis carried out for the fourth interim review in February 1992, with the planned sample size of 600 patients and the observed annual event rate of approximately 5% (as compared with the assumed 12% per year), power was estimated as 0.50 to detect the planned 50% difference in TE rates between groups. In addition, prophylaxis for TE did not appear necessary for patients taking systemic PCP prophylaxis, particularly TMP/SMX. However, the DSMB was not 100% certain about their recommendation. There were limited data on the natural history of TE and the median follow-up was less than seven months—perhaps the rate of TE would increase. Although the lower than expected rate of TE appeared to be due the type of PCP prophylaxis being used, these findings were based on observational analyses with low power. Also, there was no obvious reason for the non-significant excess mortality among those taking pyrimethamine. Thus, the DSMB decided to unblind the chair and seek his opinion.

The chair (MAJ) was unblinded and the DSMB recommended that he no longer see patients. After reviewing the data, the chair advocated continuing the study due to the uncertainties about the future TE event rate and about the association of pyrimethamine with increased mortality. The numbers of deaths were small (22/231 versus 8/120 deaths; line 2 of Table 2) and the mortality difference could be due to chance. The chair felt that the observation of a lower TE rate and death rate for those prescribed TMP/SMX as compared to dapsone and aerosolized pentamidine was important. In light of those data from the TOXO trial and a recently completed trial indicating that TMP/SMX was superior to aerosolized pentamidine in preventing

Table 2 Summary of Interim Reviews that led to Termination of the Pyrimethamine Arm of the CPCRA Toxo Study

Interim and final analyses	Pyrimethamine					Placebo for Pyrimethamine				
	No. randomized	TE		Deaths		No. randomized	TE		Deaths	
		No.	Rate*	No.	Rate*		No.	Rate*	No.	Rate*
3rd review: 29 Aug 1991	137	1	0.7	3	6.5	69	2	2.8	2	7.8
4th review: 13 Feb 1992	231	6	5.5	22	19.9	120	3	5.3	8	13.7
5th review: 17 Mar 1992	242	8	6.5	28	22.1	121	3	4.6	10	14.9
Clinical Alert: 3 Apr 1992	264	9	5.9	34	21.8	132	3	3.7	12	14.4
Final results through 30 Mar 1992	264	8	4.9	48	28.9	132	3	3.5	14	15.7

* Per 100 person years.
Note: Some TE events reported and counted in the above table were later determined to not meet event criteria according to a clinical events committee.

recurrent PCP,[9] he recommended continuing the trial but advising patients to take TMP/SMX unless they were intolerant to it.

A teleconference was scheduled in March 1992 for the DSMB to review the chair's comments on the data and the chair's recommendations. The DSMB also reviewed an updated interim analysis during the teleconference (line 3, Table 2). At this time the number of deaths was 28/242 among those assigned pyrimethamine verus 10/121 among those assigned placebo. After considering the updated data, the DSMB reaffirmed their recommendation to stop the trial.

After the teleconference on March 17, the chair and protocol team met by teleconference on March 30 and they agreed with the DSMB recommendation. A few days later, a clinical alert about the results of the trial was issued to HIV investigators. By the time the clinical alert was issued there were 34 deaths among 264 patients assigned pyrimethamine and 12 deaths among 132 patients assigned placebo (line 4, Table 2). This higher death rate in the pyrimethamine compared to the placebo group led to a recommendation to discontinue use of pyrimethamine. After the alert was issued, closeout data collection for the trial was initiated. The common calendar date chosen for counting TE events and deaths was the day the protocol team met to review the unblinded data and to discuss the DSMB's recommendation (March 30).

LESSONS LEARNED

After closeout was complete, a total of 48 deaths on pyrimethamine and 14 on placebo were identified as occurring before the common closeout date (line 5, Table 2; hazard ratio = 2.49; 95% CI for hazard ratio: 1.28 to 4.84). The final results of the study were much more conclusive than the interim analyses reviewed by the DSMB, and later by the chair. This was due to a lag in death reporting in the pyrimethamine group.

Table 3 gives the number of deaths reported for each review of the data through the cutoff date (censoring date) used for that DSMB report. These

Table 3 Deaths Reported at Interim Analyses Through Cutoff Date and Deaths Actually Occurring Through Cutoff Date

Date of interim review	Database freeze date	Cutoff date	Pyrimethamine		Placebo	
			Reported	Actual	Reported	Actual
29 Aug 1991	12 Aug 1991	31 Jul 1991	3	5	2	2
13 Feb 1992	26 Jan 1992	31 Dec 1991	22	28	8	8
17 Mar 1992	19 Feb 1992	31 Jan 1992	28	35	10	10
3 Apr 1992	24 Mar 1992	24 Mar 1992	34	46	12	14

numbers are compared with the number of deaths ultimately determined to have occurred through the cutoff dates. The cutoff dates for the third and fourth interim analyses were about 2 and 4 weeks after the "database freeze" for the interim analyses. This time period was chosen to allow some time for events to be reported and case report forms submitted. In retrospect, it was too short, at least for the pyrimethamine group. The median time for reporting deaths was approximately 1.5 weeks in both treatment groups; however, there were more extreme reporting times for patients in the pyrimethamine group. For example, nine deaths among pyrimethamine patients were reported after 90 days compared to none among patients assigned placebo. As indicated in Table 3, for each of the three interim analyses (first three lines), all deaths in the placebo group were accounted for at the time of the review. In contrast, 2, 6, and 7 deaths, respectively, had not been reported in the pyrimethamine group. This observation at the end of the TOXO study led to an increase in monitoring of the timeliness of event reporting for CPCRA studies. It also led to a policy of including a standard table in all DSMB analyses that showed the history of all previous analyses presented to the DSMB— the actual data presented and equivalent summaries using the most recent information but the same cutoff dates. Using Table 3 as an example, at the interim analysis on March 17, 1992, the first two rows of the table would be included so that the DSMB could assess how likely events were missing for the current report.

Another lesson from the CPCRA TOXO study was that statistical groups responsible for interim analyses must be able to prepare comprehensive analyses from an up-to-date database quickly. On two occasions for this study, separate interim reports had to be prepared about a month apart. Taken together with the first lesson, a more general recommendation is that the data collection system for trials like TOXO should be designed to ensure events are quickly ascertained and reported, and then quickly processed and made available for analysis.

A third lesson learned from the CPCRA TOXO trial is that procedures should be in place for unblinding the chair and adjudicating differences of opinion about early termination. While there were no notable problems with the procedures used in the TOXO study, in retrospect, it would be preferable to agree on procedures for unblinding the chair or a designated group in a DSMB charter before starting the study.

A fourth lesson from the TOXO trial was that primary endpoints like TE can be problematic. The assumption that deaths due to other causes would not be informative was wrong. While TE or death was a secondary endpoint of the trial, if it had been the primary outcome, sample size would have been much larger because a priori one would have assumed that non-TE deaths would not be related to treatment and non-TE mortality was expected to be high. In the end, this combined endpoint was the most convincing for recommending that pyrimethamine not be used as a prophylaxis for TE (hazard ratio = 2.09; 95% CI: 1.13 to 3.89).

A fifth and final lesson from the CPCRA TOXO study was that statisticians preparing reports for the DSMB must often be capable of carrying out unanticipated analyses. For the TOXO study, numerous epidemiologic analyses on the association of different PCP prophylaxes with TE and mortality were carried out, both within the TOXO study and using data from other CPCRA studies. Numerous analyses were also carried out with the aim of understanding the higher mortality in the pyrimethamine versus placebo group. Related to the latter, other CPCRA studies were used to assess whether the mortality rate observed in the placebo group was unusually low. Many of these analyses are summarized in the final report of the pyrimethamine study.[7] Thus, if recent guidance by the Food and Drug Administration to have different statisticians working with the protocol team (a blinded statistician) and DSMB (an unblinded statistician) are to be followed[10] it will be important to ensure that the unblinded statistician be very familiar with the disease, the treatments under investigation, and in some cases other relevant sources of data.

In summary, the TOXO study required a great deal of attention by the DSMB over the 1.5 years that it was ongoing. It was reviewed at three meetings and on two teleconferences. It was stopped twice—actually three times if you consider the preliminary recommendation to stop the pyrimethamine arm and unblind the chair, and the reaffirmation of that decision a month later. The finding that prophylaxis for TE was not necessary for patients already taking TMP/SMX as prophylaxis for PCP was later confirmed[11,12] and became part of the guidelines for prevention of opportunistic infections.[13] The current guidelines also do not recommend prophylactic monotherapy with pyrimethamine.[13]

REFERENCES

1. Luft BJ, Remington JS. 1992. Toxoplasmic encephalitis in AIDS. *Clin Infect Dis* 15:211–222.
2. Jones JL, Hanson DL, Dworkin MS, Alderton DL, Fleming PL, Kaplan JE, Ward J. 1999. Surveillance for AIDS-defining opportunistic illnesses, 1992–1997. *Morbidity & Mortality Weekly Report. CDC Surveillance Summaries* 48(2):1–22.
3. Neaton JD, Wentworth DN, Rhame F, Hogan C, Abrams DI, Deyton L. 1994. Considerations in choice of a clinical endpoint for AIDS clinical trials. Terry Beirn Community Programs for Clinical Research on AIDS (CPCRA). *Stat Med* 13:2107–2125.
4. Luft BJ, Remington JS: Toxoplasmosis of the central nervous system. 1985. In Remington JS, Swartz MN (eds.): *Current Clinical Topics in Infectious Disease* Vol 6., pp. 315–358, McGraw Hill, New York.
5. Haybittle JL. 1971. Repeated assessment of results in clinical trials of cancer treatments. *Br J of Radiol* 44:793–797.

6. DeMets DL, Fleming TR, Whitley RJ, Childress JF, Ellenberg SS, Foulkes M, et al. 1995. The Data and Safety Monitoring Board and acquired immune deficiency syndrome (AIDS) clinical trials. *Control Clin Trials* 16:408–421.

7. Jacobson MA, Besch CL, Child C, Hafner R, Matts JP, Muth K, et al. 1992. Toxicity of clindamycin as prophylaxis for AIDS-associated toxoplasmic encephalitis. *Lancet* 339:333–334.

8. Jacobson MA, Besch CL, Child C, Hafner R, Matts JP, Muth K, et al. 1994. Primary prophylaxis with pyrimethamine for toxoplasmic encephalitis in patients with advanced human immunodeficiency virus disease: results of a randomized trial. *J Infect Dis* 169:384–394.

9. Hardy WD, Feinberg J, Finkelstein DM, Power ME, He W, Kaczka C, et al. 1992. A controlled trial of trimethoprim-sulfamethoxazole ir aerosolized pentamidine for secondary prophylaxis of Pneumocystis carinii pneumonia in pateints with the acquired immunodeficiency syndrome. *N Engl J Med* 27:1842–1848.

10. Guidance for clinical trial sponsors on the establishment and operation of clinical trial data monitoring committees. www.fda.gov/cber/gdlns/clindatmon.htm

11. Carr A, Tindall B, Brew BJ, Marriott DJ, Harkness JL, Penny R, Cooper DA. 1992. Low-dose trimethoprim-sulfamethoxazole prophylaxis for toxoplasmic encephalitis in patients with AIDS. *Ann Intern Med* 117:106–111.

12. Bozzette SA, Finkelstein DM, Spector SA, Frame P, Powderly WG, He W, et al. 1995. A randomized trial of three antipneumocystis agents in patients with advanced immuno-deficiency virus infection *N Engl J Med* 332:693–699.

13. Masur H, Kaplan JE, Holmes KK. 2002. Guidelines for preventing opportunistic infections among HIV-infected persons-2002. Recommendations of the U.S. Public Health Service and the Infectious Diseases Society of America. *Ann Intern Med* 137:435–478.

Data Monitoring in the Randomized Evaluation of Strategies for Left Ventricular Dysfunction Pilot Study: When Reasonable People Disagree

Janice Pogue
Salim Yusuf

ABSTRACT

Randomized Evaluation of Strategies for Left Ventricular Dysfunction (RESOLVD) was a pilot study to examine the effects of various doses of an angiotensin II receptor blocker (ARB) candesartan; an angiotensin-converting enzyme inhibitor (ACE-I) enalapril; and their combination on a number of surrogate outcomes (exercise tolerance, LV function, neurohormones) in patients with congestive heart failure (CHF). A subset of patients was also randomized a second time at four months after the initial randomization to receive a beta–blocker, metoprolol CR, or placebo utilizing a partial factorial design. This pilot study was used to identify a dose of candesartan to be used in a large-scale study evaluating clinical outcomes. Toward the end of the study the External Safety and Efficacy Monitoring Committee (ESEMC) recommended that the trial be terminated. The Steering Committee (SC) disagreed with this decision and requested an external expert panel to provide further input, which led to terminating the study about four weeks prior to its scheduled end. Lessons learned by the Coordinating Center and SC are presented.

INTRODUCTION AND BACKGROUND

In 1995, apart from ACE inhibitors, no other pharmacological treatment had been shown to reduce mortality or morbidity in patients with CHF. Therefore, there was an urgent need to develop additional treatments that

330

could provide further benefits. The RESOLVD pilot study investigated the use of various doses of candesartan, an ARB; enalapril, an ACE-I; or their combination in patients with CHF. Further, the value of adding a beta–blocker was evaluated. The goal was to study the effects on exercise performance, ventricular function, quality of life, neurohormones, and tolerability. A secondary goal was to identify the optimal dose of candesartan when used alone or with an ACE-I for a large-scale study on mortality and morbidity.

PROTOCOL DESIGN

The first part of RESOLVD was a multicenter, double-blind, randomized, parallel, and placebo-controlled trial.[1] There were two stages. In stage I, participants were randomized to candesartan alone in low (4 mg/day), medium (8 mg/day), or high (16 mg/day) doses; combinations of candesartan in low (4 mg/day) or medium (8 mg/day) doses with enalapril at 10 mg/day; or enalapril alone at 10 mg/day. After 19 weeks, participants from stage I who were eligible to receive beta–blocker therapy were randomized again to either metoprolol-CR or placebo in addition to their therapies from stage I for a period of six months. Both stages I and II had run-in periods where participants received both single and combination therapy to identify and exclude those prior to randomization who could not tolerate these treatments.

The protocol required randomization into this pilot of at least 700 participants, who were in New York Heart Association functional class (NYHA-FC) II to IV with ejection fraction (EF) <0.40 and a six-minute walk distance of <500 meters. Stage I of the study was powered to detect differences in change in six-minute walk distance between the three groups of the doses of candesartan monotherapy combined (low, medium, or high dose) versus enalapril monotherapy, and the pooled combination therapy (low-dose candesartan + enalapril, medium-dose candesartan + enalapril) versus enalapril alone. With a planned sample size of 700, the study would have 80% power to detect increases in adverse event rates of between two to four times the enalapril group rate.[1] Clinical events were documented, but the investigators did not expect that the study would have adequate power to assess plausible differences in these events.

Recruitment began on February 3, 1996, and was completed in early 1997. Of the 769 patients entered into the trial, 525 were from Canada (37 centers), 100 from Italy and Switzerland (10 centers), 83 from Brazil (5 centers), and 61 from the United States (8 centers). Of these patients 327 were randomized to candesartan (111 low dose, 108 medium dose, 108 high dose), 332 to candesartan and enalapril together (165 low dose, 167 medium dose), and 109 to enalapril alone. Follow-up was scheduled to end in September/October 1997.

The External Safety and Efficacy Monitoring Committee (ESEMC) was appointed by the Steering Committee (SC) and comprised experts in cardiovascular disease, biostatistics, and bioethics. All members were independent of the study. The chairman of the SC and Coordinating Center statisticians attended the ESEMC meetings but could not vote on issues raised by the committee. The ESEMC was charged with recommending early termination or modification of the study if significant benefit or harm was detected. They were asked to meet initially to discuss monitoring policies and then subsequently at least yearly.

DATA MONITORING EXPERIENCE

The first meeting of the ESEMC was on April 1, 1996. At each meeting the committee reviewed all aspects of the study, including the progress of recruitment, data quality, compliance to study medications, tolerability, study outcomes, clinical events, and adverse events. There were subsequent meetings on September 16, 1996; December 2, 1996, January 29, 1997; and June 12, 1997. The pilot protocol did not specify any statistical monitoring boundaries to be used, but suggested that the ESEMC could recommend early termination or modification of the study if significant benefit or harm was detected. The ESEMC also did not adopt any formal monitoring boundaries during the course of the trial.

Without a formal charter agreed upon by the ESEMC and the Coordinating Center, it soon became apparent that each committee had different ideas as to the roles and function of the ESEMC. This resulted in a breakdown in communication between the two groups. This already existing gulf between them widened on December 2, 1996, when the ESEMC first expressed a safety concern in this pilot study. They requested further analysis, and the Coordinating Center questioned the rationale behind these requests. On June 12, 1997, the ESEMC met and unanimously recommended that the RESOLVD trial be terminated immediately because of concerns for the safety of the patients. Clinical events as of this date are presented in Tables 1 and 2. The letter containing this recommendation was received by the chairman of the SC on June 13, 1997 and discussed immediately in the executive of the SC. The executive of the SC reviewed the same data that the ESEMC had reviewed and disagreed with their conclusions. On June 16, 1997, they wrote back to the ESEMC indicating their reasons for disagreement. They cited issues of study power, multiple comparisons, and other factors and requested a face-to-face meeting to discuss this.

The ESEMC then responded on June 26, 1997, that the committee stood by their decision and refused to meet with the executive of the SC. Given this impasse, the SC invited a number of additional researchers who were

Table 1   Clinical Outcomes by Combined Treatment Groups Reviewed by ESEMC on June 12, 1997

| | Candesartan alone | | Candesartan & enalapril | | Enalapril alone | | p-Value | |
	N	%	N	%	N	%	Combination vs. enalapril	Combination vs. enalapril
No. randomized	327		332		109			
Mortality	20	6.1	29	8.7	4	3.7	0.335	0.081
CHF hospitalization	35	10.7	24	7.2	4	3.7	0.026	0.186
Mortality/CHF hospitalization	48	14.6	50	15.1	7	6.4	0.025	0.020

Table 2   Clinical Outcomes by Individual Doses Reviewed by ESEMC on June 12, 1997

| | Candesartan (mg) | | | Candesartan & enalapril (mg) | | Enalapril, 10 mg |
	4	8	16	4 + 10	8 + 10	
No. randomized	111	108	108	165	167	109
Mortality (%)	6.3	6.5	5.5	6.1	11.4	3.7
CHF hospitalization (%)	8.1	16.7	7.3	8.5	6.0	3.7
Mortality/CHF hospitalization (%)	13.5	18.5	11.9	13.9	16.2	6.4

experienced in heart failure clinical trials to form an expert panel. Their charge was to review the current pilot data and the positions of both committees and provide independent advice. This panel met on July 14, 1997, and concluded that there was no clear evidence of harm in the RESOLVD trial. However, they also recommended that the unanimous vote of any data monitoring board should not be overturned lightly, and that there was no compelling reason to do so in this case.

On July 15, 1997, the RESOLVD steering committee informed the investigators that the ESEMC had recommended early termination of the trial. Participants were brought back early for their last visit and the study was terminated about four weeks earlier than originally planned. The final results have been published.[2]

LESSONS LEARNED

This manuscript was not written to describe or decide who was right in this conflict. Instead, we wondered how we, at the Coordinating Center, could have been done things differently to avoid this sequence of events. Several questions arose from this discussion. Note that this manuscript represents the opinion and perspective of the Coordinating Center and not necessarily that of the ESEMC.

1. Was an ESEMC necessary to RESOLVD?

We believe that the RESOLVD study should have had an ESEMC even though it was a pilot and that many of these types of clinical trials do not require such a committee.[3] However, we felt that for this particular pilot study preliminary information on safety was being collected, and so an ESEMC would serve a necessary purpose to ensure the safety of the trial participants, in case there were unexpectedly large safety problems. Although in this case there was considerable information on each of the drugs used separately (especially in hypertension), there was little information about these combinations of therapies and their potential interactions.

2. Should we have spent more time defining roles?

The roles of an ESEMC should be clearly defined early on in a trial to try to avoid later conflict that may result from differing perceptions of the responsibilities of the ESEMC and the SC. It should be made clear in advance which outcomes will be monitored, at what frequency, and what monitoring guidelines will be used, if any. It should be decided if the recommendations of the ESEMC are advice to the SC or binding. Given an understanding of the roles to be played by the ESEMC and the Coordinating Center in a study, these two groups may be better prepared to face the sometimes challenging demands of monitoring a trial, where the emerging trends in the data are not absolutely clear and unexpected results may emerge. Further, clarifying in advance if the ESEMC is advisory as opposed to being a decision-making body would reduce the expectations of the ESEMC that the SC would automatically follow their recommendations without discussions or clarifications.

3. What did we do right?

When conflicts arose we sought the advice of an expert panel to help find a resolution. Perhaps the wisest course for both the ESEMC and the SC in situations where they do not agree is to have a face-to-face meeting with open and frank discussions, and attempt to reach a consensus. If necessary, they may co-opt one or two additional experts to assist in resolving the dilemma.

4. What do we do differently now?

Since the RESOLVD trial we have avoided designing trials with unequal randomization where more patients are included in the experimental therapy arm than the control arm to provide more information about the new therapy. Perhaps the experience in RESOLVD questions the wisdom of such an approach as chance variations in the control arm can influence all comparisons within a study. We now also present meta-analyses of all the available evidence to our ESEMCs to provide additional information of expected outcomes rates in our control arms. We also now write charters with our ESEMCs to define their roles in the trial clearly (advisory as opposed to decision-making bodies), establish the guidelines that they intend to use, and decide which outcomes are the focus of monitoring. In RESOLVD all these steps were lacking. For most studies, we ask for a consistency of treatment patterns across a range of related important outcomes in order to trigger the action of an ESEMC. We state that the advice of the ESEMC is a recommendation to the SC; the latter then makes the decision to stop or continue the trial. We now routinely discuss the possibility of how differences of opinion between the ESEMC and the SC would be resolved in all our new trials at the first meeting of the ESEMC. We mutually agree to provisions for solving disputes in the ESEMC charter. This includes an open discussion with the chair of the SC prior to formal recommendations from the ESEMC to stop the trial, inclusion of additional experts if necessary, and making every effort to reach a consensus between the ESEMC and the SC. Lastly, we endeavor to maintain good and open communication with our ESEMCs to increase the probability that we can work together effectively when difficult situations occur. Monitoring trials is complex and requires balancing multiple factors. It is therefore not surprising that at times reasonable people may disagree with one another. Planning ahead to avoid such situations, but also explicitly agreeing to a resolution process should disagreements occur, would be a wise step for most trials.

REFERENCES

1. Tsuyuki RT, Yusuf S, Rouleau JL, Maggioni AP, McKelvie RS, Wiecek EM, et al. for the RESOLVD Pilot Study Investigators. 1997. Combination neurohormonal blockade with ACE inhibitors, angiotensin II antagonists and beta-blockers in patients with congestive heart failure: design of the Randomized Evaluation of Strategies for Left Ventricular Dysfunction (RESOLVD) Pilot Study. *Canadian J Cardiol* 13(12):1166-1174.
2. The RESOLVD Pilot Study Investigators. McKelvie RS, Yusuf S, Pericak D, Avezum A, Burns RJ, Probstfield J, et al. 1999. Comparison of candesartan, enalapril, and their combination in congestive heart failure: randomized evaluation of strategies for left ventricular dysfunction (RESOLVD) pilot study. *Circulation* 100(10):1056-1064.
3. Ellenberg SS. 2001. Independent data monitoring committees: rationale, operations and controversies. *Stat Med* 20:2573-2583.

The Data Monitoring Experience in the Carvedilol Post-Infarct Survival Control in Left Ventricular Dysfunction Study: Hazards of Changing Primary Outcomes

Desmond Julian

ABSTRACT

The Carvedilol Post-Infarct Survival Control in Left Ventricular Dysfunction (CAPRICORN) study was designed to evaluate the hypothesis that carvedilol, a beta-blocker with important differences from other beta-blockers, would be effective in reducing mortality and morbidity in post-myocardial-infarction patients with poor left ventricular function. Because of slow recruitment and a lower than expected event rate, the monitoring committee was asked to advise on a change in the primary endpoint of total mortality. This it did, but the new co-primary endpoints were negative, whereas if the original primary endpoint had been retained, the result would have been strongly positive.

INTRODUCTION AND BACKGROUND

The long-term effectiveness of beta-adrenergic blocking drugs (beta-blockers) in patients who had recently sustained a myocardial infarction was firmly established in the 1980s, especially by the Norwegian timolol study[1] and the Beta-blocker Heart Attack Trial (BHAT).[2] These trials deliberately excluded patients who had experienced heart failure; indeed, the incidence of new heart failure was increased in those who received these drugs.

Since these trials, major developments have taken place in both the short-term and the long-term management of acute myocardial infarction. Trials have demonstrated the value of value of fibrinolytic therapy and aspirin in acute management. More recently, percutaneous coronary interventions (PCI) have been shown to be as effective as fibrinolysis, or even more so.

337

A further advance was the use of angiotensin-converting enzyme (ACE) inhibitors in patients with evidence of heart failure or poor left ventricular function after myocardial infarction. For decades, it had been believed that chronic heart failure was an absolute contraindication to the use of beta-blockers, although many years ago Waagstein had claimed them to be beneficial in this context if carefully used.[3]

By the late 1990s, it was unclear whether the benefits observed from the use of beta-blockers in the early 1980s were still applicable in the changed therapeutic scenario, and whether it would be safe or beneficial to use beta-blockers in those with poor left ventricular function. Carvedilol differs in important pharmacological respects from those beta-blockers used in the previous trials. Whereas timolol and propranolol are non-selective beta-blockers, and metoprolol and bisoprolol are selective β-1 blockers, carvedilol blocks β-1, β-2, and α-1 receptors. Unlike metoprolol, it increases insulin sensitivity and it has an antioxidant effect. All these characteristics suggested that it might be particularly effective in heart failure. Indeed, several small studies which predated CAPRICORN provided evidence of the superiority of this drug compared with other beta-blockers in this context.

PROTOCOL DESIGN

The hypothesis being tested in the CAPRICORN study was that the addition of carvedilol to standard modern management of acute myocardial infarction in patients with left ventricular dysfunction with or without heart failure would improve outcome in terms of morbidity and morbidity. The original primary endpoint was all-cause mortality. Secondary outcomes were defined to be (1) mortality plus cardiovascular hospitalization, (2) sudden death, and (3) progression of heart failure. Analysis was to be conducted by intention to treat, using all available follow-up on all randomized patients.

CAPRICORN was a multicenter, double-blind-randomized controlled trial of carvedilol versus placebo, involving 17 countries and 163 centers worldwide. Eligible patients were aged 18 years or older with a stable, definite myocardial infarction occurring 3–21 days before randomization.[4] Other inclusion criteria were left-ventricular ejection fraction of 40% or less by two-dimensional echocardiography or by radionuclide or contrast ventriculography, or a wall-motion index of 1.3 or less. Patients had to be receiving concurrent treatment with ACE inhibitors unless they were ACE intolerant. Patients were excluded if they had unstable angina, hypotension or uncontrolled hypertension, bradycardia, or unstable insulin-dependent diabetes. Patients with a continuing indication for beta-blockers for any clinical condition other than heart failure were also excluded.

It was intended that 2,600 patients would be recruited, and that the trial would continue until 630 deaths had occurred with a minimum follow-up of 12 months for each patient. This was based on sample-size assumptions that the 21-month mortality rate would be 29% in the control arm, with carvedilol producing a 20% reduction in mortality. The trial was designed with 90% power and a two-sided 5% significance level. Enrollment into the trial began on June 10, 1997.

DATA MONITORING EXPERIENCE

The DSMB held its first organizational meeting on June 24, 1997. It was planned to look at the first 100 patients for safety but not efficacy; four subsequent analyses were to assess both safety and efficacy. It was agreed that the sole criterion to be used for these analyses would be all-cause mortality. A statistical significance of $p \leq 0.001$ (two-sided logrank test) would be required showing evidence of benefit before early stopping would be considered.

On November 10, 1997, the next meeting was held, at which time only 47 patients had been recruited. No analysis was undertaken. However, the DSMB decided that there should be an asymmetrical monitoring guideline for harm, with a consideration for stopping for all-cause mortality at $p < 0.016$.

The next DSMB meeting was held on March 30, 1998. During the open session, the Chair of the Steering Committee raised several issues of concern. First, recruitment was much slower than had been anticipated. The Steering Committee had, therefore, discussed the possibility of modifying the primary endpoint of all-cause mortality to ones including non-fatal events such as non-fatal myocardial infarction or hospitalization for heart failure. Secondly, there was concern that the presentation of the CIBIS II trial,[5] which had shown the benefit of bisoprolol in chronic heart failure, would affect further recruitment and might also result in protocol deviation with the unauthorized use of a beta-blocker in the long-term management of patients in the placebo group. The DSMB advised that the primary endpoint should remain as all-cause mortality and did not think that CAPRICORN should be stopped or modified because of the CIBIS II findings.

The next meeting was held on September 30, 1998. No unblinded data were reviewed, but it was noted that recruitment continued to be slow. The overall death rate was low, but this might be accounted for by the fact that it appeared that a low-risk group, as judged by Killip and New York Heart Association (NYHA) classes of heart failure severity, was being recruited.

A crucial meeting took place on March 10, 1999, where two major issues emerged. First, the MERIT-HF trial,[6] testing the beta-blocker metoprolol in chronic heart failure, had recently been presented and confirmed the benefits of beta-blockade in this context. Whereas the original protocol had strongly discouraged the open use of beta-blockers in the trial population, the DSMB now considered it unethical to continue to do so in patients whose features corresponded to those shown to benefit in CIBIS II and MERIT-HF. It seemed probable that this problem would grow the longer the trial went on and the longer that patients were kept in the trial. Secondly, the DSMB, at this time, was the only group that was aware of the total number of deaths, as the Steering Committee and sponsor had not wished to be informed on this. It, therefore, fell to the DSMB to make recommendations about changes to the design of the study, based on this information. The members reviewed the mortality data blindly, and it was apparent that the death rate was so low that the target number of deaths would not occur within a reasonable time period. It was also noted that there was a high withdrawal rate from assigned treatment.

Several options were considered. First, the number of patients recruited could be increased, but it was clear that this would be very difficult to achieve and that recruitment was likely to become more difficult rather than less, as knowledge of the CIBIS II and MERIT-HF results became more widely known. Secondly, the duration of follow-up could be increased but, again, non-trial beta-blocker use would be likely to increase the longer the trial went on, and the already high withdrawal rate would increase. The third option was to change the primary endpoint from all-cause mortality so that death or cardiovascular hospitalization would be added as a co-primary endpoint. The DSMB recommended this option, albeit rather reluctantly. However, it decided to retain the stopping rules previously agreed, based on all-cause mortality.

The Executive Steering Committee considered the recommendations of the DSMB and instituted the following changes that were incorporated into a protocol amendment, dated July 27, 1999. Patients who developed heart failure during the trial were allowed to receive open-label treatment with a beta-blocker, but if they did so, they were withdrawn from trial medication.

1. A second primary endpoint of all-cause mortality or hospitalization for a cardiovascular reason was added to the original primary endpoint of all-cause mortality. It was decided to allocate a p-value of 0.045 to the new endpoint, with a p-value of 0.005 allocated to the original primary endpoint of mortality.

2. The trial would continue until 633 deaths or cardiovascular hospitalizations had occurred.

3. Because of the revised target, it was decided that it would not be necessary to recruit the 2,600 patients specified in the original protocol, and it was expected that 1,850 would be recruited by the time that 633 target events had occurred.

4. To expedite closure of the study, the minimum duration of follow-up was reduced from 12 months to 3 months.

Despite the change in the designation of the primary endpoint, the basis for early termination would still be mortality results. The anticipated treatment effect on the composite primary endpoint was assumed to be 23%, instead of the 20% reduction for total mortality.

The first DSMB meeting after this change took place on August 30, 1999. A formal interim analysis was undertaken comparing the two groups, but the treatment code was not broken. There was evidence of a difference in the incidence of death (p = 0.034), but this did not breach the trial monitoring guideline and it was agreed that no action should be taken. The DSMB recommended that the trial continue to its natural conclusion.

Final Results

The trial proceeded as planned to completion. At the conclusion of the trial, 231 placebo patients and 237 carvedilol patients had permanently discontinued study drug. One thousand nine hundred fifty-nine patients were recruited and 707 events were judged to have occurred[7] (Table 1). All-cause mortality had ensued in 12% of the carvedilol group compared with 15% in the placebo group (hazard ratio 0.77; [95% CI 0.60-0.98]), p = 0.031, (prespecified significant p-value 0.005). The second primary endpoint of all-cause mortality or cardiovascular-cause hospitalization occurred in 35% of the carvedilol group and 37% of the placebo group (hazard ratio 0.92 [95% CI 0.80-1.07]); p = 0.296 (pre-specified significant p-value 0.045). Sudden death occurred in 5% of the carvedilol group and 7% of the placebo group; hospital admission for heart failure occurred in 12% and 14%, respectively. For both primary endpoints, results trended in a favorable direction across a wide range of subgroups typically considered in post-infarction patients. In addition, results on the other secondary endpoints also trended in a favorable

Table 1 Primary Endpoints in the CAPRICORN Trial*

	Placebo group (n = 984)	Carvedilol group (n = 975)	Hazard Ratio (95% CI)	p
All-cause mortality	151 (15%)	116 (12%)	0.77 (0.60-0.98)	0.031
All-cause mortality or cardiovascular hospital admission	367 (37%)	340 (38%)	0.92 (0.80-1.07)	0.296

* Note: The original primary endpoint was for all-cause mortality only, with a significant p-value assigned at p = 0.05. The revised co-primary endpoints were all-cause mortality (assigned p-value 0.005) and all-cause mortality or cardiovascular mortality (assigned p-value 0.045).

direction, several being nominally significant. However, based on the changed criteria for significance following the creation of a second primary endpoint, the CAPRICORN did not achieve its own criteria to demonstrate a beneficial effect. Ironically, had the primary endpoint not been changed from mortality to mortality plus cardiovascular hospitalization, CAPRICORN would have achieved a significant (at the 5% level) mortality result.

Regulatory Review

Since carvedilol was a new member in the class of beta-blockers, the pharmaceutical sponsor wished to have it approved by regulatory authorities for use in the post-myocardial-infarction patients. Carvedilol had already been approved for use in chronic heart failure based on a series of small trials in the U.S. Carvedilol Program and the COPERNICUS trial,[8] both demonstrating substantial (e.g., 30% or more) reductions in total mortality. Other beta-blockers had already been approved for use in post-infarction patients to reduce total mortality. Thus, a natural question that CAPRICORN addressed was the role of carvedilol in this same population. Taking the COPERNICUS mortality results into consideration, the sponsor argued at the U.S. Food and Drug Administration (FDA) that the totality of data for carvedilol on heart failure mortality, combined with the earlier data of beta-blocker benefit on mortality reduction, provided sufficient evidence to show that carvedilol was also beneficial in the post infarction population. The argument centered on mortality being the ultimate clinical outcome and that the CAPRICORN mortality results with a p-value of 0.031 should not be dismissed because the primary endpoint had been changed. While the circumstances for this argument are somewhat unique, the FDA review panel accepted this argument.[9]

However, during the review process, one of the issues discussed was changing the primary endpoint from mortality only to mortality and mortality plus cardiovascular hospitalization. The question was, who in the trial knew the interim results and were they blinded when the decision was made to change primary endpoints? As described above, both the Steering Committee and the DSMB were blinded to treatment differences at the point of the recommendation. The letter of recommendation by the DSMB Chair to the Steering Committee was important in addressing this question.

LESSONS LEARNED

Several issues concerning the Data Monitoring Committee arose in this trial:

1. Role of the DMC in recommending changes as a result of lower than anticipated primary endpoints. It used to be not uncommon for sponsors or

steering committees to ask the DMC to advise on the need to alter the trial on the basis of the unblinded information that only they had access to. Thus, DMCs have been asked to report whether the incidence of events in the placebo group was in line with that anticipated or whether the trial should be extended if the results were promising but unlikely to be statistically significant because of a shortage of events. It is now generally accepted that the DMC should make no such recommendations on the basis of unblinded data. The situation in CAPRICORN was different in that neither the sponsor nor the Steering Committee wished to be aware of the blinded event rate. (It is unusual for the sponsor and/or Steering Committee not to be aware of the overall event rate.) This being so, only the DSMB was in a position to recommend changes based on the low number of overall events. Certainly, in this case, when seeing the overall death rate blinded, the DSMB could have recommended one of three options:

a.   Increase recruitment.
b.   Prolong the study.
c.   Change the primary endpoint

In principle, either or both of the first two options would be preferable. However, in the case of CAPRICORN, the recruitment rate was below expectations and was likely to get worse as the effectiveness of beta-blockade in heart failure became better known. Similarly, the withdrawal rate was high and was likely to get higher the longer patients were in the study. Prolongation of the trial seemed unwise; indeed, the Steering Committee not unreasonably shortened the follow-up period. Trialists are reluctant to change the primary endpoint in midstream, particularly if it means that a soft endpoint is being introduced, as in this case, but there seemed no reasonable alternative.

Should the DSMB have discussed the changed statistical considerations decided upon by the Steering Committee? They might have been in a position to do so, as the DSMB was still blinded at this time, but, in fact, they chose not to do so. In retrospect, it might have been desirable to do so because, strictly speaking, both primary endpoints were negative. Had the original primary endpoint remained unchanged, the trial could have been declared strongly positive.

Curiously, the Chairman of the CAPRICORN trial DMC was also Chairman of the DMC of the EPHESUS trial[10] with eplerenone in which a rather similar situation arose. Again, the event rate in the latter trial was less than anticipated. After nearly 2,000 patients had been enrolled, the Steering Committee decided to add a co-primary endpoint of cardiovascular mortality and cardiovascular hospitalization to the original single endpoint of all-cause mortality. However, the Steering Committee decided to test the total mortality at the 0.04 level of significance and the combined endpoint at p = 0.01. This change in the protocol was communicated to the DSMB for their comment. As the DSMB was already partially unblinded, they could not comment. In any event, the reduction in all-cause mortality was significant at p = 0.008 and the combined endpoint at p = 0.002.

These changes in protocol presented the DSMB with some difficulty. In both cases, in retrospect, it might have better not to have changed the endpoint, but, unless there is some serious ethical reason for objecting to the change, it is better for the DSMB just to assent to it.

Because the endpoints of the trial were changed following a recommendation of the DSMB, the FDA was concerned to know, as discussed, whether the recommendation had been made with knowledge of unblinded data. As meticulous minutes had been recorded at the time of the relevant DSMB meeting, it was evident that the recommendation had been made when the DSMB was unaware of the death rate in the two groups; this information was conveyed to the FDA, who were satisfied that this was so. This experience, and others which have been similar, emphasizes the need to take accurate and timely minutes of DMC meetings.

2. Role of DMCs in recommending changes as a result of information from outside the trial. An important change was made in the protocol as a result of information obtained from other trials in the same therapeutic area. The DSMB was asked at an early meeting whether such changes should be made because of the presentation of the CIBIS II trial, which had shown the efficacy of a different beta-blocker in a similar population. As the protocol then stood, patients in the placebo group would have been denied the proven benefit of beta-blockers. The usual assumption in well-conducted trials is that patients in the control group will be given the optimal contemporaneous treatment for their condition. Quite often what is optimal can change during the conduct of the trial, so it may be desirable, if the relevant information is well substantiated, to modify the protocol accordingly. When the DSMB were first consulted about this, the members felt that they would not consider that one trial, however good, should change practice, particularly as the trial had mainly been conducted in Eastern Europe on a population that was not identical to that in CAPRICORN. However, when the results of MERIT-HF became known, it was considered that the situation had changed and it would no longer be ethical to deny beta-blocker treatment to patients who fulfilled the criteria for these two trials.

This issue has arisen in a number of major trials. The DSMB surely has the responsibility in this context to recommend changes in the protocol either spontaneously or as a result of a request from the sponsor or Steering Committee.

ACKNOWLEDGMENTS

The author would like to thank Dr. Henry Dargie, Chairman of the Steering Committee of the trial, for comments and permission to publish this document.

REFERENCES

1. Norwegian Multicentre Group. 1981. Timolol induced reduction in mortality and reinfarction in patients surviving acute myocardial infarction. *N Engl J Med* 304:801–807.
2. β-Blocker Heart Attack Trial Research Group. 1982. A randomised trial of propranolol in patients with acute myocardial infarction *JAMA* 247:1707–1714.
3. Waagstein F, Hjalmarson A, Varnauskas E, Wallentin I. 1975. Effect of chronic beta-adrenergic receptor blockade in congestive cardiomyopathy. *Br Heart J* 37:1022–1023.
4. Dargie HJ on behalf of the CAPRICORN Investigators. 2000. Design and methodology of the CAPRICORN trial-a randomised double blind placebo controlled study of the impact of carvedilol on morbidity and mortality in patients with left ventricular dysfunction after myocardial infarction. *Eur J Heart Fail* 2:325–332.
5. CIBIS-II Investigators. 1999. The Cardiac Insufficiency Bisoprolol Study II (CIBIS-II): A randomised trial. *Lancet* 353:9–13.
6. MERIT-HF Study Group. 1999. Effect of metoprolol CR/XL in chronic heart failure: Metoprolol CR/XL Randomised Intervention Trial in Congestive Heart Failure (MERIT-HF) *Lancet* 353:2001–2007.
7. CAPRICORN Investigators. 2001. Effect of carvedilol on outcome after myocardial infarction in patients with left-ventricular dysfunction: The CAPRICORN randomised trial. *Lancet* 357:1385–1390.
8. Packer M, Fowler MB, Roecker EB, Coats AJ, Katus HA, Krum H, et al. 2002. Effect of carvedilol on the morbidity of patients with severe chronic heart failure: Results of the carvedilol prospective randomized cumulative survival (COPERNICUS) study. *Circulation* 106:2194–2199.
9. Department of Health and Human Services, Food and Drug Administration, Center for Drug Evaluation and Research, Cardiovascular and Renal Drugs Advisory Committee, 98th Meeting, January 7, 2003. www.fda.gov/ohrms/dockets/ac/03/transcripts/3920T2.htm
10. Pitt B, Remme W, Zannad F, Neaton J, Martinez F, Roniker B, et al. 2003. Eplerenone, a selective aldosterone blocker, in patients with left ventricular dysfunction after myocardial infarction. *N Engl J Med* 348:1309–1321.

Controversies in the Early Reporting of a Clinical Trial in Early Breast Cancer

Stephen L George

Mark R. Green

ABSTRACT

The role of adjuvant chemotherapy in the treatment of breast cancer has been the subject of intense research activity in recent years. It is now generally accepted that some types of adjuvant therapy have a positive effect on disease-free and overall survival, but the effect size appears to be modest and the optimal type of adjuvant therapy for different groups of patients remains unclear.[1,2] One major study of adjuvant therapy in breast cancer patients that generated considerable interest and controversy was an intergroup trial of the value of increasing the dose of doxorubicin or adding paclitaxel (Taxol®) to standard chemotherapy. The design was a 3 × 2 factorial design (three different doses of doxorubicin with and without paclitaxel). Based on the results of the first planned interim analysis suggesting improved disease-free and overall survival in patients receiving paclitaxel, the DSMB released the results to the study team. The events and considerations leading to the decision to release the results and some of the subsequent controversies that arose in the medical community because of this decision are discussed in this paper.

INTRODUCTION AND BACKGROUND

Since 1955, the United States National Cancer Institute (NCI) has sponsored a number of cooperative cancer research groups to carry out multi-center clinical trials and related studies in patients with cancer. The membership in these groups consists of nearly all of the major cancer centers in the country as well as a large number of smaller centers, individual physicians, and medical practices interested in cancer research. The major effort of these groups has been to conduct definitive clinical trials and the developmental studies leading to these trials. In recent years, increasing attention has been given to the "correlative sciences," relating biological findings from the basic sciences to treatment outcomes. Individually and jointly, these groups are responsible for nearly all of the large phase III trials in cancer carried out in the U.S. by the public sector. There are currently ten cancer cooperative groups involving thousands of individual investigators. Over 20,000 patients are entered annually on cooperative group studies.

The major distinction between the NCI-supported cancer cooperative groups and most other multi-center clinical trials consortia is that the cancer groups are set up as on-going organizations with funding and infrastructure not linked to specific trials. Rather, these groups carry out many trials in various diseases (e.g., breast cancer, colon cancer, leukemia and lymphoma, and so on) according to the group's focus and interest. Each group is large enough to conduct many studies within its own membership, although often the need to enter larger numbers of patients in a reasonable time period requires that the groups join together to conduct "intergroup" studies. In such cases two or more groups combine to carry out a study with one of the groups designated as a "coordinating" group for carrying out statistical design and analysis and monitoring. The trial discussed in this paper was an intergroup trial carried out by four major cooperative groups. It was coordinated by the Cancer and Leukemia Group B (CALGB), with participation by the Southwest Oncology Group (SWOG), the Eastern Cooperative Oncology Group (ECOG), and the North Central Cancer Treatment Cancer Treatment Group (NCCTG).

In 1993, when this trial was designed, it was well established that adjuvant chemotherapy was important in prolonging survival in patients with early breast cancer. In particular, the use of an alkylating agent (e.g., cyclophosphamide) together with an anthracycline (e.g., doxorubicin) was known to be beneficial. However, there was uncertainty regarding optimal drug dosing, particularly for doxorubicin, which has significant cardiac toxicity at higher cumulative doses, the types of patients who might benefit the most from therapy, and the role of a promising new agent, paclitaxel, in the adjuvant setting. To address these questions, a randomized phase III clinical trial (designated as CALGB 9344) was designed and activated in 1994.

PROTOCOL DESIGN

The CALGB study 9344 was chaired by Dr. I. Craig Henderson. Responsible statisticians were Ms. Connie Cirrincione and Dr. Don Berry. At the time of the discussions about early release of the study data, the CALGB Breast Committee was chaired by Dr. Larry Norton. The authors of this chapter served on the DSMB in the role of Group Statistician (SG) and Chair of the DSMB (MG).

The three primary objectives of CALGB 9344, as stated in the protocol, were—

1. To determine whether higher doses of doxorubicin used as an adjuvant with cyclophosphamide in patients with early breast cancer will increase disease-free and overall survival.
2. To determine whether the use of paclitaxel as a single agent after the completion of four cycles of cyclophosphamide and doxorubicin in combination will further improve disease-free and overall survival compared to cyclophosphamide and doxorubicin alone.
3. To determine whether treatment with paclitaxel will improve disease-free and overall survival regardless of the dose of doxorubicin. More specifically, to determine if paclitaxel following standard dose cyclophosphamide and doxorubicin will be as effective or more effective than cyclophosphamide and doxorubicin without paclitaxel.

In adjuvant therapy trials, disease-free survival is defined as the interval from study entry to first local or locoregional recurrence, first distant metastasis, or death as a result of any cause. In the final analysis of the results,[3] disease-free survival was treated as the primary endpoint of this study, with overall survival and toxicity assessment as secondary endpoints. In order to simplify and focus the discussion in the remainder of this paper, we will restrict our attention to the second objective (paclitaxel vs. no paclitaxel) with respect to disease-free survival. In the course of the trial, DSMB actions with regard to this objective led to the most discussion within the DSMB and to some subsequent controversy.

The key eligibility criteria on this study were—

1. Patients with operable, histologically confirmed adenocarcinoma of the female breast and histologically involved lymph nodes.
2. Performance score 0–1. These are patients who are either asymptomatic or who have minor symptoms but are fully ambulatory.
3. Normal initial laboratory values (e.g., white cell count, platelet count, hemoglobin, creatinine, bilirubin, left ventricular ejection fraction).
4. No other serious medical illness which would limit survival to less than two years or psychiatric condition which would prevent informed consent.

To achieve the objectives of this study given above, a 3×2 factorial design was employed with a stratified permuted block randomization based on the number of positive lymph nodes: 1–3, 4–9 and 10 or more. The first factor was the dose of doxorubicin given in the first phase of chemotherapy. The three possible dose levels of doxorubicin (A), each given with a fixed dose level (600 mg/M^2) of cyclophosphamide (C) for four three-week cycles were—

  i. 60 mg/m^2,
 ii. 75 mg/m^2,
iii. 90 mg/m^2.

The second factor was the administration of paclitaxel (T) as a second phase of active treatment or no further chemotherapy following AC. For patients assigned to T, four 3-week cycles infused over three hours at 175 mg/m^2 were prescribed. Thus, there were six different treatment combinations, A60C ± T, A75C ± T, and A90C ± T with randomization to one of the complete regimens taking place at study entry rather than sequentially. The randomization process was designed and managed centrally by the CALGB Statistical Center.

The eligible sample size was planned to be approximately 3,000 patients accrued over three years and followed for four years after the end of accrual, at which time an expected 1,800 events would have occurred. These calculations from the protocol were based on previous intergroup studies in node-positive breast cancer. With respect to the paclitaxel comparison, the power at 1,800 events was calculated to be in excess of 95% to detect an increase in median DFS from six months to eight months (25% decrease in hazard rate).

The primary analysis was to be based on proportional hazards models relating disease-free survival (DFS) and overall survival (OS) with doses of A and the presence or absence of T. These models were to include the main effects of A and T, the interaction of A and T, and various patient characteristics (covariates), such as number of positive lymph nodes, tumor size, and age. Estimated hazard ratios were obtained from these models. The study was not powered to evaluate effects in subsets. Further details are provided in the paper describing the outcome of this study.[3]

As the protocol was originally written, it did not include pre-planned interim analyses. These were later mandated by the CALGB DSMB, based on procedures adopted to optimize the DSMB monitoring program.

DATA MONITORING EXPERIENCE

Procedures

As with all randomized phase III trials carried out by the cancer cooperative groups, this trial was monitored by a group-specific Data and Safety Monitoring Board (CALGB DSMB). This board, composed of various medical professionals both from within and outside the CALGB, biomedical statisticians, and lay members, meets on a regular basis, twice a year, to review all phase III and selected phase II CALGB trials in active accrual or follow-up. The number of such trials reviewed at each meeting typically is between 10 and 15. The policies and procedures of the CALGB DSMB follow established NCI guidelines for monitoring. Studies are monitored by the DSMB based on reports prepared by the CALGB Statistical Center with monitoring continuing until such time as the DSMB determines the results can be revealed to the study team and committee sponsoring the study. This release is generally specified at the time in the protocol based on adequate follow-up to reach the pre-specified number of required events. Prior to the release date, all study data remain within an envelope of confidentiality restricted to the study statistician(s) and the DSMB members. In unusual circumstances, pre-specified interim analyses may indicate to the DSMB that the results are sufficiently striking that they should be released earlier than originally planned.

All recommendations of the DSMB go to the Group Chair, who has the option of requesting further information from the DSMB before accepting the recommendations. For most studies, most of the time, the recommendation is simply to continue the study accrual or follow up with no modification. These recommendations cause no particular difficulties. However, in the unusual event that a major modification to the study (early suspension or closure of accrual for toxicity or for statistically extreme findings or early release of the results to the study team) is recommended based on an interim analysis, the details behind the recommendations and the considerations which led to the decision become particularly important. The monitoring of CALGB 9344 resulted in one of these unusual events.

Outcomes

The first patient was registered to this study in May 1994 and the study was eventually closed to accrual on schedule in April 1997, at which time 3,170 patients had been randomized. Following standard CALGB procedures for monitoring, formal reports on toxicity began with the first scheduled DSMB meeting after study activation, in November 1994. However, there were no formal rules for interim analyses of efficacy in the original protocol. Following activation, the DSMB required that these be added. Thus, the study protocol was modified to include three interim efficacy analyses at 450, 900, and 1,350 events, plus a final analysis at 1,800 events. That is, the four formal interim analyses were planned to be equally spaced in terms of numbers of events (25%, 50%, 75%, and 100%). As noted earlier, it was anticipated in the protocol that the final analysis would be possible four years after the study was closed to accrual. The stopping boundaries at the earlier event milestones were based on O'Brien–Fleming rules.[4] Keep in mind that this was a test of standard versus augmented dose, number of agents, and duration of adjuvant chemotherapy. The pre-study hypothesis was that "more would be better," but that the differences would be incremental rather than dramatic. Prior to the data monitoring process discussed below, there was little expectation that clinically significant differences would emerge in the early phase of monitoring study follow up, let alone lead to consideration of early termination of accrual.

For the first five DSMB meetings from November 1994 through November 1996, the reports contained information only on toxicity, not efficacy, and need not concern us for the discussion here. However, formal early analyses of toxicity may be written into large phase III trials and were in fact an important part of early monitoring of this study. In late 1996, the study statistician reported to the DSMB chair his "concern" about "trends" in the CALGB 9344 efficacy outcomes with respect to the paclitaxel comparison. Based on these reported concerns, the DSMB chair requested a formal report of the study status for DSMB review. This was prepared in February 1997. At that time 2,951 patients had been accrued, and a total of 192 events had been reported, less than half the number of events required for the first formal pre-specified interim analysis and only 11% of the targeted number of 1,800 events. The findings of that special report, shown below, seemed to indicate an early positive effect for patients receiving paclitaxel (Figure 1).

However, the nominal logrank p-value (p = 0.0146) would not have come close to a stopping boundary even if one had been planned at this point.

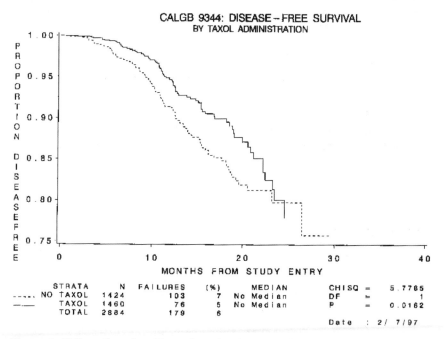

Figure 1 DFS, paclitaxel vs. No paclitaxel, February 1997.

O'Brien–Fleming rules are known to be very conservative, with little chance of stopping before a substantial proportion of events have been observed (more on this later). There was also a similar analysis of overall survival based on only 69 events (nominal p-value p = 0.0295; again far from any stopping boundary). The practical result of this special analysis was nil. The study continued to accrue patients, and the data remained fully within the envelope of confidentiality. Such early unplanned reports or analyses are often called "administrative" looks at the results, done with the intention of keeping a DSMB generally informed but without having to pay the statistical price necessary to preserve the pre-set overall error rates on which the trial is designed. This is possible only if there is no expectation of stopping accrual or confidential follow up based on the administrative looks. Arguments against such analyses have been made elsewhere.[5]

Additional administrative looks at the 9,344 data set were prepared by the study statisticians throughout 1997 and early 1998. Not all of these analyses were specifically reported to the DSMB. The results are summarized in Table 1.

Although there was considerable discussion among DSMB members about whether it was appropriate to review such non-scheduled analyses and, if so, whether or not any action should be taken, the result was that no action was taken. Instead, a special DSMB meeting was called in April 1998 to consider the results of the first formal protocol-specified interim analysis, based on 453 events, approximately the 25% point in terms of the planned number of events. This analysis occurred one year after the trial was closed to accrual with individual follow-up times between one and four years. All patients had been off all protocol-specified treatment for at least six months. The estimated DFS distributions at this time are given in Figure 2.

As in the previous "administrative" analyses, in this April 1998 analysis the DFS outcome appeared to favor the paclitaxel treatment group, although the nominal significance level (p = 0.013) still failed to reach the monitoring boundary. Nevertheless, at this point, the DSMB decided to release the results

Table 1 Administrative analyses, February 1997–March 1998

| Date | N | Failures | | | Logrank p-value |
		No paclitaxel	paclitaxel	Total	
Feb 1997	2,951	110	82	192	0.015
Apr 1997	3,170	130	100	230	0.014
Aug 1997	3,170	180	148	328	0.029
Nov 1997	3,170	215	174	389	0.009
Jan 1998	3,170	226	189	415	0.014
Feb 1998	3,170	230	194	424	0.014
Mar 1998	3,170	243	203	446	0.008

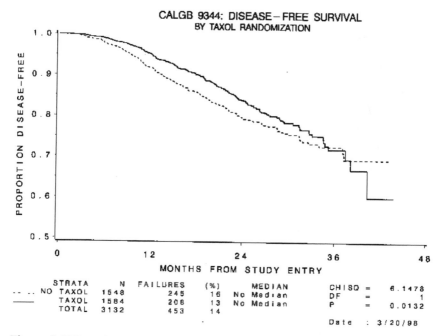

Figure 2 DFS, paclitaxel vs. No paclitaxel, April 1998.

to the sponsoring committee. This was a difficult decision for the DSMB, generating considerable internal discussion and debate, the details of which remain confidential. The general issues discussed are given in the following section.

Immediately after the results were released to the Breast Committee in April 1998, a "late-breaking" abstract was prepared and submitted for possible presentation at the upcoming American Society of Clinical Oncology (ASCO) meeting.[6] This abstract was accepted and the results were presented orally at a special ASCO session in May 1998.

There have been three subsequent substantive analyses based on additional follow up since the release of the data in April 1998. All support the original conclusions. These include an analysis prepared in December 1998 as part of a NDA for a new indication for paclitaxel in this group of patients (624 events), an analysis prepared in September 2000 for an NIH consensus conference (901 events), and an analysis prepared in May 2002 for the "definitive" publication of the results in the *Journal of Clinical Oncology* (1,054 events).[3] Figure 3 gives the DFS curves in this latter case.

In the May 2002 analysis, median follow-up was 69 months. Three-quarters of the patients had been observed for at least five years, and there were 1,054 events—approximately 58% of the expected events—and 742

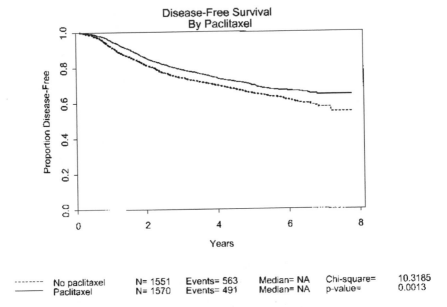

Figure 3 DFS, paclitaxel vs. No paclitaxel, May 2002.

deaths. The analysis indicates that adding paclitaxel to the CA combination yields estimated hazard reductions of 17% for recurrence and 18% for death. The estimated percentage of patients alive and recurrence free at five years was 65% for patients assigned to CA alone and 70% for patients assigned to CA plus paclitaxel. The percentages for overall survival were 77% and 80%, respectively. Whether similar benefits will be observed at longer times (e.g., ten years and beyond) is unknown at present, but the five-year results will obviously not change much with further follow-up. Using the O'Brien-Fleming boundaries and assuming that this represents a second formal look at 58% of the total expected events, the O'Brien-Fleming Z-value would be 2.4 and the pvalue 0.0087, so the O'Brien-Fleming boundary was crossed at this point.

It is of interest to recall that at the time the protocol document was written, the final analysis was projected to occur four years after the study closed to accrual, with 1,800 events expected at that time. However, in May 2002, more than five years after the study closed to accrual, the actual number of events observed (1,054) was only 58% of the "targeted" number of events due to better than expected overall outcomes.

Issues in the DSMB Deliberations

No *post hoc* report of the deliberations of a DSMB, particularly those leading to a difficult and controversial recommendation, can hope to capture completely the richness and interactive nature of the discussions. The confidential nature of the deliberations further restricts full disclosure. Nevertheless, it is possible to identify some of the key topics informing the discussion. For CALGB 9344, some of these were—

- *Effect on patients enrolled on the study.* At the time of the first planned interim analysis, accrual had been completed one year previously and all patients had completed all protocol-specified therapy at least six months prior to the analysis date. Thus, the release of preliminary information on outcome would not be expected immediately to influence therapy for the patients in this study, the patients of most concern to the DSMB.
- *Effect on the medical and research community.* The effect on scientific opinion and on other on-going studies of releasing the results early was perhaps the major topic of discussion. Was it more important, both for researchers and patients, for the early results to be known, with the clear understanding that further follow-up might reveal less of a long-term effect, than to keep the early results confidential awaiting the long-term outcome? Was it not true that clinicians and researchers should be able to understand the limitations of the results of early results? Or would the potential criticism of "premature" release of the results lead some to conclude that the results were unreliable, thus failing in an important purpose of a clinical trial: to change medical practice? Were the results strong enough to convince reasonable skeptics? What impact might early release have on the ability of on-going studies of similar design to reach their accrual goals? Was it possible that early release of 9,344 information might lead to inadequate accrual and early closure of these other trials?
- *Stopping rules versus stopping guidelines.* It is often stated that statistical stopping rules in clinical trials should be treated as guidelines, not as fixed immutable rules, but what does that mean in practice? For example, in this trial it was decided to release the results at a time when the stopping rule had not been met. Such decisions will inevitably increase the error rates, so under what conditions are they defensible? Later, the boundary was hit, but that of course could not have been known at the time and in any case is irrelevant for a discussion of the decision process at the time. Another point of discussion was whether the rules applied simply to stopping the study (i.e., stopping accrual or follow-up) or, rather, applied to reporting and release of results as well. In the present example, accrual was already completed and follow-up would have continued in any case, so the issue was primarily one of reporting or release of the results beyond the DSMB. In addition, the DSMB, in accordance with its operating poli-

cies and procedures, does not review or comment on protocols before they are activated. The O'Brien–Fleming stopping rule adopted for this study was considered by some DSMB members to be rather extreme in the early time periods. A truncated rule, using a nominal p = 0.005, say, when the unadjusted OBF rule required a more extreme p-value, would have satisfied most members, but this is not the way the design was written.

- *Early versus late outcomes.* The early results (i.e., an early difference in DFS distributions) were based on solid evidence that would not change with further follow-up. But the longer-term outcome was of course unknown. The discussion centered on whether it is it reasonable to report a relatively conclusive finding of early differences without knowing whether these early differences would translate into longer-term differences as well. Stated another way, is it essential to know the long-term results before one can interpret the short-term results? Prior adjuvant trials in breast cancer have often first shown early disease-free survival differences that later were sustained and accompanied by evidence of overall survival differences. Some DSMB members may have felt the same pattern was likely enough in this study to enhance their comfort level with "early release" of the information to the CALGB Breast Committee.

- *Statistical predictions.* Could one offer more than a gestalt of individual DSMB members concerning the probability that the results would or would not change with further follow-up? Various calculations, including Bayesian calculations based on predictive distributions[7] as well as frequentist conditional power calculations, indicated that the overall results would be unlikely to change substantially with further follow-up. These calculations of course depended on assumptions but, in the event, the predictions have been remarkably accurate for the subsequent results based on additional follow-up.

- *Crossovers.* If results were made public now, what was the potential for "crossovers," patients switching to paclitaxel, to contaminate the results? Since all patients had been off protocol-specified treatment for at least six months, this was considered unlikely. In fact, no patients randomized to AC alone had "delayed crossover" to paclitaxel following release of the study data.

- *Role of the DSMB.* Although not a topic peculiar to this study, the considerations above led to a more general discussion of the proper role of the DSMB, particularly with respect to keeping a study "under wraps" after accrual has ended, all patients have completed protocol-specified therapy, and there is little chance for crossover contamination. One view was that there should be an automatic release of the data at this point to the study team, regardless of the results. The study team would then be responsible for how the information should be handled and when it should be openly reported. This view was partially based on a feeling that holding the data beyond this point was paternalistic and failed to credit the investigators with the maturity and judgment to decide how to proceed. The alternative, more traditional, view was that the investigators were so heavily invested in the study, that an independent DSMB should make these decisions.

- *Role of repetitive exposure of DSMB members to administrative ("non-actionable") interim analyses.* There may be a real difference in the psychological response of DSMB members to provocative but not "statistically significant" differences first seen at a pre-specified interim analysis compared to more frequent exposure to a sequence of administrative analyses leading to the same point. Perhaps a DSMB can develop a comfort level with data generated by administrative looks seen repetitively over time, but does this pervert the objectivity or evidence base of the DSMB deliberations over time? Is there a similar danger for study statisticians in slipping from objective stewards of the study data to advocates for a specific interpretation of the findings? These issues are addressed elsewhere.[5]

All of the issues noted above, and others, were thoroughly discussed by the DSMB. In the end, the recommendation was made to release the results to the study team for their use. Note that there was no recommendation for a release to the broader medical community. However, the study team decided to immediately write a "late-breaking" abstract for presentation at the upcoming American Society of Clinical Oncology (ASCO) meeting in May 1998. This presentation generated considerable discussion about the merits of releasing the results at this time, mostly unpublished, although there was one written commentary.[8] However, it can be argued that this trial was highly successful in changing medical practice, both with respect to delivery of adjuvant paclitaxel and with respect to not requiring higher than necessary doses of doxorubicin. The latter result was not described in this paper but was an important result because of the significant cardiac and other toxicities that can result from higher doses of doxorubicin.

LESSONS LEARNED

Several lessons can be learned from this experience that, had they been followed, would have simplified some of the deliberations, although it is unclear whether the outcome would have been any different in this particular case. Some of these are—

- *Flexible interim analyses are required in the protocol and these should be followed in practice.* This may seem like an obvious point, but some plans for interim analyses as described in clinical protocols either leave room for interpretation of the intent or are so inflexible that it isn't clear how to apply them if there is any deviation from the plan. For example, the timing of interim analyses is not an issue if a spending function approach is used. Even though other considerations will be involved in any DSMB decision, it is important to have the statistical rules clearly described in advance and followed in the execution of the trial.
- *Careful and pre-specified procedures are needed after DSMB release.* Given that results for a minority of studies will warrant early release, the rules and procedures for such eventualities need to be carefully delineated beforehand.
- *Administrative looks at efficacy data should be dropped.* There are significant problems in preparing so-called administrative looks at the efficacy results outside of planned interim analyses.[5] Instead, the use of flexible interim analysis approaches, clearly defined in the protocol as mentioned above, that allow for proper interpretation should be used. These are easily available.[9] In contrast to efficacy analyses, it should be noted that in cancer trials it is routine to carry out safety analyses quite frequently, generally without any pre-planned stopping rules.
- *Use the device of imaginary results.* In designing the study, a useful device is to consider "imaginary" results. That is, consider various scenarios that might unfold to see if the design chosen is appropriate and acceptable to the study team and the DSMB. One example is with respect to the stopping rules. It would be worthwhile to calculate items such as the minimum differences in numbers of events that would cause a stopping boundary to be reached at various times. Also, if an unexpectedly long time between analyses results under plausible scenarios, this might cause a rethinking of the design. Although the use of a suitably flexible design addresses the issue in a statistical manner, there are options in choosing among candidate designs, so a prior review of outcomes that would lead to stopping or continuing is instructive and might lead to design modifications.

In the final analysis, the judgments of a DSMB will always be difficult in studies where some type of emerging trend, either positive or negative, is seen relatively early in the study. However, the judgment that must be made can be facilitated by careful attention beforehand to those issues likely to arise in the course of study monitoring.

REFERENCES

1. Piccart M. 2003. The role of taxanes in the adjuvant treatment of early stage breast cancer. *Breast Cancer Research and Treatment* 79:S25–S34.
2. Cardoso F, Lohrisch C, Piccart MJ. 2003. Landmark adjuvant randomized clinical trials of systemic therapy in early breast cancer. *Drugs of Today* 39:399–414.
3. Henderson IC, Berry DA, Demetri GD, Cirrincione CT, Goldstein LJ, Martino S, et al. 2003. Improved outcomes from adding sequential Paclitaxel but not from escalating Doxorubicin dose in an adjuvant chemotherapy regimen for patients with node-positive primary breast cancer. *J Clin Oncol* 21:976–983.
4. O'Brien PC, Fleming TR. 1979. A multiple testing procedure for clinical trials. *Biometrics* 35:549–556.
5. George SL, Freidlin B, Korn EL. 2004. Strength of accumulating evidence and data monitoring committee decision making. *Stat Med* 23:2659–2672.
6. Henderson IC, Berry DA, Demetri GD, Cirrincione CT, Goldstein LJ, Martino S, Ingle JN, et al. 1998. Improved disease-free (DFS) and overall survival (OS) from the addition of sequential paclitaxel (T) but not from the escalation of doxorubicin (A) dose level in the adjuvant chemotherapy of patients with node-positive primary breast cancer. *Proc ASCO* 17:390a.
7. Qian J, Stangl DK, George SL. A Weibull model for survival data: Using prediction to decide when to stop a clinical trial. 1996 In Berry DA, Stangl DK (eds.): *Bayesian Biostatistics*, pp. 187–205. Marcel Dekker, New York.
8. Piccart MJ, Lohrisch C, Duchateau L, Buyse M. 2001. Taxanes in the adjuvant treatment of breast cancer: Why not yet? *J Natl Cancer Inst Monogr* 30:88–95.
9. Freidlin B, Korn EL, George SL. 1999. Data monitoring committees and interim monitoring guidelines. *Control ClinTrials* 20:395–407.

Making Independence Work: Monitoring the Bevacizumab Colorectal Cancer Clinical Trial

Janet Wittes
Eric Holmgren
Heidi Christ-Schmidt
Alex Bajamonde

ABSTRACT

Genentech's phase III study of colorectal cancer aimed to show that administration of bevacizumab, its recombinant human anti-vascular endothelial growth factor antibody, to patients with metastatic colorectal cancer would reduce mortality. The four-member DMC was responsible for reviewing real-time safety data, selecting the experimental arm of the study at an interim analysis, and assessing efficacy at a second interim analysis. Genentech and the entire study team remained blinded to treatment allocation during the course of the trial. The study, which proceeded to its planned end, showed an estimated hazard ratio for death of 0.66 (p < 0.001). On the basis of this study, the FDA approved bevacizumab for patients with metastatic colon cancer. This example shows how a DMC can make complicated decisions and recommendations even when neither it nor the statisticians reporting to it participate in any other way with the conduct of the study.

INTRODUCTION AND BACKGROUND

The late 1990s saw the refinement of our biological understanding of angiogenesis, the development of blood vessels. Because angiogenesis contributes to the growth of human cancers, scientists theorized that interfering with angiogenesis should retard tumor growth. This theory led various drug companies to develop monoclonal anti-vascular endothelial growth factor antibodies as potential treatments for cancer. One such antibody is Genentech's bevacizumab [Avastin®], which showed promising effects when administered with fluorouracil plus leucovorin in a phase II trial of colorectal cancer.[1] Some early-phase studies with the product in other cancers had suggested serious toxicities associated with its use, in particular, excess major bleeding, thrombosis, hypertension, proteinuria, and severe diarrhea. Thus, proceeding with a phase III study required careful monitoring of these safety events. Genentech chose a four-member Data Monitoring Committee (DMC) and asked it to review safety data in essentially real time to ensure that the rate of serious adverse events in patients given bevacizumab was not unacceptably high.

When the study was being designed, the standard of care for the treatment of metastatic colon cancer had been a combination of two chemotherapeutic agents, fluorouracil and leucovorin (FL). Genentech had studied bevacizumab in colorectal cancer in a phase II trial with the FL regimen as background therapy. In 2000, when Genentech was ready to initiate its phase III study to demonstrate the effect of bevacizumab on mortality in colorectal cancer, optimal care had changed to a regimen consisting of irinotecan, fluorouracil, and leucovorin (IFL).[2] The designers of the phase III trial selected the IFL regimen as the control arm because its efficacy was superior to that of FL; however, the IFL regimen was considerably more toxic. The choice of experimental regimen then became problematic. To start a large phase III3 trial comparing the IFL regimen plus bevacizumab to IFL alone was risky, for if the combination proved unacceptably toxic, the study would stop early without adequately testing the effect of bevacizumab. On the other hand, selecting FL plus bevacizumab as the experimental arm could produce ambiguous results. If the study showed FL plus bevacizumab to be less effective than IFL, the oncologic community would not be able to distinguish between the inferiority of the FL regimen or the lack of efficacy of bevacizumab. If the experimental arm demonstrated superiority over the IFL regimen, oncologists would not know whether combining IFL with bevacizumab would be even more effective.

PROTOCOL DESIGN

The sponsor and the investigators designed a study in colorectal cancer that started with a control group given IFL and a bevacizumab placebo. It had two experimental arms, one that combined the antibody with FL and one that combined it with IFL. The primary endpoint was mortality; the secondary endpoint was time to progression. The study began, therefore, as a three-arm trial of patients with metastatic colorectal cancer. The two IFL arms were blind; however, because the schedule of administration of the FL arm differed from the schedule for the IFL alone arm, the FL plus bevacizumab arm could not be blinded.

Integral to the design of the study was the DMC, which was to select the experimental arm during the course of the study. When approximately 100 patients had been randomized to each of the three treatment arms, the DMC would review all data on safety. The DMC would then select either the bevacizumab plus FL or the bevacizumab plus IFL as the experimental arm; it was to select the combination with IFL as long as that arm was "not unsafe." Having made the decision, the DMC would recommend randomizing only to the ILF alone and to the selected experimental arm. The total sample size would be approximately 900 patients—400 each in the control and selected experimental arm, 100 in the arm not selected. After determination of the experimental arm, the study was to continue until 385 deaths had occurred unless the DMC recommended stopping the study at its single efficacy interim analysis. The interim analysis for efficacy was to occur halfway through the trial, that is, when a total of 193 deaths had occurred in the control (IFL) and the selected treatment arm. The DMC would use an O'Brien-Fleming[3] spending function to assess whether to stop for efficacy.

The study design specified a log-rank test to compare mortality in the two groups with a two-sided type 1 error rate of 0.05. This design had approximately 80% power to detect a hazard ratio of 0.75 for death in the group given the experimental treatment compared to the control group.

DATA MONITORING EXPERIENCE

Genentech established a Data Monitoring Committee composed of three medical oncologists, all of whom treated patients with colorectal cancer and were involved in clinical trials of the disease. In addition, the DMC had one statistician. The DMC reviewed concurrently this trial and a phase II trial in patients with colorectal cancer who were too fragile to be given the IFL regimen. This second trial was two-arm study of bevacizumab plus FL compared to FL alone. While the data from this second trial played no formal role in judgments about the phase III trial, the DMC used the data, especially the data on safety, in statistically informal ways to provide additional insight into the use of bevacizumab in colorectal cancer. The statistician on the committee also was the statistician for a concurrent study of bevacizumab in breast cancer; again, while he did not use the data from the breast cancer study explicitly in reviewing the phase III trial in colorectal cancer, the information provide additional qualitative insights into the use of the product.

Statistics Collaborative, a statistical consulting firm with no other relationship to the three studies, presented data to the DMC for each study. Therefore, like the statistician on the DMC, staff at Statistics Collaborative had access to information from all three ongoing studies. Genentech and the investigators in all three studies were blind to treatment allocation (except for the FL and bevacizumab arm in the phase III study) at the individual patient level. Importantly, they remained blind to summary data by treatment, even for the FL and bevacizumab arm.

During the trial, the DMC had three distinct roles. First, it was charged with monitoring safety. In light of observations from early-phase studies, the DMC was to review data on specific adverse events every two weeks until it met to choose the experimental arm. At that point, the DMC would review safety data monthly. Genentech designed four special case report forms, one for each of the following events: (a) thromboembolic events, (b) major bleeding, (c) severe hypertension, and (d) severe diarrhea. The DMC was to monitor these so-called "targeted events" as well as all serious adverse events. Every two weeks, Genentech downloaded a database with information from these forms and Statistics Collaborative prepared a brief report for the DMC. The DMC met by telephone to review the data and to decide whether to recommend continuation of the trial.

Second, the DMC was to choose the experimental arm on the basis of safety. Genentech and the investigators did not provide the DMC with formal guidelines for this decision; rather, it was to use its collective judgment to assess whether the bevacizumab plus IFL regimen was "not unsafe."

Finally, it was to review efficacy. The predefined statistical guideline for stopping for efficacy specified the DMC was to look formally at efficacy at the halfway point in the trial. If at that time the p-value for benefit was 0.0018, the DMC could recommend stopping for efficacy.

The first patient was randomized in September 2000.

Each in-person DMC meeting began with an open session with the sponsor to report on the status of the trial. The representatives from the sponsor were staff directly involved in the design and conduct of the study. At the closed session, attended only by the DMC and the statisticians reporting to it, the DMC reviewed the data. At the end of the meeting, the DMC reported its recommendations by telephone and in writing to a committee at Genentech composed of clinical experts—a statistician and physicians—with no direct responsibility for the conduct of the study. This Data Review Board, which served as a buffer between the DMC and the study team, had the authority to review unblinded data if the DMC made a recommendation to stop the study early.

The study had three such meetings. The first, or introductory meeting, dealt with the design of the study, the hypothesized action of bevacizumab, and the DMC's charter. At the second in-person meeting, the DMC met to select the experimental arm. The third meeting dealt with the formal interim analysis for safety. In addition, the board met monthly by telephone with Statistics Collaborative to discuss safety data.

The real-time reporting of the data made the process complex. Data came from Genentech to Statistics Collaborative in several different streams and structures. Because Statistics Collaborative was not involved in collecting the data and Genentech was blind to treatment allocation, the two groups met by telephone weekly to discuss procedures and the data themselves. For the interim in-person meetings Genentech provided Statistics Collaborative with all the data from the study, not just the data planned for the DMC. This procedure, although quite labor intensive, allowed Statistics Collaborative to understand the nature of the data adequately enough to report accurately to the DMC.

Early Real-Time Safety Data

Almost from the beginning of the study, the serious and targeted adverse event rates were higher in the IFL arms than in the bevacizuman plus FL; however, because the rates in the bevacizumab plus IFL arm were very similar to the rates in the placebo plus IFL arm, the DMC did not recommend any change in protocol or issue any statement about adverse events. The biweekly reports changed in character over time. At first, the reports used graphs we all dubbed "LJ Pictures," after LJ Wei, the statistician on the DMC. These pictures displayed, on a patient-by-patient basis, the time course of all serious and targeted adverse events. As the weeks progressed and the dataset grew, the format of the reports changed to summarize more succinctly the patterns of events.

The 300-Patient Meeting: Choosing the Treatment Arm

At its 300-patient in-person meeting, the DMC reviewed data on safety for the three arms. Although patients in the bevacizumab plus IFL arm had somewhat higher adverse event rates than did those in the bevacizumab plus LF arm (Table 1), the DMC judged the arm as "not unsafe." Consistent with its charge, it recommended proceeding with the bevacizumab plus IFL arm and not randomizing further to the bevacizumab plus LF arm. It did make two recommendations related to safety for both IFL arms. It recommended that the General Medical Concerns section of the exclusion criteria indicate that patients older than 65 years are at increased risk of irinotecan-associated diarrhea. It also recommended that the study exclude patients whose total bilirubin exceeded 1.6 mg/dl because other studies had shown that patients with Gilbert's syndrome, who have elevated bilirubin measurements, are at higher risk of adverse events when they are on the IFL regimen.

While its charter had specified that real-time safety monitoring would end after the first in-person meeting, the DMC opted to continue its real-time monitoring monthly because it felt that 100 patients in the bevacizumab plus IFL arm constituted an insufficient safety database.

Table 1 Estimated Percentage of People Experiencing Specific Adverse Events Within the First Five Months of Therapy

People with at least one—	Experimental arm 1: bevacizumab plus IFL (n = 113)	Experimental arm 2: bevacizumab plus FL (n = 112)	Control arm: IFL (n = 110)
Serious or targeted adverse event	45	35	29
Serious adverse event	27	25	20
Grade 3 or 4 bleeding	3	0	3
Grade 3 or 4 diarrhea	23	15	20
Thromboembolic event	6	12	2
Episode of serious hypertension	0	0	0
Grade 3 or 4 proteinuria*	0	0	0

* Note: Grades 3 and 4 refer to serious adverse events and life-threatening adverse events, respectively.

The Efficacy Analysis

At its third in-person meeting, the DMC reviewed data from the two enrolling arms to judge whether to recommend stopping the study on the basis of efficacy of the bevacizumab plus IFL arm. The estimated hazard ratio for mortality was 0.64. The DMC, impressed with the large reduction in mortality, considered recommending stopping for efficacy, but decided that because the data had not crossed the prespecified boundary for efficacy (observed $p = 0.003$; critical $p = 0.0018$), a recommendation for early stopping would jeopardize the study because the results would not be statistically convincing.

The DMC also reviewed safety data of all patients enrolled in the study, including the bevacizumab plus FL arm that was closed to enrollment. This review was the last safety review for this study.

Ending the Study

The last patient entered in May 2002. The study ended as planned. The median duration of survival was 20.3 months in the IFL plus bevacizumab group and 15.6 months in the IFL plus placebo group for an estimated hazard ration of 0.66 for death ($p < 0.001$).[4] In 2004, the FDA granted approval for bevacizumab in the treatment of metastatic colorectal cancer.[5]

LESSONS LEARNED

This happy case history may appear boring; it may remind the reader of Tolstoy's introduction to Anna Karenina: "Happy families are all alike; every unhappy family is unhappy in its own way." The retelling sounds as if the study, from the vantage point of the DMC, proceeded smoothly. The DMC had three responsibilities, all of which it discharged responsibly. The antibody was highly effective so that at the end of the study everyone—sponsor, investigators, the DMC, the patients, and the oncology community at large—benefitted from the successful implementation of the trial. But the calm, orderly history masks difficulties that occurred with the DMC during the study.

1. Managing real-time data from a study with many centers poses huge logistical challenges for the sponsor and for the reporting statistician. The successful monitoring of a trial of this type requires that the sponsor and the reporting statistician develop mutual trust. Because the patients in this trial came from 164 clinical sites, the logistics of implementing this study required considerable effort on the part of the sponsor. The sponsor necessarily focused on the implementation of the study. To pretend that all interactions among the two pairs of authors of this paper were smooth during the years of the study would be to ignore the inevitable tensions that arise when two groups are working together with complementary but very different roles. Because Genentech remained blind to the effects of treatment, it often found Statistics Collaborative's requests, which echoed the questions from the DMC, unreasonable. For its part, Statistics Collaborative found Genentech's reluctance to comply with requests frustrating. The basic problem we both faced was that Statistics Collaborative could not tell Genentech the reason for its requests and Genentech could not tell Statistics Collaborative about some of the constraints under which it operated. The two groups had to develop enough trust to allow us to proceed as each party thought best even though we were ignorant of the reasons for the other's needs. At one point, two of us (J.W. and A.B.) took a long walk along a Pacific beach knowing that the calm lapping of the waters would lead us to better cooperation during the course of the study.

2. In trials of toxic therapy, a DMC with direct experience treating patients of the type being studied provides invaluable insight into safety. In many disease areas, a DMC can look at safety infrequently. Because of the toxicity of chemotherapy, trials in cancer require frequent monitoring of safety. Part of the success of this DMC was the expertise of the clinicians on the DMC and their direct experience with patients of the type under study. They were able to assess the importance of the particular events that were occurring in the context of knowledge of other chemotherapeutic regimens.

3. A statistician experienced in DMCs and intellectually engaged in the study can contribute greatly to the process of safety monitoring. The statistician on this DMC played a crucial role. He pushed for various ways of looking at the data. Of particular interest to him, and ultimately to rest of the DMC, was the time course of adverse events.

4. The reporting structure for a DMC, in bypassing the study team, can afford an extra level of protection of the integrity of the study.

5. Independent data monitoring of a complex protocol requires considerable work and expense.

In retrospect, everyone involved in the DMC for this study believes the charge to, and the actions of, the DMC strengthened the study. In particular, the ability to proceed without having selected the final experimental arm saved many months over alternative designs. Only the use of a DMC, and the separation of it from the operation of the study, could have allowed this selection during the course of a study. Nonetheless, this study showed all of us involved how time-consuming and labor-intensive—and hence expensive—this type of activity can be. Before embarking on such a large undertaking, the sponsor should satisfy itself of the necessity of such a structure.

ROLES AND ACKNOWLEDGMENTS

The authors of this chapter included two statisticians at Genentech, the study statistician (E.H.) and the head of oncology statistics (A.B.) as well as the two statisticians at Statistics Collaborative (H.C.S. and J.W.) who presented the data to the DMC. The DMC was composed of three oncologists— Richard Schilsky, M. D. (chair), Robert Mayer, M.D.; Alan Venook, M.D.—and one statistician (Lee-Jen Wei, Ph.D.). Herbert Hurwitz, M.D., was the principal investigator, and William Novotny, M.D., was the medical monitor.

REFERENCES

1. Kabbinavar F, Hurwitz HI,. Fehrenbacher L,. Meropol NJ,. Novotny WF, Lieberman G, et al. 2003. Phase II, randomized trial comparing bevacizumab plus fluorouacil (FU)/leucovorin (LV) with FU/LV alone in patientts with metastatic colorectal cancer. *J Clin Oncol* 21:60–65.
2. Saltz LB, Cox JV, Blanke C, Rosen LS, Fehrenbacher L, Moore MJ, et al. 2000. Irinotecan plus fluorouracil and leucovorin for metastatic colorectal cancer. *N Engl J Med* 343:905–914.
3. O'Brien P, Fleming T. 1979. A multiple testing procedure for clinical trials. *Biometrics* 35:549–556.
4. Hurwitz H, Fehrenbacher L, Novotny W, Cartwright T, Hainsworth J, Heim W, et al. 2004. Bevacizumab plus irinotecan, fluorouracil, and leucovorin for metastatic colorectal cancer. *N Engl J Med* 350:2335–2342.
5. Genentech, Inc. Label for AvastinTM (Bevacizumab). U.S. BLA Amendment: Bevacizumab— Genentech, Inc. Februrary 2004, 27pp. http://www.fda.gov/cder/foi/label/2004/125085lbl.pdf

Data Monitoring Committee Members

The following individuals have served on one or more monitoring committees

Abeloff, Martin
Applegate, William
Armstrong, Paul W.
Ayers, Stephen M.
Ballintine, Elmer
Bearman, Jacob, E.
Berge, Kenneth
Berry, Donald A.
Blackburn, Henry
Blum, Ronald H.
Boissel, Jean-Pierre
Boyle, Edwin
Bristow, J. David
Brown, B. William
Bruce, Robert
Buring, Julie
Cairns, John
Califf, Robert
Campbell, Ronnie
Canner, Paul L.
Carleton, Richard
Carter, Michele
Cassel, Cristine
Chalmers, Thomas
Chatterjee, Kashinath
Childress, James F.
Clark, Charles
Clements, Rex S. Jr.
Cody, Robert J.

Cohen, Lawrence M.
Collins, Rory
Colton, Theodore
Cooper, Edward
Cornfield, Jerome
Cowles, Andrus
Crofford, Oscar
Cryer, Henry M III
Cutter, Gary
Davis, C. Edward
Davis, Matthew
DeMets, David L.
Deykin, Daniel
Dickstein, Kenneth
Ederer, Fred
Erban, John Kalil
Feigl, Polly
Ferdinand, Keith
Ferris, Frederick
Fisch, Charles
Fisher, Lloyd
Fisher, Marian
Fleming, Thomas R.
Ford, Ian
Fost, Norman
Francis, Gary
Freedman, Laurence
Friedewald, William T.
Friedman, Ephraim

Friedman, Lawrence M.
Furberg, Curt D.
Gent, Michael
Gifford, Raymond
Gillette, James
Goldstein, Sidney
Grant, Igor
Hainline, Adrian
Halperin, Max
Hamilton, Michael P.
Harrington, David
Harris, Jay R.
Hart, Robert
Hennekens, Charles H.
Higgins, Millicent
Hillis, Argye
Hirsh, Jack
Hochman, Judith
Hulka, Barbara
Hutchison, George B.
Iber, Frank
Johnson, Susan
Johnstone, David
Judd, Howard
Julian, Desmond G.
Kimbel, Philip
Klatskin, Gerald
Kligfield, Paul D.
Klimt, Christian R.
Knatterud, Genell
Krome, Ronald
Kulbertus, Henri
Lachin, John
Lasagna, Louis
Lebovitz, Harold
Lee, Stephanie J.
Levy, Robert
Lewis, Roger J.
Lilienfeld, Abraham
Malchon, Jean K.
Massie, Barrie
Mayer, Kenneth H.

Mayer, Robert
Meinert, Curtis L.
Menkes, Harold
Miller, Anthony
Miller, Dayton T.
Miller, Max
Miller, William F.
Naughton, John
Newman, Elliot
Nies, Alan
Norton, Edward
Packer, Milton
Palmberg, Paul
Patz, Arnall
Pitt, Bertram
Pocock, Stuart
Pollard, James
Pollard, Richard B.
Pratt, Lois
Prineas, Ronald
Prout, Thaddeus
Rahal, James J.
Rapaport, Elliot
Rosner, Bernard
Ruskin, Jeremy
Ryan, Thomas
Sackett, David
Sackner, Marvin A.
Saudek, Christopher
Schiffrin, Alicia
Schilsky, Richard
Sears, Marvin
Sheps, Sheldon
Smith, William M.
Snapinn, Steven
Sobel, Burton
Stamler, Jeremiah
Stone, Neil
Strauss, Harold
Thompson, Simon
Tilley, Barbara
Turner, Robert

Vachon, Louis
Venook, Alan
Walters, LeRoy
Wang, Dualo
Washington, Geraldine
Wedel, Hans
Wei, Lee-Jen

Whitley, Richard J.
Wilhelmsen, Lars
Wilkens, Robert
Williams, O. Dale
Wittes, Janet
Wyse, D.G.
Zukel, William

Case Study Acronym Key (Title)

ACTG:	AIDS Clinical Trials Group Study #981
ALLHAT:	Antihypertensive and Lipid-Lowering Treatment to Prevent Heart Attack Trial
BCPT:	Breast Cancer Prevention Trial
BHAT:	Beta-Blocker Heart Attack Trial
CALGB:	Cancer and Leukemia Group B
CAPRICORN:	Carvedilol Post-Infarct Survival Control in Left Ventricular Dysfunction Study
CARET:	Carotene and Retinol Efficacy Trial
CAST:	Cardiac Arrhythmia Suppression Trial
CDP:	Coronary Drug Project
CHARM:	Candesartan in Heart Failure Assessment of Reduction in Mortality and Morbidity
CONSENSUS II:	Cooperative New Scandinavian Enalapril Survival Study II
CURE:	Clopidogrel in Unstable Angina To Prevent Recurrent Ischemic Events Trials
DCCT:	Diabetes Control and Complications Trial
DCLHB	Diaspirin Cross-Linked Hemoglobin Trial
DRS:	Diabetic Retinopathy Study
HERS:	Heart and Estrogen/progestin Replacement Trial
HOPE:	Heart Outcomes Prevention Evaluation
MERIT-HF:	Metoprolol CR/XL Randomized Intervention Trial in Chronic Heart Failure
MOXCON:	Moxonidine Congestive Heart Failure Trial
NOTT:	Nocturnal Oxygen Therapy Trial
PHS:	Physicians Health Study
PROMISE:	Prospective Randomized Milrinone Survival Evaluation
RALES:	Randomized Aldactone Evaluation Study
RESOLVD:	Randomized Evaluation of Strategies for Left Ventricular Dysfunction Pilot Study
SPAF I:	Stroke Prevention in Atrial Fibrillation I Trial
TOXO:	AIDS Toxoplasmic Encephalitis Study

INDEX